Bottom Line's
HEALTH
BREAKTHROUGHS
2017

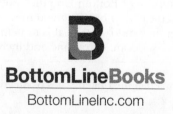

BottomLineBooks
BottomLineInc.com

10 9 8 7 6 5 4 3 2 1

ISBN 0-88723-754-1

HealthDay

Selected articles in this book were written by reporters for HealthDay, an award-winning international
daily consumer health news service, headquartered in Norwalk, Connecticut.

Bottom Line Books® publishes the advice of expert authorities in many fields.
These opinions may at times conflict as there are often different approaches to solving problems.
The use of this material is no substitute for health, legal, accounting or other professional services.
Consult competent professionals for answers to your specific questions.

Telephone numbers, addresses, prices, offers and websites listed in this book are accurate
at the time of publication, but they are subject to frequent change.

Bottom Line Books® is a registered trademark of Bottom Line Inc.
3 Landmark Square, Suite 201, Stamford, Connecticut 06901

www.BottomLineInc.com

Bottom Line Books is an imprint of Bottom Line Inc., publisher of print periodicals,
e-letters and books. We are dedicated to bringing you the best information from the most
knowledgeable sources in the world. Our goal is to help you gain greater wealth,
better health, more wisdom, extra time and increased happiness.

Printed in the United States of America

Contents

Contents

Contents

11 • GET THE BEST MEDICAL CARE

12 • HEART AND STROKE

13 • INFECTIOUS DISEASES

Contents

17 • MEN'S HEALTH

18 • NATURAL CURES

19 • PAIN NEWS

Contents

Preface

We are proud to bring you the all-new *Bottom Line's Health Breakthroughs 2017*. This collection represents a year's worth of the latest health news and scientific discoveries in a broad spectrum of fields.

When you choose a Bottom Line book, you are turning to a stellar group of experts in a wide range of specialties—medical doctors, alternative practitioners, renowned nutrition experts, research scientists and consumer-health advocates, to name a few.

We go to great lengths to interview the foremost health experts. Whether it's cancer prevention, breakthrough arthritis treatments or cutting-edge nutritional advice, our editors talk to the true innovators in health care.

How do we find all these top-notch professionals? Over the past 40 years, we have built a network of leading physicians in both alternative and conventional medicine. They are affiliated with the world's premier medical institutions. We follow the medical research, and with the help of our partner HealthDay, an award-winning service that reports on evidence-based health news, we bring the latest information to our readers. We also regularly talk with our advisers in teaching hospitals, private practices and government health agencies.

Bottom Line's Health Breakthroughs 2017 is a result of our ongoing research and contact with these experts, and is a distillation of their latest findings and advice. We hope that you will enjoy the presentation and glean helpful information about the health topics that concern you and your family.

As a reader of a Bottom Line book, please be assured that you are receiving reliable and well-researched information from a trusted source. But, please use prudence in health matters. Always speak to your physician before taking vitamins, supplements or over-the-counter medication… changing your diet…or beginning an exercise program. If you experience side effects from any regimen, contact your doctor immediately.

The Editors, Bottom Line Books, Stamford, Connecticut.

CHAPTER 1

Allergies, Asthma and Respiratory Disorders

The Allergy-Fighting Diet

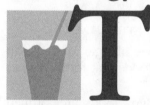

The right diet can help relieve your allergies whether you're allergic to pollen, dust, mold, certain foods or other allergens. And it can relieve symptoms that you might not even know come from allergies—including fatigue, weight gain and depression. The key is to use foods to improve your immune response. *Here's how…*

BOOST YOUR T-REGS

Immune cells known as regulatory T-cells, or T-regs, limit inflammation and dampen the allergic response. The cells don't function properly in people with allergies, which can lead to a host of allergic symptoms.

If you know you're allergic to something, avoidance is an obvious solution. But many people don't know what they're allergic to—or even if they are allergic. You can use dietary changes to increase T-regs and dampen any allergic response.

STEP 1: THREE-DAY POWER WASH

I advise patients to completely give up the foods that commonly aggravate allergies. These include dairy (including yogurt), wheat, seafood, eggs, soy, nuts, peanuts, yeast (found in bread, alcohol, vinegar, commercial fruit juice and commercial soups and sauces) and nightshade vegetables (such as tomatoes, bell peppers, potatoes and eggplant).

This is not meant to be a permanent diet. You have to give up these foods for three days (unless you discover that you're allergic to a particular food, in which case you'll give it up altogether). Taking a break from likely offenders resets the immune system—it clears your body of potential allergens and lets you start with a clean slate.

Leo Galland, MD, director of the Foundation for Integrated Medicine in New York City. He has held faculty positions at Rockefeller University, Albert Einstein College of Medicine and State University of New York, Stony Brook. He is coauthor of *The Allergy Solution: Unlock the Surprising, Hidden Truth About Why You Are Sick and How to Get Well.* DrGalland.com

For three days, you'll consume only the soup and the smoothie (see below) that I developed for blunting the immune response (you'll also drink oolong tea). Have the smoothie for breakfast and a midafternoon snack. The soup is lunch and dinner. Eat until you are satisfied but not too full. Have your doctor look at the recipes to make sure that they are appropriate for you.

•**Immune Balance Smoothie.** In a blender, combine one cup of strawberries, one medium avocado, one cup of chopped arugula, one-half head of chopped romaine lettuce, two tablespoons of ground chia seeds and one cup of brewed green tea. If desired, add one medium banana.

Blend until smooth. The smoothie will become thicker and creamier if you refrigerate it after blending.

If you happen to be allergic to any of the ingredients, just leave it out.

•**Immune Balance Soup.** This is one of the Galland family's favorite recipes.

Sauté three cups of sliced carrots in three tablespoons of extra-virgin olive oil for 10 minutes. Add one cup of chopped parsley, two cups of chopped scallions (green parts only), 12 ounces of chopped broccoli, three ounces of chopped baby kale, one teaspoon of turmeric powder and one-quarter teaspoon of ground black pepper. Add salt to taste. Cook and stir for one minute. Add 12 cups of water, and bring to a boil. Cover and simmer for 20 minutes.

Add one tablespoon of shredded daikon radish just before serving.

•**Organic oolong tea.** I emphasize this tea for a specific reason. It's very high in catechins, which are flavonoids that inhibit allergic reactions—they're even stronger than the compounds in green tea. One study found that a majority of patients with allergic eczema who didn't respond to medications had significant improvements after drinking oolong tea for one to two weeks. Drink four cups daily (no more) during the Three-Day Power Wash and a cup or two daily after that.

STEP 2: REINTRODUCTION

After three days, continue to enjoy the homemade smoothie and soup and organic oolong tea as you gradually reintroduce foods from your regular diet—a new food or food group each day. Start with foods that are less likely to provoke allergic reactions such as rice or free-range poultry, and gradually move toward the more allergenic foods such as nuts, seafood, eggs and dairy products, one group at a time. Keep notes about what you're eating and symptoms (if any) that you experience—including symptoms you don't typically associate with allergies. This will help you determine whether particular foods—or ingredients in packaged foods—are triggering symptoms.

I've found that patients who give up problem foods for at least six months can sometimes eat them again, in small amounts, without having symptoms return. This doesn't apply to things such as sodas, candies or other junk foods, including commercially prepared pastries. These foods always contribute to allergies (including common dust and pollen allergies) by increasing inflammation and should be avoided.

Important: Consult your doctor before reintroducing foods, especially if you suffer from anaphylaxis or asthma or if you previously have experienced an adverse reaction to any of the foods.

STEP 3: IMMUNE BALANCE

No matter what you're allergic to, make an effort to eat healthier foods that fortify T-regs. *Most important…*

•**Natural folate.** Many foods are fortified with folic acid, an important (but synthetic) B vitamin. Natural sources of folate are better for T-reg function.

Examples: Leafy vegetables, legumes, peas, asparagus, cauliflower and brussels sprouts.

•**More flavonoids.** I believe that many of the inflammatory disorders that plague Americans, including allergies and asthma, are due in part to flavonoid deficiencies. Flavonoids, an important family of plant compounds, have anti-inflammatory and antioxidant effects. A Tufts University study found that animals given a flavonoid-enhanced diet had an increase in T-regs and a decrease in Immunoglobulin E (IgE) antibodies—molecules involved in the allergic response.

The flavonoids in tea are particularly helpful. But you'll get healthy amounts from many different plant foods, including onions, blueberries, sweet potatoes, apples and bell peppers.

•**Lots of strawberries.** Strawberries are the richest food source of *fisetin*, a type of flavonoid that helps preserve T-regs. Fisetin blunts the allergic response and has been shown in laboratory studies to help prevent allergic asthma.

Important: Organic strawberries, fresh or frozen, have more vitamin C and other antioxidants than conventionally grown berries.

•**Put parsley on your plate.** It's more than just a garnish. It's high in *apigenin*, a flavonoid that decreases the activity of allergy-inducing lymphocytes and reduces levels of IgE. The carotenoids in parsley (it has more than carrots) also are helpful.

•**Eat seafood twice a week** (as long as you're not allergic). A lack of omega-3 fatty acids can cause or aggravate allergy symptoms. People with allergies actually need more of these fats because their cells don't metabolize them efficiently.

•**Broaden your palate.** While tea, parsley and strawberries are among the allergy-fighting stars, all plant foods can help balance the immune system and reduce symptoms. I'm a big fan of legumes (such as black beans, garbanzo beans and lentils), along with carrots, sweet bell peppers, spinach and brussels sprouts. Most of your diet should consist of these and other healthful plant foods. (For more on testing for food allergies, see page 5.)

HIDDEN ALLERGY SYMPTOMS

Here are allergy symptoms that aren't typically associated with allergies…

- •**Anxiety**
- •**Bloating**
- •**Brain fog**
- •**Constipation or Diarrhea**
- •**Depression**
- •**Fatigue**
- •**Headaches**
- •**Insomnia**
- •**Joint pain**
- •**Muscle aches**
- •**Stomachaches**
- •**Weight gain**

Hidden Allergies

Richard Firshein, DO, founder and director of the Firshein Center for Integrative Medicine in New York City. A leading authority in preventive and nutritional medicine that integrates Eastern and Western medical practices, he is the author of Reversing Asthma *and* The Vitamin Prescription (for life).

I f you escaped allergies as a child or a young adult, then you're home free now, right? Well…maybe not. And if you have had allergies for years, then you surely know exactly what triggers a reaction, right? Not necessarily.

These are just two of the instances when people can get walloped by hidden allergies.

NEVER TOO OLD

Contrary to popular belief, a first-time allergy can occur at any age. While the reasons are not completely understood, it's believed that adult-onset environmental allergies can occur when people move to a new area (and get exposed to different allergens)…or when a genetic predisposition to react to an environmental or food allergen finally kicks in after years of being exposed to it.

Takeaway: If you have typical allergy symptoms, including sneezing, coughing and itchy eyes (telltale signs of, say, springtime allergies)…or nausea, diarrhea and itchy hives (common red flags for food allergies), do not rule out allergies just because you've never suffered from them before. See your doctor for advice and possible allergy testing.

COMMON ALLERGY MIX-UPS

Allergies are a tricky health problem—largely because people tend to self-diagnose based on what they believe to be their allergic trigger. *But that can lead to mix-ups, as allergies, related to those below, go undetected…*

•**Tree pollen.** While most hay fever sufferers have zeroed in on tree pollen as the culprit, they often fail to realize that having this allergy means that they may also react to tree fruits, such as apples, pears or peaches, and tree nuts, such as walnuts. For these people, exposure to tree fruits or tree nuts can set off the same immune response as pollen. This so-called oral allergy syndrome (OAS) may cause swelling and irritation in the mouth, lips and throat.

What to do: Cooking these fruits may help. Otherwise, avoiding these fruits and nuts (as well as melons, which also may cause symptoms) is the simplest solution.

•**Pet fur.** People who get watery eyes or start sneezing around pets often assume that they're allergic to the pet's fur…and look for a dog or cat breed that's touted as "hypoallergenic"—a loosely defined term that usually suggests the animal's fur produces fewer allergens.

But this often does not help, because animal fur is typically not the allergen—it's almost always pet dander (shedding skin flakes) and/or saliva, each of which contains proteins that trigger the allergic immune response. Even hypoallergenic pets produce at least some dander—and all pets groom themselves, leaving bits of saliva on their fur.

What to do: If you are allergic but want a pet, try grooming the animal frequently, isolating the pet to certain areas of the house and using a high-efficiency particulate arresting (HEPA) air-filtration system.

•**Chocolate.** If a piece of chocolate causes symptoms, such as a rash or trouble breathing, the actual culprit may be one of its ingredients, such as soy lecithin, milk or nuts.

What to do: Get checked to see if you're allergic to cocoa, the health-promoting substance in chocolate. If you're not, get further testing to reveal the true source of your allergy, which then can be avoided.

•**Alcohol.** Many people who drink wine, beer and/or hard liquor experience flushed skin, itching, nasal congestion and even an elevated heart rate. For some individuals, protein residues from the alcoholic beverage cause the reaction.

But for many others, the trigger is actually sulfites, chemicals that act as a preservative and prevent the growth of mold or bacteria.

Other examples of foods and drinks that may contain sulfites: Dried fruits…soft drinks …cookies…crackers…noodle or rice mixes…and shellfish.

For a more detailed list, go to: *Sulfites. org/sulfite-foods/.*

What to do: If testing shows that you are allergic to sulfites, read labels and avoid products that contain this additive. It can also be listed on the label in one of various forms, such as potassium bisulfate…sulfur dioxide…and potassium metabisulfite.

Note: Alcoholic beverages also may contain contaminants, such as gluten and yeast, that may require further testing by a doctor.

BEST TESTING OPTIONS

The only way to know for sure that you have an allergy is to undergo allergy testing. If you are truly allergic to something, your immune system mistakes an otherwise harmless substance for an intruder, producing immunoglobulin E (IgE) antibodies. *Two main types of tests identify environmental allergies (such as pollen, dust, mold, etc.) and food allergies (such as peanuts, eggs, soy, milk, etc.)…*

•**Skin tests.** A suspected allergen is introduced into the body by pricking, scratching or injecting it into the skin—or by applying a skin patch coated with it.

•**Blood tests.** These tests can be used if the doctor is concerned about a dramatic skin reaction that could cause a severe allergic response…or if a person has psoriasis or some other skin condition that could be aggravated by skin testing.

For example, with the *radio allergosorbent test* (RAST), a sample of your blood is exposed to a suspected allergen.

Note: Sometimes you may not have an actual allergy, but rather a sensitivity that produces allergy-type symptoms when you are exposed to the substance. A separate test is needed to identify an environmental or food sensitivity.

THE RIGHT DOCTOR TO SEE

To get an accurate diagnosis, it's fine to start with a family physician who is well versed in allergies. If you suspect a food allergy, be sure the doctor is experienced in this problem. *Other options…*

•**Allergists/immunologists may be the best choice for difficult cases.** To find one near you, consult the American Academy of Allergy, Asthma & Immunology, *AAAAI.org.*

•**Integrative medicine physicians,** who identify allergies as an aspect of overall health, are another choice. To find one near you, check the American Board of Integrative Holistic Medicine website, ABIHM.org, and search "allergy/immunology" in the specialty field.

•**Naturopathic physicians can also be helpful,** especially in offering guidance on diet and the use of supplements (such as butterbur and quercetin). To find a naturopathic physician, consult the American Association of Naturopathic Physicians, *Naturopathic.org.*

How to Find Your Food Triggers

Maggie Moon, MS, RDN, registered dietitian nutritionist, Los Angeles, and author of *The Elimination Diet Workbook: A Personal Approach to Determining Your Food Allergies.*

Food is medicine. But it can also be poison. It depends on the food—and the person. For some people, with certain conditions, specific "trigger" foods can bring on symptoms such as skin rashes, wheezing, bloating, diarrhea, constipation, cramps, headaches, fatigue and mood swings.

The best way to identify your trigger foods? An elimination diet, a kind of experiment-of-one, conducted hand-in-hand with a health professional.

HOW ELIMINATION DIETS WORK: THE BASICS

An elimination diet is the classic way to identify food allergies, which can bring on symptoms such as hives, often soon after the food is eaten. It can also identify more subtle food intolerances—to lactose sugar in dairy foods, for example, or gluten protein in wheat—which can cause immunological and digestive problems that may take hours, even days, to cause symptoms. If you have irritable bowel syndrome (IBS), for example, you may want to begin eliminating "FODMAP" foods, a class of hard-to-digest carbohydrates (see pages 142–144) that often are at the root of the problem—to find out which ones are your triggers. Elimination diets can often help improve symptoms for conditions as different as migraines, chronic sinus congestion, adult acne, rheumatoid arthritis and asthma.

The goal of an elimination diet is to identify your specific problem foods by removing possible triggers and then slowly reintroducing them—while monitoring your symptoms. That way, you find out which foods are really causing your symptoms—and which ones you can safely eat.

A HEALTH COACH CAN GUIDE YOU THROUGH

Before you get going, check with your doctor. That's especially important if you've ever had a life-threatening allergic reaction (anaphylactic shock), have battled an eating disorder or are on medications that are diet-sensitive, such as the heart drug *warfarin* (Coumadin).

Even if you don't have such a medical concern, the best way to be successful is to work with a qualified health professional such as an allergist, gastroenterologist, integrative physician or naturopath. He or she may refer you to a nutritionist, such as a registered dietitian nutritionist—or you may start with a nutritionist—who can be your coach through the process, providing support and making sure you're meeting your nutritional needs.

A few more tips for success…

•**Be honest.** First, you'll need to be scrupulous as you keep track of what you eat and how you feel for several weeks, before you start the diet.

•**Accept change.** The new way of eating will restrict your choices and limit your options, and it can be a challenge to learn how to cook different foods than you are used to—and then make time to cook them—and to adjust to a new way of eating out.

•**Get support.** Your spouse, partner, kids and friends will be affected by your new diet, so you'll need to explain what you plan to do and why.

FIVE STAGES TO A SUCCESSFUL ELIMINATION DIET

1. Assess. During this phase, assess your dietary habits by writing down what you eat and how it makes you feel. Your record needs to be as honest, detailed and accurate as possible.

You can track food and symptoms with a spreadsheet. Make four columns, labeled "Meal," "Food/Drink (How much)," "Ingredients" and "Symptoms." For the symptoms column, describe when they start and when they end and rate the intensity on a scale of 1 to 10. Keeping track for two to four weeks should allow you to note immediate and delayed symptoms.

Helpful: The mySymptoms Food & Symptom Tracker app from SkyGazer Labs. Available on iTunes and on Google Play for Android devices, it allows you to enter foods, ingredients, supplements, medications and drinks—as well as different kinds of exercise—and track your symptoms.

Tip: This needs to be an honest baseline, so eat the way you normally would. While symptoms may persist during this time, keep in mind that soon you'll be able to say good-bye to them.

2. Get Ready. Once you've identified possible food triggers remove them from your kitchen, pantry, office and car to make it easier to stick to your "safe" foods and avoid temptation. If that's not feasible (because you live with others, for example), try to put the "safe" foods you'll be eating now in a separate place.

Prepare yourself, too, by acknowledging that the elimination diet is not an easy process and you will have ups and downs. Symptoms could flare up and might even seem worse at the start of an elimination diet. Have patience—the end results will be worth it. Just knowing this will enable you to follow through.

Tip: This is a good time to create meal plans and grocery lists of allowed foods.

3. Avoid (Eliminate). Now it's time to stop eating all the possible trigger foods. Continue to keep track of what you eat and how you feel, along with overall levels of energy, body aches, etc.

After a week, if symptoms have improved, you can move to the challenge phase. However, if symptoms persist after two to four weeks, it's time to take a closer look at your food and symptom tracker. Circle foods that precede

symptoms, and eliminate the foods that show up most often first.

Tip: If you still experience symptoms after eliminating possible food triggers, consider the possibility that food is not the reason for your symptoms after all. Make an appointment with your health-care professional to pinpoint the problem.

4. Challenge. In this step, you'll reintroduce foods to confirm that they are safe for you through a food challenge. You'll test one and only one potential trigger food in the morning and then monitor for symptoms.

Here's how: Put a tiny amount of the food inside your lower lip for two minutes, and monitor for a half hour before trying a small amount, which varies by food. For example, if the food challenge is milk, and you normally drink eight ounces a day, a small amount would be about an ounce.

Assuming there are no symptoms, you can increase the amount of the same food at lunchtime, while again monitoring how you feel. Repeat at dinner with an even larger portion if there were no symptoms after lunch. Keep track of what you're eating and how you feel to get the most accurate picture of which foods are causing you to feel ill.

To monitor for any delayed symptoms that don't show up right away, use a "washout" period of two weeks, which means going back to the baseline elimination diet in Step 2. If all goes well, you can add the "challenge" food to your list of "safe" foods. Keep in mind that the challenge phase can last for several weeks or more depending on how many challenge foods you need to test.

Tip: Test foods one at a time, but keep even the foods that tested "safe" out of your diet until all of the food challenges are done. This assures that only one variable is being tested at a time without potential confounding factors.

5. Change. In this step, you learn how to follow a maintenance diet. The elimination diet plus your list of "safe" foods can be used as a foundation for a long-term maintenance diet. Using a list of all your safe foods, the easiest way to plan meals is to identify a protein, vegetables and a grain or starch per meal.

Tip: It varies by individual, but a good rule of thumb is to add a new food for two to four weeks and see how you react.

MAKING PEACE

The ultimate purpose of an elimination diet is to reestablish a friendly and healthy connection with food instead of having an adversarial relationship with what you're eating. It can enable you to live a healthier life by teaching you how to make and eat food that is healthier for you. You may even lose weight. It's time to make peace with the food you eat.

Reaction to Mangoes Could Mean Other Allergies

Michael Lewin, MD, an allergist in New York City and Wilton, Connecticut. He is a leading expert in sublingual immunotherapy.

Mango tree sap, which is on the skin of the fruit, contains an oil called *urushiol* (also in poison ivy and poison oak). Urushiol can cause mild to severe skin reactions, including hives, blistering and/or itching.

In some instances, it is the fruit of the mango that triggers a reaction, which can range from mild to extremely severe, causing gastrointestinal discomfort, itching in the mouth, swelling, hives and, in rare instances, throat swelling. People with this allergy may also react to cashews and pistachios, and similar fruits, such as papaya.

Mango sensitivity has also been linked to latex allergies, so your health-care providers should be advised to use nonlatex gloves.

An allergist can determine if you are allergic to the mango peel or fruit as well as check for other food sensitivities with skin or blood tests.

Papain: The Dark (and Allergenic) Side of a Skin-Care Ingredient

Study titled "Papain Degrades Tight Junction Proteins of Human Keratinocytes In-Vitro and Sensitizes C57BL/6 Mice via the Skin Independent of Its Enzymatic Activity or TLR4 Activation" by researchers at the Messerli Research Institute of the University of Veterinary Medicine Vienna, Austria, published in *Journal of Investigative Dermatology*.

What's sweet to your gastrointestinal tract may not be so kind to your skin. Papain, an enzyme derived from the papaya fruit, has long been relied upon, in supplement form, to aid the digestive process, especially the breakdown and absorption of proteins. It's generally considered to be a safe digestive aid, although there can be some allergic reactions, especially in people allergic to mangoes or kiwis. If most people can put the stuff inside their bodies, you might figure there should be no problem putting it on skin, right? Well, think again!

REMOVING DEAD SKIN...AND CAUSING ALLERGIES

The cosmetic industry uses papain in many different skin-care products, shampoos and conditioners and even in enzymatic contact lens cleaners to remove protein deposits. When it's applied to the skin, it helps remove dead cells from the surface, revealing fresh, healthy cells that lie beneath and improving skin texture and appearance. It may also open clogged pores. No wonder it's used in exfoliating products such as facial scrubs, body cleansers, facial masks and peels. In hair-care products, papain conditions and softens dry or damaged hair, but there's a dark side.

In a recent study, researchers in Vienna, Austria, put papain directly on the skin of mice as well as on human skin cells in the petri dish. *Within a short time (30 to 120 minutes), the papain...*

•**Compromised the integrity of the skin barrier by degrading the "tight junctions" that join skin cells together.** That makes it easier for other compounds...including nasty ones...to penetrate your skin's natural protective barrier.

•**Increased water loss,** contributing to drier skin.

•**Induced vasodilation**—a widening of blood vessels—which can cause skin to become warm, red and itchy.

•**Stimulated the release of inflammatory cells in the skin** (which can lead to irritation)...including mast cells, which release histamine as part of allergic reactions.

After repeated exposure, the mice developed antibodies to papain—a sure sign of an allergic response. (Papain, it turns out, is structurally very similar to a very common dust mite allergen.) All of these effects are problematic on their own but, adding insult to injury, compromising the skin barrier function could allow other chemicals to penetrate the skin more deeply, setting the stage for further irritation or allergic responses. This is a particular concern for people who have eczema, whose skin is already susceptible to bacteria, fungi and viruses.

The researchers' conclusion: Papain has all the characteristics of a strong allergen.

The FDA, it turns out, already strongly warned manufacturers against selling unapproved ointments that contain papain as a treatment for serious skin conditions such as diabetic ulcers and traumatic wounds, based on allergic reactions. That was back in 2008. The new research makes us wonder if its place in everyday cosmetics, should be revisited, too.

Take-home message: If you have sensitive skin or you're prone to skin redness or irritation, especially after using new products, read product ingredient lists and steer clear of skin- and hair-care products that contain papain. The allergy is related to latex allergies, the researchers find, so that if you're allergic to latex, you should also avoid papain-containing products. (Look for other names as well—papainase, papaine, summertrin, tromasin, vegetable pepsin, velardon.)

If your skin is at all sensitive, you are prone to allergic skin reactions or you have a skin condition such as eczema, there's no need to take a chance on papain.

Natural Relief from Asthma

Jamison Starbuck, ND, is a naturopathic physician in family practice and a guest lecturer at the University of Montana, both in Missoula. She is a past president of the American Association of Naturopathic Physicians and a contributing editor to *The Alternative Advisor: The Complete Guide to Natural Therapies and Alternative Treatments.*

Asthma is a disease that begins in childhood, right? Well, not always. Though many adult asthma sufferers have struggled with the condition since childhood, research shows that up to 40% of new asthma patients are over age 40 when they have their first asthma attack. Some of my patients are surprised when I explain to them the role that a naturopathic physician can play in helping them prevent and control mild-to-moderate asthma. While patients with severe or unresponsive moderate asthma need conventional medical attention, natural medicine has a lot to offer.

First, it's important to recognize which adults are at increased risk of developing asthma. This includes people who suffer from frequent and recurrent upper respiratory infections, such as colds, sinusitis and the flu. When these illnesses occur too frequently (once a month or more often), inflammation can damage the respiratory tract—a perfect setup for asthma. Asthma is also closely linked to allergies (due, for example, to certain food preservatives, such as sodium bisulfate, and inhaled irritants, such as pollen and mold) as well as exposure to pollutants and toxins, including cigarette smoke. Research now shows that severe stress can also trigger an asthma attack.

There's no one-size-fits-all approach to treating asthma. In general, I recommend approaches for my patients that will reduce inflammation and enhance their lung and immune health. Asthma-fighting supplements that I recommend (all can be used with asthma medication, if needed)...*

•**Fish oil.** Research has found that these oils reduce bronchial inflammation that often accompanies asthma.

*Consult your doctor to find out if this asthma-fighting protocol is right for you.

Typical dose: 2,000 mg daily.

•**Antioxidants.** Vitamin C—2,000 mg per day—and vitamin E—400 international units (IU) daily. Both improve immune health and reduce the allergic response that so often triggers an asthma attack.

•**Magnesium.** Use of this mineral (300 mg to 500 mg daily) can reduce bronchospasm (a tightening of the airways that makes breathing more difficult).

•**Botanicals.** One of my favorites is astragalus. It supports both lung and immune health.

Typical dose: Use one-quarter teaspoon of tincture in two ounces of water, daily until asthma symptoms improve. Repeat when needed.

Also helpful: Deep-breathing exercises and/or yoga help prevent asthma attacks by calming the nervous system and increasing lung capacity.

Because all asthma patients have different needs, I recommend seeing a naturopathic doctor (ND) to help create a personalized natural regimen. To find an ND near you, consult The American Association of Naturopathic Physicians, Naturopathic.org. But remember, not all asthma can be well controlled with natural medicine. If you have more than mild-to-moderate asthma, you should also be under the care of an allergist or pulmonologist and not shirk any prescription drugs, such as inhalers, that he/she has prescribed for you.

Combining natural medicine with prescription medication (when needed) gives you the best chance of keeping your asthma well controlled!

Can Salt Rooms Really Help Asthma?

Leonard Bielory, MD, chair, American College of Allergy, Asthma & Immunology (ACAAI) Integrative Medicine Committee, professor and director, STARx Allergy and Asthma Center, Springfield, New Jersey and research associate, Rutgers University, Center of Environmental Prediction, New Brunswick, New Jersey.

At the very same time that we're being inundated with advice on restricting salt intake, we're also hearing about a new type of therapy based on the claim that spending time in a salt room, breathing in moist, salty air, can help ease chronic respiratory problems such as asthma. Based on a centuries-old Eastern European curative therapy, spalike salt rooms are beginning to appear around the country. Are the benefits for real?

THE SALT ROOM EXPERIENCE

The quasi-medical term for this treatment is "halotherapy." It involves sitting in a smallish room lined with blocks of salt mined from ancient salt caves. A generator (like a steam vaporizer) emits vapor containing about one-half cup of salt during a 45-minute session. People remain clothed for the treatment but often bring a clothing change for afterward since the salt tends to leave a residue.

It sounds like "a day at the beach"—but does halotherapy help your health in any meaningful way? To find out, we spoke with asthma and allergy specialist Leonard Bielory, MD, chair of the American College of Allergy, Asthma & Immunology (ACAAI) Integrative Medicine Committee and director of the STARx Allergy and Asthma Center in Springfield, New Jersey.

NICE BUT…

Dr. Bielory calls salt rooms a "nice concept"—but voices some concerns. He agrees that the salt particles may help skin conditions such as acne or eczema but he worries that salt therapy may prove detrimental to some people with asthma. He pointed out that asthma is the result of constriction in the respiratory tract, which can be caused by excess mucus or by spasms. Breathing salt-infused air might help break up mucus and therefore help some folks to breathe better, but others may find that the salt is an irritant that triggers spasms.

Dr. Bielory's objections don't stop there. There's no way to guarantee the purity of the air in the rooms, he said—pointing out that, theoretically at least, salt attracts certain bacteria and that each person coming for treatment brings a fresh supply of additional bacteria that might evolve in the environment. Other worries relate to the length of time and at what temperature it is safe to stay in the rooms, and whether salt rooms may be dangerous for people with other health conditions, such as cardiac problems.

Offering a different perspective, naturopath Andrew L. Rubman, ND, was less dismissive. While agreeing with some of Dr. Bielory's concerns, he pointed out that this therapy has hundreds of years of successful use in Europe behind it, and he knows naturopathic physicians who treat patients with inhaled salt therapy for such things as chronic bronchitis, asthma and chronic fatigue syndrome. "There is potential benefit for some patients under the supervision of a skilled doctor with experience," he said. Dr. Rubman agrees with Dr. Bielory that medical oversight is imperative because there is potential for harm.

Is it worth a try? Maybe, but don't be casual about it. If you are interested in exploring the use of halotherapy for a particular medical concern, make sure you find a doctor "worth his salt":…in other words, one who knows the way around this particular block.

What Really Works to Clear Your Sinuses

Study titled "Medical Therapies for Adult Chronic Sinusitis: A Systematic Review" by Luke Rudmik, MD, MSc, director of the Endoscopic Sinus and Skull Base program, and colleagues, University of Calgary, Canada, published in *The Journal of the American Medical Association*.

If you're one of the millions of Americans who suffer from chronic sinusitis, with that nasal discharge, painful pressure and congestion that builds up in your head and just won't go away, you may have tried just about anything to get relief—antibiotics, decongestants, pain relievers, saline sprays, steroid sprays, steroid pills…you name it. You may have even considered surgery.

You can stop now. We know what *really* works.

While chronic sinusitis was until recently believed to be basically an infection, it's now recognized as primarily an inflammatory disease…similar to asthma.

To find out what works best, researchers at University of Calgary in Canada and the Medical University of South Carolina performed a systematic review of more than 40 clinical studies. They found out that antihistamines, antibiotics and other common treatments didn't work very well.

Here's what probably will: A combination of saline nasal irrigation and prescription corticosteroid sprays.

A GREAT COMBINATION

Saline irrigation doesn't mean those low-volume saline nasal sprays or mists you can buy in the pharmacy—which only help a little—but a product such as a neti pot. These vessels look like tiny teapots or squeeze bottles, and they make it easy to pour salt water into one side of your nose and let it drain out the other side. They've been used for centuries but have only recently become a part of mainstream Western medicine. Saline irrigation helps clean the sinuses by removing mucus and irritants that contribute to inflammation. According to the new analysis, saline irrigation improves sinusitis symptoms—and quality of life.

Cortocosteroid nasal sprays are prescription-only topical medicines that reduce inflammation and reduce symptoms such as nasal congestion and nasal discharge. Steroid sprays by themselves have been shown to be more effective than nasal irrigation by itself.

While there haven't been studies of using the two approaches together, these were the only

Foods for Better Breathing

A diet high in fiber—especially from fruits and vegetables—can protect against such lung conditions as chronic obstructive pulmonary disease (COPD) and asthma.

New study: Spirometry tests found that among more than 1,900 adults, those who ate the most fiber every day had the best lung function.

Possible reason: Inflammation underlies many lung diseases, and fiber has anti-inflammatory properties. Fiber also changes the composition of the gut microbiome, which may release lung-protective compounds.

Corinne Hanson, PhD, RD, associate professor of medical nutrition, University of Nebraska Medical Center, Omaha.

two treatments that scored the highest rating (A-1) based on the American Heart Association Grade of Evidence and Recommendation Grading Scale. They also work in a true complementary fashion—nasal irrigation clears out the sinus passages while corticosteroids fight the inflammatory process.

Based on the strength of the evidence, the researchers recommend a combination of the two treatments as the best first therapy for most people with chronic sinusitis.

FINDING OUT WHAT WORKS FOR YOU

If you're concerned about using a steroid medication, it's important to realize that a topical spray is much safer than a steroid pill. Corticosteroid sprays are considered safe for all adults, although pregnant women should discuss this treatment option with their physicians before using it. It typically takes two to three weeks before symptoms start to improve, and that depends on how severe your sinusitis is. Some patients use the sprays for a few months during seasons when their symptoms are the worst, while others need to be on them indefinitely.

As for using a neti pot, you can do that once or twice a day. However, some research has found that using a neti pot every day can lead to more infections—after all, there's a reason your body produces mucus, which has antimicrobial properties. So removing your mucus all the time isn't ideal. If you don't have symptoms, you may not want to use a neti pot preventively. You can use it when you do get symptoms, such as when you have a cold. But if you have daily symptoms of chronic sinusitis, then the benefit of using daily saline irrigations often outweighs the small risks.

Since several other conditions can mimic sinusitis, including sinus migraines, if your symptoms don't improve after about two to three months, check back in with your doctor to rule out other conditions. If you're seeing your primary care doctor, he or she may send you for a CT scan of your sinuses or to an otolaryngologist for more detailed evaluation.

Finally, no one study can replace individualized medical care. For example, many people with chronic sinusitis have nasal polyps—noncancerous, teardrop-shaped growths that form in the nose or sinuses. For them, according to

Luke Rudmik, MD, lead author of the study and clinical associate professor at the University of Calgary, best treatment is often to take an oral corticosteroid pill (such as prednisone) for one to three weeks, to take a course of the antibiotic doxycycline for three weeks or to use a leukotriene receptor antagonist, such as *montelukast/ (Singulair)*, a drug that blocks inflammation.

If you don't want to use any medications at all, there's no harm in trying a neti pot for a few weeks and seeing if that works for you. Make it part of your preventive strategy. Since sinus infections typically follow a cold or other upper respiratory infection, use your neti pot at the first sign of an infection coming on. Avoid cigarette smoke, which can irritate nasal membranes, and consider getting a humidifier at home to increase the moisture in the air.

But if preventing colds plus saline irrigation isn't enough help for a chronic sinus condition, talk to your doctor about adding a corticosteroid spray to the mix.

New Drug Shows Promise Against Severe Sinusitis

Claus Bachert, MD, PhD, head, Upper Airway Research Laboratory (URL), and chief, clinics ENT department, University Hospital Ghent, Ghent, Belgium.

Mark Glaum, MD, PhD, associate professor, medicine and pediatrics, division of allergy and immunology, Morsani College of Medicine, James A. Haley Veterans Hospital and the University of South Florida, Tampa, and vice chair, rhinitis, rhinosinusitis and ocular allergy committee, American Academy of Allergy, Asthma and Immunology.

Journal of the American Medical Association.

An experimental drug for the treatment of nasal polyps has shown promise in a small, preliminary trial involving a group of patients struggling with chronic sinusitis.

Dupilumab, which is injected, is aimed at helping those patients who do not respond well to current first-line treatments, such as corticosteroids.

"The more severe patients are the target of the new treatment option," explained study author Claus Bachert, MD, PhD, head of the Upper Airway Research Laboratory at Ghent University Hospital in Belgium.

The study was funded by Sanofi and Regeneron Pharmaceuticals, Inc., the manufacturers of dupilumab.

Chronic sinusitis is a common ailment, affecting an estimated 12% of those living in Western nations.

Roughly one-third of those patients have a specific form of chronic sinusitis characterized by the presence of nasal polyps. Though the polyps vary in size, such growths are typically small, benign and teardrop-shaped. They take root in the mucus membrane lining of the sinus region and/or nasal cavity, the researchers said.

Patients suffering from chronic sinusitis with polyps often struggle with a long-lasting range of symptoms, which can include nasal obstruction and congestion, drip, discharge, headaches, facial pain and pressure, and a diminished sense of smell.

Standard treatment aims to reduce tissue inflammation and usually involves corticosteroids, antibiotics and/or oral steroids. Surgery is an option in some cases.

"Even after oral steroids, polyps recur after just a few weeks, and also after surgery. The recurrence rate is as high as 80 percent over 12 years," said Dr. Bachert.

Surgery also raises the risk for serious complications, he added, while oral steroids can end up weakening bones and boosting the risk for developing diabetes.

With that in mind, the Belgian researchers decided to test the potential of dupilumab, an experimental medication that has already shown promise as a treatment for both severe asthma and the skin rash known as eczema.

The research team focused on a pool of 60 patients, average age about 48, who were being treated at 13 different health care centers in the United States and Europe.

Half of the participants received a 16-week regimen of dupilumab injections, while the other half received a dummy drug (placebo). All patients were additionally prescribed a nasal spray, the study authors said.

After comparing results among the 51 patients who completed their respective course of treatment, the investigators concluded that dupilumab triggered a significant and lasting elimination of polyps, and/or reduction in size. Patients who received the drug also appeared to see benefits in terms of an improved sense of smell, a drop in nasal congestion and obstruction, and improved sleep, the findings showed.

No serious side effects were reported.

"The effects of dupilumab are comparable or better than oral corticosteroids, but last much longer," said Dr. Bachert.

He added that, in some cases, eliminated polyps didn't return for several months following the termination of treatment. However, he said that patients would ultimately require continued treatment.

According to experts, the cost of dupilumab will likely be high, typically thousands of dollars per month. So the cost/benefit analysis will have to be tailored to patients who are still symptomatic after failing to improve with standard therapies.

Air Pollution: The Invisible Kind Is the Deadliest

Study titled "Ambient Particulate Matter Air Pollution Exposure and Mortality in the NIH-AARP Diet and Health Cohort" by researchers at New York University School of Medicine, University of California, Berkeley, Washington University School of Medicine, St. Louis, and National Cancer Institute, Bethesda, Maryland, published in *Environmental Health Perspectives*.

Fine particulates kill. They're so tiny—less than 2.5 micrograms (about 1/10,000th of an inch). Because they're too small to be coughed out of your lungs like other irritants, these deadly particles, which often contain toxic compounds such as mercury and arsenic, slip deep into the tissues of the lungs…and eventually into the bloodstream.

Environmental researchers have been concerned about them for years. But now a large new study of more than 500,000 Americans reveals just how nasty they are. People who live in areas with the highest levels were 3% more likely to die from any cause, 10% more likely to get heart disease and, among nonsmokers, 27% more likely to get respiratory diseases, compared with people who live in the cleanest areas.

Want to know where your part of the country stands? See "Check Your Air Quality" below.

Check Your Air Quality

Neil Schachter, MD, medical director of the respiratory care department at Mount Sinai Hospital and the Maurice Hexter Professor of Pulmonary Medicine at the Icahn School of Medicine at Mount Sinai, both in New York City. He is the author of *The Good Doctor's Guide to Colds and Flu* and serves on the American Lung Association's Northeast Board of Directors.

In the American Lung Association's recent report *State of the Air 2015*, six cities were ranked as having the cleanest air in the nation. They had no days when the air quality reached unhealthy levels for ozone or short-term particle pollution and had the best records for year-round particle pollution. The cities, listed alphabetically, are Bismarck, North Dakota…Cape Coral-Fort Myers-Naples, Florida…Elmira-Corning, New York…Fargo-Wahpeton, North Dakota…Rapid City-Spearfish, South Dakota…and Salinas, California.

To check the air quality in your county, go to *StateoftheAir.org*.

Inform Airlines ASAP About Allergies

Tell the airline if you are allergic to animals as far in advance as possible. Airlines are required to accommodate passengers with service animals, and ordinary pets now are traveling in passenger cabins as well. Airlines can make arrangements for passengers who are highly allergic by rearranging seating or moving you to a different flight. If you are only mildly allergic, take allergy medicine such as Benadryl with you—and bring a dose of epinephrine in your carry-on bag if you might need it.

Roundup of experts on airline travel involving animals, reported in *USA Today*.

Are You Allergic to the Gym?

Jane Wilkens Michael, nationally syndicated radio host and author of *Long Live You! Your Step-by-Step Plan to Look and Feel Better Than Before* and host of *The Jane Wilkens Michael Show* on iHeart Radio Talk. JaneWilkensMichael.com

Allergens that cause coughing, sneezing, wheezing, rashes and/or watery eyes can be found in health clubs.

Common culprits: Pool—some people are sensitive to chlorine. Shower immediately after swimming, or try a saltwater pool, which may be less irritating. Locker room—a recent study found a link between allergies and triclosan, a common ingredient in antibacterial soaps, which often are found in gyms. Bring along your own products. Mats—most mats contain allergy-inducing latex or PVCs. If you have had allergic reactions to these, bring your own mat made of hemp or organic cotton. Workout clothes—polyester and nylon and anything "odor-free" or "antimicrobial" can cause itching. Opt for natural fiber.

Kid Peanut Allergy Cure

Study of 640 children led by researchers at King's College London, UK, and funded by the National Institute of Allergy and Infectious Diseases, published in *The New England Journal of Medicine*.

Kids who eat peanuts from infancy are less likely to develop peanut allergies. Babies regularly given small amounts of peanuts for at least four years had 81% lower risk, on average, for peanut allergies, compared with babies not given peanuts. This means the long-standing medical advice to keep peanuts away from kids to prevent allergies is wrong.

Caution: Young children should be given peanuts only under a doctor's supervision to prevent possibly life-threatening allergic reactions.

Are E-Cigarettes Ever a Good Idea?

Article titled "Evidence, Policy, and E-Cigarettes—Will England Reframe the Debate?" by Sharon H. Green, MPH, project coordinator, Mailman School of Public Health, Columbia University, New York City, and colleagues, published in *The New England Journal of Medicine.*

If you smoke and want to start an argument, here's how—just tell your friends that you're switching to e-cigarettes.

Some might applaud you for taking a positive step—and even suggest the best brands to try. Others will warn you that you're jumping from the frying pan into the fire, falling prey to a new and largely unknown harm—and a new addiction.

The news that the FDA will now regulate e-cigarettes only deepens the debate.

To understand what this means for our readers, we spoke with Sharon H. Green, MPH, a researcher at Columbia University's Mailman School of Public Health, who recently covered e-cigarette controversies in *The New England Journal of Medicine.* Are e-cigs merely a new way for Big Tobacco to keep people hooked...or could they play a role in helping some people quit? Do they benefit health even if you don't quit?

In short, do e-cigarettes ever make sense?

Green believes that for some people, they do.

NEW FDA REGULATIONS...AND NEW CONTROVERSY

Until now, electronic cigarettes have been entirely unregulated—a true Wild West. They can include any of hundreds, even thousands, of ingredients—including flavorings such as "gummy bear" that appeal to kids. Some of these flavorings and other ingredients have been shown to pose health risks—butter flavor, for example, has been linked to a lung disease called popcorn lung.

The new FDA regulation means that e-cigarettes—along with cigars, pipe tobacco and hookahs—are banned for sale to minors. Over the next two years, manufacturers with products that are on the market now are required to divulge all ingredients and submit any health claim to the FDA for approval. These are positive steps,

says Green. Among public health advocates, she says, "Everyone agrees about banning sales to minors—and registering ingredients. Quality control is a good thing."

Many American health groups, however, remain skeptical that e-cigarettes can play a positive role in helping people quit smoking. The Centers for Disease Control and Prevention focuses almost entirely on the health risks of e-cigs, and the American Lung Association argues that there are FDA-approved ways to quit smoking without resorting to e-cigs.

But the Truth Initiative (formerly the American Legacy Foundation), the nation's largest nonprofit anti-tobacco group, argues that e-cigarettes are less harmful than tobacco cigarettes and may help some people quit smoking. To add to the confusion, Public Health England, the British counterpart to our CDC, and the Royal College of Physicians, a British professional medical body, strongly support encouraging smokers to turn to e-cigarettes—even if they aren't able to quit smoking entirely.

BALANCING RISKS

Green readily agrees that e-cigarettes may pose small adverse health effects, that we don't know exactly what the risks are and that, "it will be years before we do know—especially for long-term use." That's why she's sure of one thing. "I would not advise anyone who is not a current smoker to take up e-cigarettes."

On the other hand, she argues, while e-cigarettes have possible risks, which according to the current state of the evidence is a tiny fraction of the risk of combustible cigarettes, tobacco products have proven risks. "Tobacco products kill 480,000 Americans a year," she says. And while research hasn't proven e-cigarettes help people quit smoking, there is evidence that they do help some people—and she weighs that against the frustration most smokers have in quitting. "Seventy percent of smokers say that they want to quit—but only 6% of those who want to quit do quit that same year," she says. "Not only is it extremely difficult to quit this addiction, but the smoking-cessation tools that we have haven't proven to be effective enough.

"We need a new approach," she says. "So anything that smokers find useful and is less damaging to their health—including e-cigarettes—we should embrace." Inhaled nicotine, as in e-cigs, reaches the brain faster than the nicotine in patches and gums, she notes, which can help people fighting nicotine cravings. Some brands of e-cigarettes allow smokers to taper down the level of nicotine, which some smokers may find helpful in reducing dependency.

If you are trying to quit, or know someone who is, by all means work with a doctor so that you can try a combination of approved prescription aids such as nicotine patches, gums, and prescription inhalers—along with quit-smoking counseling available in free call lines, texting apps and more.

But if these approaches don't work, "e-cigarettes can be an effective way to reduce your risk from the harmful effects of tobacco smoking while still satisfying a nicotine addiction," Green says.

Most Smokers Have Impaired Lungs

Study of almost 9,000 current and former smokers by researchers at National Jewish Health, a respiratory hospital in Denver, published in *JAMA Internal Medicine*.

Smokers whose lungs appear all right often have respiratory impairment. When long-term smokers and ex-smokers who passed lung-function tests were evaluated through lung imaging, walking and quality-of-life tests, 55% had some breathing-related difficulty, such as emphysema.

The New Anti-Snoring Workout

Murray Grossan, MD, a board-certified otolaryngologist at Tower Ear, Nose & Throat at Cedars-Sinai Medical Center in Los Angeles. He is also the author of *The Whole Person Tinnitus Relief Program* (DrGrossanTinnitus.com) and founder of Hydro Med Inc.

Snoring can be a nightmare—both for the sufferer and his/her bed partner. But until recently, the treatments have been limited. A snorer might be told to lose weight, for example, wear a mouth guard or a mask (part of a continuous positive airway pressure, or CPAP, system) that delivers a steady stream of air at night…change his sleeping position…or, in severe cases, get surgery.

New development: In a 2015 study of 39 men who snored or had mild obstructive sleep apnea (OSA), a common cause of snoring, scientists found that performing mouth and tongue exercises reduced the frequency and intensity of snoring by up to 59%—a reduction on par with other therapies, including mouth guards or surgery.

And while snoring may seem like more of an annoyance than a health problem, that is simply not true. Snoring has been linked to medical conditions, including heart attack, stroke and glaucoma. *How mouth and tongue exercises can help…*

SIT-UPS FOR YOUR THROAT

If your bed partner has complained of your snoring or you have unexplained daytime sleepiness, consider trying the following exercises.

About half of my patients improve enough after doing these exercises (think of them as "throat sit-ups") for five minutes three times a day for six weeks to avoid surgery or other inconvenient

Dry Eye Link to Seasonal Allergies

Dry eye and seasonal allergens may be linked. Dry eye—a condition of red, watery, gritty-feeling eyes—peaks each year in April, the same month as pollen. Dry eye affects about 20% of women and 10% of men. The correlation between dry eye and the peak in pollen may mean that people with dry eye would benefit from allergy-prevention approaches in addition to current treatments, such as artificial tears.

Examples: Wearing goggles outside when doing yard work…using air filters indoors.

Study of 3.4 million visits to Veterans Affairs eye clinics between 2006 and 2011 by researchers at Bascom Palmer Eye Institute, University of Miami, Florida, published in *Ophthalmology*.

therapies such as wearing a mouth guard or using CPAP. They also awaken feeling more refreshed and reduce their odds of developing OSA.

Here are the main exercises included in the recent study mentioned above (led by Geraldo Lorenzi-Filho, MD, PhD)—along with some slight variations that I have found to be effective for my patients. The tongue positions for these exercises strengthen your tongue muscle and the sides of your throat. However, my variations give these muscles a more rigorous strength-training workout.

●**Tongue Push.**

What to do: Push the tip of your tongue forcefully behind your upper front teeth and move it all the way back along the roof of your mouth (palate) 20 times.

My variation: Say the vowel sounds "A, E, I, O, U" while doing the exercise.

●**Flat Tongue Press.**

What to do: Suck your tongue up against the roof of your mouth, pressing the entire tongue against your palate 20 times.

My variation: Repeat "A, E, I, O, U" while doing the exercise.

●**Say "Ahhh."**

What to do: Focus on raising the back of the roof of the mouth and uvula (the fleshy appendage in the throat that's responsible for the rattling sound made by snorers) 20 times.

My variation: Say the vowel "A" (or "Ahhh") while doing the exercise.

THESE THERAPIES HELP, TOO

Colds, allergies and sinus infections can cause nasal congestion and/or postnasal drip—two common conditions that can make your throat swell, increasing your risk for snoring. *What helps…*

●**Nasal lavage** (using a saline solution to irrigate and cleanse the nasal cavity) helps clear nasal congestion and postnasal drip. Subjects in the study mentioned above performed nasal lavage three times a day. Based on my clinical experience, once a day does the job.

A product that I created called The Hydro Pulse Sinus System ($77.95, *HydroMedOnline. com*) works well. It includes a special throat attachment that directs pulsating irrigation to the tonsils and throat to ease swelling. But you could also use a neti pot (typical cost: $10)—just be sure to keep it clean and sanitized between uses and use distilled or sterile water to prevent a sinus infection. Or you can buy sterile squeeze bottles filled with nasal saline.

●**Nose taping.** With age, the tip of one's nose naturally begins to droop some. This can obstruct the nasal valve, which impedes breathing and contributes to snoring.

Try this simple test: Use your finger to press the tip of your nose up. If breathing feels easier when you do this, try taping your nose up before bedtime.

What to do: Cut a three-inch strip of one-half-inch medical grade tape. Place it under the nose at the center, without blocking the airway. Gently lift the nose as you run the tape up the midline of the nose to the area between the eyes. The taping should be comfortable and is for use during sleep.

Important: Commercial nasal strips, such as Breathe Right, spread the sides of the nose apart. Taping up the nose, as described above, also does this, with the additional advantage of opening the nasal valve.

Depression-Apnea Link

Sleep apnea may worsen depression. Nearly 300 depressed men and women with sleep apnea who successfully received continuous positive airway pressure (CPAP) treatment for their sleep disorder reported that they no longer had feelings of depression after three months.

Why: Disrupted sleep cycles can worsen depression.

If you have symptoms of depression and snore or have disturbed sleep: Ask your doctor to evaluate you for sleep apnea.

David Hillman, MD, clinical professor, The University of Western Australia, Perth.

Big Lung Cancer Risk

Ann Olsson, PhD, MPH, epidemiologist, International Agency for Research on Cancer, Lyon, France, and coauthor of an analysis of seven studies, published in *American Journal of Respiratory and Critical Care Medicine*.

Common respiratory diseases are linked to lung cancer. People who have chronic bronchitis or emphysema were 30% to 50% more likely to have lung cancer than people without the disease. Co-occurring bronchitis, emphysema and pneumonia were associated with twice the lung cancer risk. This increased cancer risk may be related to chronic inflammation.

Exercise May Extend Lives of People With COPD

Alan Mensch, MD, chief, pulmonary medicine, Northwell Health's Plainview Hospital, Plainview, New York
ERJ Open Research, news release.

Regular exercise could help boost the survival of people who've left the hospital after battling chronic obstructive pulmonary disease (COPD), a new study finds.

COPD includes emphysema, chronic bronchitis or a combination of the two, and is often related to smoking. Common symptoms include difficulty breathing, chronic cough, wheezing and phlegm production. Over time, the condition can prove fatal.

One expert, Alan Mensch, MD, noted, "COPD is estimated to affect up to 7% of adults and is a leading cause of death worldwide."

He explained that "difficulty breathing often leads to a sedentary lifestyle in COPD patients, resulting in deconditioning of multiple organ systems, including the heart and muscles.

"Improving muscle function with exercise has been demonstrated to decrease the use of health services in patients with COPD," said Dr. Mensch, who is chief of pulmonary medicine at Northwell Health's Plainview Hospital in Plainview, New York.

The new study's authors also said that the risk of hospital readmission and death is especially high after a person has been hospitalized for COPD.

Could exercise help lower that risk? To find out, Harvard medical school researchers looked at the medical records of almost 2,400 people in California who were hospitalized for COPD.

The researchers found that those who did any amount of moderate to vigorous physical activity were 47% less likely to die in the 12 months after hospitalization than inactive patients.

In fact, low levels of physical activity reduced the risk of death by 28%, the researchers report.

Because of the observational nature of the study, the findings can't prove cause and effect. However, the researchers believe that tracking physical activity levels might be a good way for doctors to pinpoint those COPD patients at high risk for death after hospitalization.

Play the Harmonica to Strengthen Your Lungs

Missy Von Luehrte, RN, pulmonary rehabilitation nurse, El Camino Hospital, Mountain View, California. She participates in the harmonica therapy program for lung patients.
John Schaman, MD, Ontario Aerobics Centre, Canada.

Blowing the blues is good for your lungs. So is just about anything else you play on a harmonica. Whether your tastes run to "Love Me Do," "Sweet Home Chicago" or that 19th-century nonsense ditty "Oh! Susanna," as little as 10 minutes a day playing a harmonica may give you better breathing. In fact, what they're calling "harmonica therapy" is gaining steam in pulmonary-rehabilitation programs across the country for people with asthma, COPD and even lung transplants. But don't let the word "therapy" put you off. Playing the harmonica is a ton of fun, and it's good exercise for healthy lungs, too.

Whether your lungs are compromised or in good shape, you should try it—here's why.

TOE-TAPPING MUSIC-MAKING CLINICAL THERAPY

How does harmonica playing strengthen the lungs? Experts say that it mimics the inspiratory (inhaling) and expiratory (exhaling) breathing exercises taught by pulmonary rehabilitation staff.

When you play a harmonica, you create sounds by the resistance of your breath against the instrument's reeds. Unlike, say, the clarinet, you're working against that reed resistance when you're exhaling and when you're inhaling. That strengthens the diaphragm (the largest muscle of the respiratory system), encourages deep breathing, and may help clear mucus from the lungs. While scientific studies haven't specifically validated therapeutic harmonica playing, it mimics… and encourages…the breathing exercises that have been shown to improve lung function.

FOR PEOPLE WITH HEALTHY LUNGS, TOO, IT'S INTERNAL POWER LIFTING

Some experts believe that playing a wind instrument such as the harmonica can benefit everyone, especially as we age. After about the age of 30, most people begin to lose lung function. By age 50, even people with healthy lungs may lose 50% of their younger capacity, says John Schaman, MD, Ontario Aerobics Centre, a cardiac rehabilitation center in Ontario, Canada. "There is considerable anecdotal evidence that those who use their lungs in more extraordinary ways have less decline," he says.

Sure, you can get deep breathing in other ways, such as meditation practice and yoga, and that's great. What harmonica adds is resistance, says Missy Von Luehrte, RN, a pulmonary rehabilitation nurse at El Camino Hospital in Mountain View, California. "It's like lifting weights for your lungs."

DO YOU NEED A SPECIAL TYPE OF HARMONICA?

Some medical experts recommend harmonicas specifically developed for lung therapy. The Pulmonica (*pulmonica.com*), for example, is designed to create more resistance than a standard harmonica, promoting the clearance of secretions. It makes a pleasant sound, but you can't as easily use it to play songs. The Seydel Medical Harmonica (available at *harmonicamd. com* and other online outlets), which Dr. Schaman helped develop, uses chords rather than single notes, so it may be easier for some people to learn than a standard harmonica.

Others prefer everyday harmonicas. Von Luehrte thinks devices such as the Pulmonica and the Seydel can take the fun out of a simple, joyful musical experience, making harmonica play more like other physical therapy exercises and less of a relaxing, social activity. And while playing chords may be easier and create more resistance, it hasn't been shown that one way of playing is better, healthwise, than another.

So go play…a minimum of 10 minutes a day—more is better. Many pulmonary centers across the country have harmonica therapy groups, which can make it a more social—and musical—experience.

Plus the instructors can teach patients the basics of proper breathing and playing. Some senior centers are getting into the act, too. The most important skill to learn is to breathe with your diaphragm to help your lungs expand, according to nurse Low. If you want to explore a musical approach, check out the book and CD *Harmonica for Fun and Health* to get you started. Or you can Google "harmonica therapy" or "learn to play harmonica" to find a number of instructional sites.

Tai Chi for COPD

W. Darlene Reid, PhD, professor and chair of physical therapy, University of Toronto, Ontario, Canada.

Tai chi helps those with chronic health conditions, such as lung disease. A review of health data for more than 1,500 adults with osteoarthritis, heart failure and/or chronic obstructive pulmonary disease (COPD) found that 30- to 90-minute sessions of tai chi (an ancient Chinese exercise of slow, fluid movements) two to three times a week led to improved strength, balance and posture with no increase in pain or breathlessness in most participants.

To find a tai chi class: Go to *AmericanTai Chi.net.*

Implanted Lung Valves Show Promise in Some Emphysema Patients

Gary Hunninghake, MD, assistant professor, Harvard Medical School, Boston.

Dirk-Jan Slebos, MD, PhD, associate professor, department of pulmonary diseases, and Karin Klooster, graduate student, University of Groningen, the Netherlands.

New England Journal of Medicine.

New research suggests that more careful selection of patients could help improve the success rate of valves implanted into the lungs of people with emphysema.

The valves aim to improve breathing, allowing patients with the chronic lung disease to be more active and to perhaps survive longer. Previous research into the valves has been mixed, but the new Dutch study found that they work more effectively if physicians are more selective about which patients get them.

However, the valves come with a risk of serious side effects, the study authors noted, and the treatment appears to be expensive. It's also not clear whether the valves actually extend lives.

ABOUT EMPHYSEMA

Emphysema is a type of chronic obstructive pulmonary disease (COPD) that damages the airways and makes it difficult for people to breathe. Smoking is the main cause.

Treatment may help patients. But the prognosis can be grim for some people, with death expected within a few years.

In patients with emphysema, pockets filled with air can develop in the lungs and disrupt breathing. The pockets may push on other areas of the lung, causing it to expand in an unhealthy way.

NEW VALVE TREATMENTS

Scientists have developed one-way "endobronchial valves," which are implanted in the lung and allow air to get out of the pockets but not get back into them, said Gary Hunninghake, MD, assistant professor at Harvard Medical School. "It's a way of reducing the volume of these areas without doing surgery on them," he added, and patients may have several valves implanted.

Some physicians have wondered if they don't work as well in certain patients because air finds other ways to re-enter the pockets. In those patients, it appears that "the valve doesn't shut down the problem," Dr. Hunninghake said.

The new study aimed to eliminate these kinds of patients from the research. The study authors recruited 68 patients with severe emphysema, average age 59, to get valves implanted or regular treatment.

In general, those who received the valve treatment were able to breathe better and walk 243 feet farther in six minutes. Seventy-five percent of the patients who got the devices responded to the treatment, said study co-author Dirk-Jan Slebos, MD, PhD, associate professor with the department of pulmonary diseases at the University of Groningen, in the Netherlands.

Will more doctors embrace this treatment? Maybe, Dr. Hunninghake said, if the findings can be confirmed. More research is under way, said study author Karin Klooster, a graduate student at the University of Groningen.

But doctors will have to consider the side effects, Dr. Hunninghake said, including those that occurred in this study—an 18% chance of a collapsed lung and a 15% chance that the valve would have to be removed. It's possible, however, that the side effect rate will improve as surgeons get better at implanting the valves, he said.

CHAPTER 2

Blood Pressure and Cholesterol

7 Little Ways to Keep Your Blood Pressure Down All Day Long

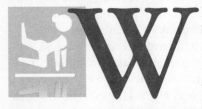**W**hether your blood pressure is normal, borderline or high, you probably think of it as a Big Number. If it's less than 120/80, it's normal. If it's between that and 139/89, it is considered prehypertension. If it's 140/90 or higher, that's hypertension/high blood pressure.

To lower the number, we think of doing Big Things—changing our diet, losing weight, getting regular exercise and, if needed, taking medication. They are important.

But so are some of the little things we do every day. *Here are seven simple lifestyle changes that can help...*

STOP

•**Pouring that extra drink.** Moderate consumption of alcohol actually lowers systolic blood pressure by 2 to 4 millimeters. But if you have more than one drink a day for women, two drinks for men, it can raise blood pressure. Binge drinking—four or more drinks for women, five or more for men, within two hours—is even worse. It not only raises blood pressure in the short term, but it's associated with an increased risk of developing chronic high blood pressure.

•**Drinking lots of coffee—if you're a slow metabolizer.** The jury is out on whether coffee—or caffeine in general—raises blood pressure significantly, but some studies show that drinking a lot of it (about 24 ounces a day)

Samuel J. Mann, MD, professor of clinical medicine, New York-Presbyterian Hospital/Weill-Cornell Medical College, New York City. He is a nationally recognized hypertension specialist and author of *Hypertension and You: Old Drugs, New Drugs, and the Right Drugs for Your High Blood Pressure*.

Health Insider research (*Health Insider* is a free e-newsletter published by *Bottom Line Inc.*)

can raise it. One study published in *Journal of Hypertension* found that coffee raised adrenalin levels and blood pressure—but only in people whose bodies were slow to metabolize caffeine.

Self-test to see if you are a slow metabolizer: Check your blood pressure for a baseline reading. Then drink some coffee, and check your blood pressure again an hour later. If systolic goes up five to 10 millimeters you should cut back on caffeine.

START

•**Taking mini exercise breaks.** Blood pressure actually rises slightly while exercising, but studies consistently show that it goes down soon after exercising, and the results last for as much as eight hours. If a long morning run or gym session isn't in the cards, there's good news—spreading your exercise out over the day has blood pressure benefits. One study in *Medicine & Science in Sports & Exercise* of men with borderline high blood pressure (aka, prehypertension) showed that taking three 10-minute walks throughout the day was more effective at preventing increases in blood pressure than working out for 30 minutes once a day.

•**If you can't exercise, get up and stretch.** If exercise lowers blood pressure, the reverse—being sedentary—keeps it high. Just standing up can help. Another study in *Medicine & Science in Sports & Exercise* of overweight volunteers with prehypertension found that those who stood up for a total of two-and-a-half hours over an eight-hour day had better blood pressure readings than those who sat continuously for an eight-hour workday.

•**Calm yourself.** When stressors hit—whether you're fighting with your spouse or coping with a demanding boss—it's easy for blood pressure to rise. "Anger raises your blood pressure in the moment," says Samuel Mann, MD, professor of clinical medicine at New York Presbyterian Hospital/Weill-Cornell Medical College. "So does fear." Stress hormones raise levels of epinephrine and norepinephrine, which boost heart rate and constrict blood vessels. The stress surge will subside on its own…but you can speed the process by using relaxation techniques. Just five minutes of deep breathing, for

example, has been shown to lower blood pressure. So can short bouts of meditation. This is especially true if you practice meditation—then you can elicit the "relaxation response" in just two or three minutes. Transcendental meditation, for example, has been shown to lower blood pressure by about three points.

•**Take a midday snooze.** Getting a good night's sleep—especially the deeper, restorative, "slow wave" phase—helps keep blood pressure lower during the daytime. But if you didn't get your proper ZZZs, consider an afternoon nap, which has been shown to lower blood pressure in people with hypertension.

According to one study presented at a European Society of Cardiology conference, habitual mid-day snoozers (average nap was one hour) had blood pressure readings that were about 4% lower than people who didn't nap. Nappers also had greater nighttime drops in blood pressure, and they needed less hypertension medication.

•**Breathe in the scent of lemon or lavender.** Aromatherapy can quickly lower blood pressure, although it hasn't been shown to have long-term benefits.

Most effective scents: Lemon, lavender, peppermint, chamomile, neroli. In one study published in *Physiology & Behavior*, simply smelling oil of lemon for 15 minutes reduced blood pressure by about five millimeters systolic (the upper number) and three millimeters diastolic (the bottom number). Try putting two to four drops of essential oil on a cotton ball and keeping it in your office or at home…or putting just a drop or two on your pillow at night. You don't have to take a whiff to have the effect…just having it in the room helps.

Doing these little things doesn't get you off the hook to tackle big issues such as losing weight, eating a healthy diet, getting regular exercise and, if you have high blood pressure that doesn't respond to these lifestyle changes, taking medication.

But sometimes the best way to accomplish the Big Things is to start with little things.

Acupuncture Can Reduce High Blood Pressure

John C. Longhurst, MD, PhD, is a professor of cardiology at Susan Samueli Center for Integrative Medicine, University of California, Irvine, and leader of a study published in *Medical Acupuncture*.

A cupuncture can lower blood pressure for up to a month and a half in patients with mild-to-moderate hypertension.

Recent finding: 70% of patients given acupuncture had systolic (top number) pressure reductions averaging 6 mmHg to 8 mmHg and diastolic (bottom number) reductions averaging 4 mmHg. They also had significant declines in blood levels of *norepinephrine*, which constricts blood vessels and increases blood pressure.

Are Your Blood Pressure Readings Fooling You?

Samuel J. Mann, MD, a hypertension specialist and professor of clinical medicine at New York-Presbyterian Hospital/Weill-Cornell Medical College in New York City. He is also the author of *Hypertension and You: Old Drugs, New Drugs and the Right Drugs for Your High Blood Pressure*.

W hen your blood pressure is taken at the doctor's office, it is good news when it's normal. But a growing body of scientific evidence now shows that these readings may be giving you only part of the picture.

New finding: Studies have reported that about 10% to 20% of people who have normal blood pressure in a doctor's office actually have elevated blood pressure when outside the doctor's office—a condition known as masked hypertension.

Why this is important: Like traditional hypertension (140/90 mmHg or higher), masked hypertension increases risk for coronary artery disease and stroke. In fact, people with masked hypertension may face even more risk because they don't know they have it—leaving them

Watch the Highs and Lows

Big variations in blood pressure increase risk for cardiovascular disease.

Recent finding: People whose systolic pressure (top number) varies by more than 14 mm Hg between one doctor visit and the next are 46% more likely to have a stroke and 30% more likely to have a heart attack or fatal coronary artery disease.

Theory: Big swings may indicate stiff arteries.

Paul Muntner, PhD, is vice chair and professor of epidemiology at University of Alabama at Birmingham and leader of a study of 25,814 patients, published in *Annals of Internal Medicine*.

without a diagnosis or the necessary treatment. *What you need to know...*

HYPERTENSION AT HOME

Many people have heard of white-coat hypertension, the surge in blood pressure that occurs at medical offices when otherwise healthy people see a doctor and get their pressure tested. The theory behind this is that blood pressure rises because you're anxious about having it measured.

Masked hypertension poses a different challenge. Because there's no evidence of high blood pressure at the doctor's office, blood pressure can remain elevated and untreated if it is not checked at home in those who have this condition.

How then can you tell if you have masked hypertension and need to be treated? Should everyone check his/her blood pressure at home, even if it was normal at the doctor's office?

Watching for the danger zone: If your office systolic (top number) blood pressure reading is less than 120, you're not likely to develop hypertension in the near future, since studies show that few people in this range have elevated pressure at home.

But if it is in the 130s, particularly in people under the age of 60, it would be considered borderline hypertension (also called prehypertension) and needs to be followed—both at home and in the doctor's office. Most masked hypertension is actually borderline hypertension, a warning sign that you may need to improve your diet, get more exercise, lose weight and reduce excessive sodium intake.

The risk: Research has found that patients with masked hypertension have more than twice the cardiovascular risk—including risk for heart attack and atherosclerosis—as patients with normal blood pressure. Meanwhile, a recent study presented at an annual meeting of the American Society of Hypertension found that the risk for cognitive dysfunction in people with untreated masked hypertension was twice as high as for those who had controlled hypertension.

Of course, everyone's blood pressure does naturally vary, depending on age, activity levels, stress and other factors. That's why doctors should take at least two or three office readings, during separate appointments, before diagnosing traditional hypertension.

For a more complete picture, your physician might ask you to also take home readings (see below for details) to better assess your blood pressure and check for masked hypertension.

DO YOU NEED HOME-TESTING?

If your systolic readings are in the 130s in the doctor's office, talk to your doctor about at-home blood pressure monitoring.

The main options for home blood pressure testing are either ambulatory or self-monitoring. Ambulatory monitoring, in which you wear a blood pressure monitor for 24 hours, provides a more reliable picture of your blood pressure and is considered a better predictor of cardiovascular risk than office measurements.

Self-monitoring allows you to check your blood pressure over time. *To get the most accurate readings when self-monitoring, be sure to follow these tips…*

•**Don't check every day.** I tell patients not to check their blood pressure every day. It can become an obsession that can even affect your blood pressure readings. Your doctor can guide you on how often to check, depending on your readings and overall health. People with severe hypertension (frequent systolic readings of 160

or higher) or who have recently changed medications and/or doses may need to check their pressure more often until it is stable.

•**Use an arm cuff.** It's more reliable than a wrist or finger device. I recommend Omron automated blood pressure monitors, which hypertension specialists consider to be reliable. Depending on the device, the cost can range from about $50 to $110.

What to do: Put the cuff in place with the bottom of the cuff about one-half to one inch above the elbow crease, then sit and relax for five minutes.

Next, take three readings a minute or so apart to obtain your resting blood pressure. Because the first reading can be unreliable, I recommend averaging the other two. As long as your doctor has found that your blood pressure is about the same in both arms, you need to check only one arm.

•**Test at different times of day.** It will help you get a sense of what your usual blood pressure is. However, you don't want to test immediately upon awakening. Blood pressure is commonly elevated when you first wake up, so wait half an hour or so.

Also important: Keep a written or digital record of your readings, and share them with your doctor. If your systolic blood pressure average is 135 or higher, your doctor may want to begin treatment with medication…and should also talk to you about better diet and exercise habits.

Blood Pressure Too Low?

Mark Houston, MD, director, Hypertension Institute of Nashville, and coauthor of *What Your Doctor May Not Tell You About Hypertension*.

Exercise dilates arteries and can reduce blood pressure by as much as five to 15 points after a workout. Low blood pressure is technically defined as a systolic (top number) of less than 90 and diastolic (lower number) of less than 60. But if you take blood pressure medication and your readings are below 100/69 (or hovering in that general area), your numbers are too low. Ask your doctor to review your medication and possibly adjust the dosage and when you take it.

The High-Fat Path to Low Blood Pressure... and a Healthier Heart

Study titled "Comparison of the DASH (Dietary Approaches to Stop Hypertension) diet and a higher-fat DASH diet on blood pressure and lipids and lipoproteins: a randomized controlled trial" by researchers at Children's Hospital Oakland Research Institute, Oakland, California, and College of Pharmacy, Touro University California, Vallejo, published in *American Journal of Clinical Nutrition*.

The DASH diet is one of the most healthful diets ever created. But it's not that easy to stick to.

One reason that it's so tough is that it's low in fat, especially the saturated fat found in "real" dairy foods that we love so much. In particular, you're supposed to give up full-fat cheese and yogurt and whole milk in favor of low-fat and fat-free versions.

Not very tasty.

And, according to the latest study, not at all necessary.

MORE SATURATED FAT, LESS SUGAR

The DASH diet started out as a way to lower blood pressure—hence the name, an acronym for "Dietary Approaches to Stop Hypertension." That it does well. People who follow the diet have also been found to have less risk for heart disease, stroke, diabetes, kidney stones, colon cancer and dementia. Oh, yes, it's also great for weight loss.

The diet emphasizes plenty of fruits and vegetables, whole grains and low-fat dairy, along with lean poultry and fish, nuts, beans and seeds.

But it's also a low-fat diet, with a particular emphasis on keeping saturated fat low.

Here's the problem: Saturated fat, especially the kind found in dairy foods, doesn't appear to

Almonds Lower Blood Pressure

Men who ate a handful of almonds daily for four weeks had lower blood pressure and improved blood flow.

Study by researchers at Aston University in Birmingham, UK.

be bad for the heart. Meanwhile, sugar is—and the diet allowed sugar-laden fruit juices to be counted toward the fruit servings.

So the researchers wondered: What if we allowed DASH dieters to eat full-fat cheeses, high-fat yogurt and whole milk—while asking them to cut back on fruit juices and other sugar sources?

Bingo.

A TASTIER, HEALTHIER DIET

To test out the idea that full-fat dairy could make DASH both more palatable and just as healthy, researchers put 36 men and women on different diets over about two-and-a-half years—a control diet, similar to the standard American diet...a traditional low-fat DASH diet...or a high-fat DASH diet. By letting dieters have whole-fat dairy, the total fat went up from 27% in the traditional DASH to 40%...and saturated fat nearly doubled, from 8% to 14%. By cutting back on sugar, mainly from fruit juice, daily consumption went down from 158 grams a day on the traditional DASH to 93 grams.

No doubt, the high-fat DASH was tastier. But it was also just as effective at lowering blood pressure, both systolic and diastolic, as the low-fat DASH.

Plus, it had extra benefits: Compared with the low-fat, higher-sugar traditional DASH diet, it lowered triglycerides—blood fats that raise the risk for heart disease and diabetes. The high-fat DASH also was better at reducing very low density lipoprotein (VLDL), which is particularly associated with heart disease risk.

That makes this already heart-healthy diet even heart-healthier.

And more enjoyable.

Juice Up Your Heart!

Drinking a 2.4-ounce glass of beet juice daily reduced systolic (top number) blood pressure by five to 10 points in a small, week long study of older patients with a common form of heart failure that affects the pumping ability of the left ventricle. A 24% boost in aerobic endurance was also reported. Beet juice tastes sweet and is packed with inorganic nitrate, a nutrient that has been shown to improve vascular health and oxygen metabolism.

Dalane Kitzman, MD, professor of cardiology, Wake Forest Baptist Medical Center, Winston-Salem, North Carolina.

Got High Blood Pressure? Cut Your Diabetes Risk by 57%

Study titled "Bedtime ingestion of hypertension medications reduces the risk of new-onset type 2 diabetes: a randomised controlled trial" by researchers at University of Vigo, Spain, published in *Diabetologia*.

If you are on high blood pressure medications, you might want to take your pills at night rather than in the morning. In a study, doing that improved all-day blood pressure control and reduced the risk of developing diabetes by 57%.

Possible reason: Bedtime meds lead to a more normal nighttime "dip" in the hormone angiotensin, which affects both blood pressure and blood sugar. Talk to your doctor before changing your medication schedule.

Get It Down After 50

The New England Journal of Medicine, Hypertension and *The New York Times*.

Aim for much lower blood pressure if you are over age 50. The government now says that the longstanding recommendation of 140/90 is too high. Instead, people over age 50 should have blood pressure of 120/80 or lower. Those with high blood pressure who reduced the systolic (top) number to 120 had a 30% bigger drop in stroke risk and a 25% bigger reduction in risk for death than those who lowered it to 140.

Shake Your Way to Lower Blood Pressure

Study titled, "Whole-body vibration exercise training reduces arterial stiffness in postmenopausal women with prehypertension and hypertension" by Arturo Figueroa, MD, PhD, associate professor of vascular exercise physiology at Florida State University, Tallahassee, and colleagues, published in *Menopause*.

"Jiggle" machines to lose weight—those belts that vibrate around your middle while you just stand there—go back to the 19th century.

News flash: They don't work too well…for weight loss, that is. The best that can be said is that they may help with weight loss…if you also cut calories. Thanks a lot.

But a new generation of "whole-body vibration" (WBV) machines is showing up in some gyms, in physical therapy clinics and even as home fitness equipment. What gives? It turns out that new research is uncovering other health benefits. They help build muscle, and there is some evidence that they may help build bone, too.

The latest benefit—lowering elevated blood pressure.

To learn more, we spoke to Arturo Figueroa, MD, PhD, associate professor of exercise physiology at Florida State University in Tallahassee who has been researching these new machines.

KEEPING YOUR ARTERIES FLEXIBLE

In his research, Dr. Figueroa has shown that 30-to-40-minute sessions three times a week with WBV brought down blood pressure by an average of 12 mmHg systolic and 6 mmHg diastolic over a three-month period.

That's enough to bring you down an entire blood pressure category. That is, if you are "prehypertensive" (aka "borderline"), with a reading between 120/80 and 139/89, WBV treatment could bring you into the "normal" category—below 120/80. If you are hypertensive, with a reading of 140/90 or higher, you could drop down to prehypertensive—and you might no longer require medication. Dr. Figueroa's research has been on women after menopause, when risk for high blood pressure increases, but he believes that the blood pressure–lowering effects are likely to apply to older men as well.

How does jiggling work therapeutically? WBV has been shown to make the arteries more flexible—less stiff—Dr. Figueroa said. "Arterial stiffness is a process in which the arteries lose their elasticity," he explains. "A stiffer artery makes the heart work harder, raising blood pressure and cardiovascular risk." WBV may make arteries—including the peripheral ones that go throughout the body—more flexible by improving the functioning of their lining cells (the endothelium) and by stimulating production of nitric oxide, which helps arteries contract and dilate more efficiently.

READY TO RUMBLE?

To put this research into perspective, remember that regular exercise also reliably lowers high blood pressure, although not as dramatically. Exercise with WBV is no substitute for aerobic exercise and strength training, which have many more benefits for the body and the mind than can be expected from WBV. Indeed, these machines often are used in physical therapy clinics for people who can't do conventional exercise, such as someone recovering from a stroke or with severe arthritis.

Want to add WBV to your exercise routine? First, if you're being treated for hypertension or other ailments, get an OK from your doctor—and don't stop taking any medications without his or her approval. Next, try out one of these machines at a gym or physical therapy clinic that has one—especially before sinking hundreds or thousands of dollars into buying one for home use.

Be aware of possible side effects. As with any exercise, you can experience fatigue and muscle soreness. You may also experience skin redness and itching during the initial sessions due to the increased blood flow to your legs. These are minor. Swelling (edema) in the legs also can happen, but it is rare—if you experience this, tell your doctor.

The most important advice: Whether you use a WBV machine at a gym or get one for home use, Dr. Figueroa advised that you'll get the most benefit if you first get trained by someone who knows how to work with WBV, such as an exercise physiologist. In fact, he said, gyms that have these machines often stick them in an out-of-the-way room because no one knows how to use them properly. "There are many personal trainers who are not prepared to provide advice for WBV training," warns Dr. Figueroa. "Personally I have seen physical therapists use them with patients who wear shoes during the vibration exercise. That dampens the beneficial effects, negating some of the benefits." There are other subtleties such as how to bend your knees to get the best benefit, but they're easy to learn from a trained instructor the first time you use one of these machines.

Beta-Blocker Warning

Mads Emil Jørgensen, MB, is a researcher at Copenhagen University Hospital Gentofte, Hellebæk, Denmark, and leader of a study published in *JAMA Internal Medicine*.

People taking beta-blockers for high blood pressure are more likely to have complications such as heart attack or stroke within 30 days after noncardiac surgery, warns Mads Emil Jørgensen, MB. If you are scheduled for noncardiac surgery, ask your doctor if you should switch to a different blood pressure drug or temporarily stop taking medication before surgery. Never stop taking a blood pressure drug on your own. Beta-blockers include drugs such as *metoprolol* (Lopressor), *nadolol* (Corgard) and *propranolol* (Inderal).

Si, Siesta!

Manolis Kallistratos, MD, cardiologist, Asklepieio Voulas General Hospital, Athens, Greece.

Middle-aged adults with high blood pressure who took a 60-minute afternoon nap every day had average blood pressure readings that were four points lower (which correlates to a 20% reduction in cardiovascular disease risk) than those who didn't nap.

Theory: Napping seems to calm the sympathetic nervous system, which controls heart rate and blood pressure.

Caveat: A nap of more than an hour may not have the same beneficial effect.

No Statins Before Heart Surgery, Study Suggests

Barbara Casadei, MD, professor, cardiovascular medicine, University of Oxford, U.K.
Gregg Fonarow, MD, professor, cardiology, University of California, Los Angeles.
New England Journal of Medicine.

Taking cholesterol-lowering statins right before heart surgery, once touted as a way to prevent common postoperative complications, has no benefit and may even cause harm, a recent study suggests.

In that setting, *rosuvastatin* (Crestor) did not prevent either the abnormal heart rhythm known as atrial fibrillation or heart damage, and it was linked to a slightly increased risk of kidney damage, researchers said.

"There are many valid reasons why one may want to take statins, but prevention of postoperative complications in cardiac surgery is not one of them," said lead researcher Barbara Casadei, MD. She is a professor of cardiovascular medicine at the University of Oxford in England.

STUDY DETAILS

"Our study is consistent with the idea that well-established beneficial effects of statin therapy, such as the reduction in heart attacks and strokes, are only achieved by long-term treatment with these drugs," she added.

For the study, Dr. Casadei and her colleagues randomly assigned more than 1,900 patients who were having elective heart surgery to take Crestor or a placebo before surgery.

The researchers found that patients given Crestor had lower levels of cholesterol and C-reactive protein (another marker for heart trouble) after surgery, compared with patients given a placebo.

However, the percentages of those who developed atrial fibrillation were essentially the same in patients given Crestor (21.1%) and those given a placebo (20.5%), the investigators found.

And further analyses showed that Crestor was associated with a 5.4% greater chance of mild kidney damage, when compared with a placebo.

The cause of the kidney damage isn't known, said Dr. Casadei, since the study was not designed to show cause-and-effect. However, her team plans to study that issue further, she added.

"The risk of kidney injury is relatively small, but considering that the benefit of statin treatment before a heart operation is zero, one may well consider stopping statins for a few days before surgery," Dr. Casadei said.

The report was published in the *New England Journal of Medicine.*

EXPERT COMMENTARY

Gregg Fonarow, MD, a professor of cardiology at the University of California, Los Angeles, said the study findings should not deter patients from taking statins to prevent heart attacks and strokes.

New Screening for High Blood Pressure?

A modified version of the troponin T test, long used to identify heart attacks, can predict the risk for hypertension years before it actually occurs. More research is needed.

Circulation

"Current guidelines recommend that all patients with cardiovascular disease, including patients after coronary artery bypass surgery, receive statins to lower the risk of fatal and nonfatal heart attacks and strokes," he said.

Beyond the intermediate and long-term benefits of statins, a number of small clinical trials have suggested an additional short-term benefit of starting or continuing statin therapy before heart surgery. However, many of these studies may have had problems that clouded the findings, Dr. Fonarow noted.

"This new trial suggests that there is no compelling reason to initiate statin therapy just before cardiac surgery," he said.

"However, long-term treatment with statins is essential to lower the intermediate and long-term risk of fatal and nonfatal cardiovascular events in patients with cardiovascular disease," Dr. Fonarow added.

Visit the American Heart Association website, Heart.org, for more on statins.

Get This Scan First

Khurram Nasir, MD, MPH, cardiologist, Baptist Health South Florida, Miami Beach.

Simple scan tells whether you really need a statin.

Recent finding: Coronary calcium scans given to nearly 5,000 adults revealed that almost half of those considered candidates for statins had no plaque in their coronary arteries, and their risk for heart attack and/or stroke in the next 10 years was much lower than previously thought.

If you're unsure about taking a statin: Ask about getting this test (which checks for calcifications in the walls of coronary arteries) first. It costs $99 and up (which could be covered by insurance) and typically uses a low dose of radiation, about 3 mSv, a little more than the amount used for a film mammogram.

Statins and Aggression

The popular cholesterol-lowering statins *simvastatin* (Zocor) and *pravastatin* (Pravachol) were found to increase aggressive acts (such as slapping someone or self-harm) in postmenopausal women but reduced aggression in men in a recent six-month study of 1,000 adults.

Theory: Statins not only reduce cholesterol but may also influence testosterone levels and sleep patterns, which affect men and women differently.

Beatrice Golomb, MD, PhD, professor of medicine, University of California, San Diego.

Forget "Bad" Cholesterol: Here's the Number You Should Really Worry About

Stephen T. Sinatra, MD, assistant clinical professor of medicine, University of Connecticut School of Medicine, Farmington, Connecticut, clinical assistant professor of family medicine, University of New England College of Osteopathic Medicine, Biddeford, Maine. He is coauthor of *The Great Cholesterol Myth: Why Lowering Your Cholesterol Won't Prevent Heart Disease—and the Statin-Free Plan That Will.*

Study titled "Study of the Use of Lipid Panels as a Marker of Insulin Resistance to Determine Cardiovascular Risk," by Ruth Ann Bertsch, MD, PhD, Sacramento Medical Center, California; Maqdooda A. Merchant, MSc, MA, Kaiser Permanente, Oakland, California, published in *The Permanente Journal.*

Old habits die hard. For several decades, doctors have focused on low-density liprotein (LDL), the so-called "bad cholesterol," as a key indicator of a person's risk for heart disease.

But another readily available measurement usually ignored by doctors is much better—the ratio of triglycerides, a kind of fat found in the blood, to high-density lipoprotein (HDL), the "good" cholesterol. The lower the ratio, the better.

And now a new study has confirmed that the triglyceride/HDL ratio, as opposed to LDL levels, is far more predictive of heart disease risk.

That would be bad enough if it meant that many doctors are missing a prime driver of heart disease in their patients. But the real effects actually are much worse—they're missing the right prescription for heart disease prevention and often prescribing the wrong one...statins.

To find out about the latest study—and the very different approach to heart disease prevention that it supports, we spoke with cardiologist Stephen Sinatra, MD, an assistant clinical professor of medicine at University of Connecticut School of Medicine and coauthor of *The Great Cholesterol Myth.*

A BETTER MEASURE OF HEART RISK

The triglyceride/HDL ratio has shown up as a big risk factor in small studies, so researchers at Kaiser Permanente Northern California, one of the country's largest health-care providers, analyzed data from more than 100,000 healthy men and women between ages 50 and 75 over about eight years to see which ones developed ischemic heart disease. That's the most common form of heart disease, caused by narrowing of the arteries.

The researchers checked these outcomes against lab values available in the typical "lipid profile." For LDL, they looked at people with levels above 160 mg/dL, which is officially "high" according to national guidelines. For the triglyceride/HDL ratio, they looked at people within the top third of trigylcerides and the bottom third of HDL levels.

Here's what they found...

•**Those with high LDL cholesterol were 19% more likely to develop heart disease.**

•**Those with high triglyceride/HDL ratios were 68% more likely to develop heart disease**—more than triple the risk of those with high LDL.

The new research strengthens the growing body of evidence that LDL cholesterol levels aren't the main drivers of heart disease. Here's the big concern—one in four Americans is currently taking cholesterol-lowering prescription medication, primarily statins, which reliably lower LDL levels but do little or nothing to prevent a first heart attack. (To learn more, see Bottom Line's "What the Research Really Shows About Cholesterol-Lowering Drugs" on page 31.)

The triglyceride/HDL ratio, on the other hand, can indicate something completely different—potential insulin resistance, the ability of the body to metabolize carbohydrates. Insulin resistance, Dr. Sinatra explains, a well-known risk factor of type 2 diabetes, also is a main driver of metabolic syndrome—a constellation of risk factors that may include high blood pressure and being overweight, especially with a big belly, that greatly increases heart disease risk.

"If you have insulin resistance and you cannot metabolize sugar effectively, the calories are not burned up but stored as fat in the form of triglycerides," Dr. Sinatra explains. "If you look at love handles on men and women, that's a visual of triglycerides," he says. "Visceral belly-fat tissue is a hotbed of inflammatory chemicals, and studies show that inflammation is a key cause of plaque buildup in blood vessels."

Paying attention to the more significant triglyceride/HDL ratio leads to a very different treatment plan—lose weight, increase exercise and change your diet. Instead of statins, says Dr. Sinatra, "What these patients really need is to treat the insulin resistance with a low-carbohydrate, low-sugar diet and exercise."

HOW TO LOWER YOUR RATIO—AND PROTECT YOUR HEART

To find your ratio, divide your triglyceride level by your HDL level. For instance, if your triglyceride level is 150 and your HDL is 50, your ratio is 150/50 or 3. A ratio of 2 or less is considered ideal. In the Kaiser study, the cut-off for being in the top third of trigylcerides and lower third of HDL turned out to be 2.7.

"Anything over 3, I tend to get a little concerned about," says Sinatra. "If you're 5 or over, I'm very aggressive at reducing it." *To improve your ratio, he recommends...*

•**Reducing your intake of sugar and processed carbohydrates,** which break down quickly into blood sugar and raise triglyercides.

•**Adding healthy fats including olive oil, coconut oil and avocados.**

•**Including foods rich in omega-3s,** such as fish and fish oil, flaxseed, walnuts and fermented soy. (He often recommends squid or fish oil supplements to his patients with poor ratios.)

•**Getting regular exercise,** which helps boost HDL among many other heart benefits.

How Statin Makers Skew the Truth

David M. Diamond, PhD, professor, departments of psychology and molecular pharmacology and physiology and director of the USF Neuroscience Collaborative Program and the USF Center for Preclinical and Clinical Research on Post-Traumatic Stress Disorder, University of South Florida, Tampa. His article appeared in *Expert Review of Clinical Pharmacology*.

Those so-called "wonder" drugs that help reduce cholesterol—the statins (Lipitor, Crestor and Zocor, to name a few)—aren't anywhere close to being all they're hyped up to be. Sure, they reduce cholesterol, but their use is fraught with questions. In fact, the hype on statins can be considered a statistical deception.

A review of several statin studies found that the results are often framed in ways that make them seem much more promising or beneficial than they really are. A major study called JUPITER, for example, shows how statistical data can be reported to overexaggerate benefit. JUPITER, stands for "Justification for the Use of Statins in Primary Prevention: An Intervention Trial Evaluating Rosuvastatin." The results of this study were used back in 2008 to get FDA approval to use *rosuvastatin* (Crestor) to help prevent heart disease in healthy people. Before that time, it was approved for use only in people who were known to be at high risk for heart attack and stroke.

The JUPITER trial compared Crestor to a placebo in 17,800 healthy people. The study results showed that, overall, a mere 0.76% of people taking the placebo had heart attacks, strokes or other major cardiovascular events compared with 0.35% of people taking Crestor—in both groups, less than 1% of participants. But in a press release about the study, the manufacturers of Crestor reported that the statin reduced the risk of heart attack "by more than half" because the percentage difference between 0.76 and 0.35 is 54 ("more than half"). Results were then framed in a similar way at a major medical meet-

ing and published in the journal *Circulation*. Although the percentage of risk reduction was technically accurate, it alone completely failed to convey the fact that the absolute amount of risk even for the group that didn't take the drug was very small—les than 1%!

Other major studies engendered similar overstatements about the benefits of one or another statin. Take, for example, the study results that the manufacturer of Lipitor emblazoned on ads placed in medical journals—that Lipitor (known generically as atorvastatin) "reduces risk of heart attack by 36% in patients with multiple risk factors for heart disease." In the Lipitor study, which included 10,305 people who had high blood pressure and at least three other risk factors for heart disease, 3% of the people on placebo had heart attacks within three years versus 1.9% of the people on Lipitor, leading to a risk reduction rate of 36% using the same math as was used in the JUPITER study. A similar scenario was illustrated in a major study of simvastatin, marketed as Zocor.

THE CHOLESTEROL MYTH

Profit may be a driving force behind America's "high cholesterol" epidemic and drugs to keep it under control. Consider that more than 200 million statin prescriptions are written in the US each year—we're talking $26 billion in revenue for pharmaceutical companies. And if the updated clinical guidelines from the American College of Cardiology and American Heart Association are followed, 46 million more Americans may end up on statins. These guidelines recommend statin treatment for diabetics and almost all of the elderly. Not surprisingly, eight of the 15 panelists who created these guidelines have extensive ties to the pharmaceutical industry.

Doctors are pushing statins on us based on the fact that cholesterol is found in tissue that has become atherosclerotic, but there's no concrete evidence that cholesterol causes coronary heart disease. In older adults, atherosclerosis is found equally in those with high and low cholesterol. And you can have high levels of "bad" cholesterol (low-density lipoproteins) and not be at increased risk of heart disease and vice versa.

Lipoproteins (cholesterol and other blood fats called triglycerides) play a major role in our immune systems, and it's perhaps inaccurate to label them "good" or "bad." Low cholesterol levels have been linked to viral infection and cancer—there are several large and long-term studies showing associations between low cholesterol levels, use of statins as well as other cholesterol-lowering drugs and cancer risk. There are also several studies showing that low cholesterol is associated with neurological and mood disorders, including violent behavior, depression, suicide and dementia. In fact, there are two studies that showed that cognitive function improved in adults with memory problems or dementia when statin medication was stopped and returned when it was restarted.

THE ALTERNATIVE

You won't find good health in a pill. For the vast majority of people, the secret to longevity and to reducing the risk of heart disease is in weight and stress control, moderate exercise and maintaining a healthy diet. This means reducing the amount of sugar and fried foods you eat and, if you eat red meat or dairy, choosing natural sources of saturated fats that are free from antibiotics and hormones that can wreak havoc on your metabolism. These include grass-fed beef, eggs from free-range chickens, and butter and cheese from grass-fed cows.

Statins and Memory Loss

Linda L. Restifo, MD, PhD, is professor in the department of neurology at University of Arizona, Tucson.

Statins can cause memory loss in some patients, despite a recent study that found they don't have cognitive side effects,. The study was a generalized statistical study—not a personalized look at vulnerable patients. Some people who are susceptible do have "statin brain." Symptoms stop when the drug is stopped. These patients should talk to their doctors. Anyone considering starting a statin should ask about every-other-day rather than daily dosing.

What the Research Really Shows About Cholesterol-Lowering Drugs

Barbara H. Roberts, MD, director of the Women's Cardiac Center at The Miriam Hospital and a clinical associate professor of medicine at Alpert Medical School of Brown University, both in Providence. She is author of *The Truth About Statins: Risks and Alternatives to Cholesterol-Lowering Drugs.*

Under recent controversial guidelines from the American Heart Association, nearly half of all American adults between the ages of 40 and 75 would be advised to take a cholesterol-lowering statin drug. This class of drugs includes *simvastatin* (Zocor), *atorvastatin* (Lipitor), *rosuvastatin* (Crestor) and others. About 25% of adults are taking a statin now.

Statins do an impressive job of lowering LDL "bad" cholesterol—by up to 50% in some cases. How well do they achieve the real goal of reducing the risk for heart attacks? That evidence isn't impressive. And statins can have serious side effects.

IS LDL REALLY THE ENEMY?

For decades, the public-health message hasn't changed. High cholesterol—particularly high levels of LDL cholesterol—leads to atherosclerosis, blood clots and heart attacks.

Yet many important studies, including the Framingham Heart Study, have shown that most patients who have had a heart attack have cholesterol levels that are nearly identical to those who haven't. Further, many experts believe that HDL "good" cholesterol is a more important predictor of heart disease than LDL.

Statins can lower the risk for recurrent heart attack by a small amount in people who already have had one. But most studies of statins have not shown a reduction in mortality. And way too often, they're used for primary prevention—to lower LDL in those who haven't been diagnosed with heart disease.

In people who haven't been diagnosed with cardiovascular disease, the use of statins reduced the risk for heart attacks and other cardiovascular events by a paltry 1% to 2%.

SERIOUS SIDE EFFECTS

Statins are not the benign drugs that they're made out to be. About 20% to 25% of patients experience side effects, some of which are serious. For example, statins reduce blood levels of CoQ10, which is involved in energy production inside cells. Low CoQ10 has been linked to heart failure, hypertension, fatigue and "mental fog."

The most common side effect of statin therapy is myalgia, or muscle pain. The pain usually is mild, but the risk—and severity—increases at higher doses. Rhabdomyolysis is a severe form of statin-related muscle damage that can lead to kidney failure, which can be fatal.

Side effects are an acceptable trade-off when drugs truly save lives. This isn't the case for the vast majority of patients who take statins.

Two exceptions: If you have high LDL and have had a heart attack…or if you've been diagnosed with cardiovascular disease (or diabetes if you are a man), a statin can make sense. I also recommend statins to patients who have familial hypercholesterolemia, sky-high cholesterol caused by a genetic abnormality.

A BETTER APPROACH

I advise most patients to work on their diets before resorting to statins. *Dietary changes can increase HDL and reduce triglycerides, which is more important than reducing LDL…*

•**Mediterranean diet.** The Lyon Diet Heart Study showed conclusively that heart attack patients who followed a Mediterranean-type diet (more whole grains, vegetables, fruit and fish, and less beef, lamb and pork, among other factors) greatly improve their odds of never having another heart attack. Compared with those who followed a "prudent" Western diet, they were 56% less likely to die from any cause…65% less likely to suffer cardiac death…and 70% less likely to have a heart attack.

You might assume patients in the Mediterranean diet group had lower LDL. Not so. Their LDL was roughly the same as that of people in the control group—further proof that you don't need to reduce LDL to improve cardiovascular risks. For more on the Mediterranean diet, read my book or the book *Low-Fat Lies, High-Fat Frauds and the Healthiest Diet in the World* by Kevin Vigilante, MD, MPH, and Mary Flynn, PhD.

Why was the Mediterranean diet so effective? Some credit goes to olive oil and fish (see below) and antioxidant-rich fruits and vegetables, which reduce inflammation and blood clots. The diet also is low in pro-inflammatory omega-6 fatty acids (from corn and other vegetable-based oils) and high in fiber.

•**More olive oil.** Extra-virgin olive oil is rich in phytochemicals, many of which inhibit oxidation. Oxidized cholesterol increases atherosclerosis and the "stiffening" of arteries that leads to higher blood pressure. Olive oil also has been shown to increase HDL.

I advise patients with low HDL to have three to four tablespoons of olive oil daily in addition to the small amounts that are used in cooking. Use it in salad dressings, or drizzle it on fish or poultry.

•**Don't worry about saturated fat.** Patients with high cholesterol usually are advised to consume less saturated fat. It's true that saturated fat raises LDL—but only the "fluffy" LDL particles that are largely benign. Saturated fat, such as dairy fat, is an effective way to increase HDL. There's some evidence that the saturated fat found in milk and other dairy foods reduces diabetes risk.

•**Seafood a few times a week.** In parts of the world where people eat a lot of fatty fish (such as salmon and tuna), the risk for cardiovascular disease tends to be lower. The omega-3 fatty acids in fish reduce triglycerides and inflammation.

•**Enjoy your wine.** Moderate drinking (no more than two drinks a day for men and one for women) has been shown to reduce the risk for heart disease. Red wine may be particularly helpful because it is high in antioxidants.

Be wary of "white" foods—simple carbohydrates such as white bread, white rice, white pasta and some breakfast cereals. These are essentially sugar and cause a surge of insulin, which increases the risk for cardiovascular disease. Insulin also increases fat storage, particularly in the abdomen. Abdominal fat is a leading risk factor for heart disease.

•**Don't forget to exercise.** You already know the importance of regular exercise, but it is worth repeating. Everyone should get at least 150 minutes of moderate-intensity exercise a week with brisk walking, biking, swimming, etc. It is among the best ways to lower the risk for diabetes, hypertension and heart disease.

Snooze Your Way to Better Cholesterol

Study titled "Prolonged sleep restriction induces changes in pathways involved in cholesterol metabolism and inflammatory responses" by researchers at University of Helsinki, Finland, published in *Scientific Reports*.

A high level of HDL, the good kind of cholesterol, protects your heart and your brain. You've heard plenty about how to get that level up—exercise, drink red wine, eat HDL-boosting foods such as nuts and avocados.

Now two studies by researchers at University of Helsinki have uncovered another way to boost HDL—getting enough sleep. In fact, a little less than one week of skimping on sleep triggered a worrisome trend.

First study: Fourteen volunteers had their sleep restricted to only four hours a night for five days, while seven other volunteers were allowed to sleep normally. Compared to the well-rested volunteers, the sleep-deprived ones had a significant drop in the activity of genes that regulate cholesterol.

The researchers confirmed their results in a second study: They used data from 2,739 participants who filled out questionnaires about their sleep habits. Just like the sleep-deprived volunteers in the first study, those who reported that they regularly didn't get enough sleep (less than seven hours) had less expression of cholesterol-regulating genes—and their HDL levels were lower than those who reported that they got sufficient sleep.

So keep up your heart-healthy lifestyle—exercise, red wine, a cardio- and brain-protective diet. But make sure to also get to bed at a reasonable hour.

Genetic High-Cholesterol Condition More Common Than Thought

Sarah de Ferranti, MD, MPH, assistant professor, pediatrics, Harvard Medical School, and director, preventive cardiology clinic, department of cardiology, Boston Children's Hospital Boston.
Gregg Fonarow, MD, professor, cardiology, University of California, Los Angeles.
Circulation.

Twice as many people as previously thought are genetically predisposed to develop dangerously high cholesterol levels, new research suggests.

Familial hypercholesterolemia, as this condition is called, significantly ups the risk for an early heart attack. The study found it affects about one in every 250 American men and women, rather than one in 500.

The new numbers don't reflect a problem on the rise, however, said study author Sarah de Ferranti, MD, PhD, an assistant professor of pediatrics at Harvard Medical School. Instead, the condition was previously "under-recognized," she explained.

For those who have this potentially deadly condition, "it is extremely important to get early, consistent preventive care," Dr. de Ferranti said.

"The key is for you and your clinician to understand and distinguish between mild to moderately high cholesterol that comes on in middle age related to a less than ideal lifestyle, and very high cholesterol that has been present since birth, which has allowed the high cholesterol to build up over decades," she explained.

If a close relative has a heart attack or chest pain before age 50, consider having other family members checked, she suggested.

Preventive measures include medication and lifestyle modification, Dr. de Ferranti noted. "We have very effective medications to lower cholesterol that we believe can reduce heart disease rates to the level of people without [familial hypercholesterolemia] if taken early enough and with good consistency," Dr. de Ferranti noted.

It's also important to maintain a healthy weight, watch what you eat and control blood pressure, she said. Not doing so can make your situation worse, she explained.

"Up to now, we really haven't had a good estimate of how common familial hypercholesterolemia is in the U.S.," said Dr. de Ferranti. One reason for this is the diversity of the United States, she said. Rates of the genetic disorder vary based on racial/ethnic background, but most studies had focused on specific population groups, she explained.

The current effort, she noted, set out to rectify that problem.

STUDY DETAILS

The researchers analyzed data concerning nearly 37,000 American adults enrolled in the 1999-2012 National Health and Nutrition Examination Survey.

To determine rates of familial hypercholesterolemia, they looked at levels of "bad" (LDL) cholesterol. Then they looked for evidence of early heart disease, such as a heart attack or stroke at a young age, in individuals or their close relatives. The cutoffs were before 55 for men and before 60 for women.

Using a statistical model, the team concluded that roughly 834,500 Americans have this inherited condition.

Risk varied considerably depending on ethnicity: about one in 414 for Mexican-Americans; one in 249 among whites; and one in 211 among blacks.

Risk also appeared to differ with age, rising from one in every 1,557 adults in their 20s to about one in every 118 men and women in their 60s.

Obesity also boosted risk, the researchers found.

The new estimate includes both severe forms of the condition and potentially under-the-radar cases. That's because even relatively mild forms convey a "substantially higher risk for early heart disease," Dr. de Ferranti said.

EXPERT COMMENT

Gregg Fonarow, MD, a professor of cardiology at the University of California, Los Angeles, agreed that while the risks are serious, good treatment is at the ready.

"Without treatment," he said, "men who have familial hyperchosterolemia frequently have heart attacks in their 40s and 50s, and women with familial hypercholesterolemia frequently have heart attacks in their 50s and 60s."

Once detected, "there are a number of very effective treatments that can lower the LDL cholesterol and prevent heart attacks and stroke in individuals with familial hypercholesterolemia," added Dr. Fonarow.

These include statin medications, medications that block cholesterol absorption, and the new PCSK9 inhibitors, he said. These are once- or twice-monthly injectable medications that help bring cholesterol levels under control.

The study results appear in *Circulation*.

Good News for High Cholesterol

Michael D. Ozner, MD, is medical director of wellness and prevention at Baptist Health South Florida, Miami, and author of *Heart Attack Proof* and *The Complete Mediterranean Diet*.

New cholesterol-lowering drug is best for high-risk individuals. An FDA advisory panel has recommended approval of two PCSK9 inhibitors—*alirocumab* (Praluent) and *evolocumab* (Repatha). These drugs are for people with a genetic condition that causes LDL "bad" cholesterol to be extremely high and for others at high risk for heart disease who can't tolerate statins. Unlike statins, which reduce LDL by curtailing its production in the liver, PCSK9 inhibitors remove cholesterol from the bloodstream. Side effects are minor—mostly injection-site irritation. They can be used alone or in combination with statins—the combination can cut cholesterol 50% to 70% more than statins alone.

CHAPTER 3

Brain and Memory Health

Dr. Kosik's Alzheimer's Prevention Plan

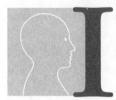If someone told you that there was a pill with no side effects and strong evidence showing that it helps prevent Alzheimer's disease, would you take it? Of course, you would!

The truth is, there's no such "magic bullet," but most adults do have the ability to dramatically decrease their risk for this dreaded disease.

A window of opportunity: According to the latest scientific evidence, slowing or blocking Alzheimer's plaques (buildups of dangerous protein fragments), which are now known to develop years before memory loss and other symptoms are noticeable, could be the key to stopping this disease.

To learn more, we spoke with Dr. Kenneth S. Kosik, a renowned neuroscientist who has researched Alzheimer's for 25 years. He shared with us the habits that he incorporates into his daily routine to help prevent Alzheimer's...

STEP 1: Make exercise exciting. You may know that frequent exercise—particularly aerobic exercise, which promotes blood flow to the brain—is the most effective Alzheimer's prevention strategy. Unfortunately, many people become bored and stop exercising.

Scientific evidence: Because exercise raises levels of brain-derived neurotrophic factor, it promotes the growth of new brain cells and may help prevent shrinkage of the hippocampus (a part of the brain involved in memory).

What I do: Most days, I spend 35 minutes on an elliptical trainer, followed by some weight training (increasing muscle mass helps prevent diabetes—an Alzheimer's risk factor). To break up the monotony, I go mountain biking on sunny days. I advise patients who have trouble sticking to an exercise regimen to try out the

Kenneth S. Kosik, MD, the Harriman Professor of Neuroscience Research and codirector of the Neuroscience Research Institute at the University of California, Santa Barbara, where he specializes in the causes and treatments of neurodegeneration, particularly Alzheimer's disease. Dr. Kosik is coauthor of *Outsmarting Alzheimer's.* KennethSKosikMD.com

new virtual-reality equipment available in many gyms. While riding a stationary bike, for example, you can watch a monitor that puts you in the Tour de France!

Also helpful: To keep your exercise regimen exciting, go dancing. A recent 20-year study found that dancing reduced dementia risk more than any other type of exercise—perhaps because many types of dancing (such as tango, salsa and Zumba) involve learning new steps and aerobic activity. Do the type of dancing that appeals to you most.

STEP 2: Keep your eating plan simple. A nutritious diet is important for Alzheimer's prevention, but many people assume that they'll have to make massive changes, so they get overwhelmed and don't even try. To avoid this trap, keep it simple—all healthful diets have a few common elements, including an emphasis on antioxidant-rich foods (such as fruit and vegetables)…not too much red meat…and a limited amount of processed foods that are high in sugar, fat or additives.

Scientific evidence: Research has shown that people who consume more than four daily servings of vegetables have a 40% lower rate of cognitive decline than those who get less than one daily serving.

What I do: I try to eat more vegetables, particularly broccoli, cauliflower and other crucifers—there's strong evidence of their brain-protective effects.

Helpful: I'm not a veggie lover, so I roast vegetables with olive oil in the oven to make them more appetizing. Whenever possible, I use brain-healthy spices such as rosemary and turmeric.

STEP 3: Guard your sleep. During the day, harmful waste products accumulate in the brain. These wastes, including the amyloid protein that's linked to Alzheimer's, are mainly eliminated at night during deep (stages 3 and 4) sleep.

Scientific evidence: In a long-term Swedish study, men who reported poor sleep were 1.5 times more likely to develop Alzheimer's than those with better sleep.

Regardless of your age, you need a good night's sleep. While ideal sleep times vary depending on the person, sleeping less than six hours or more than nine hours nightly is linked to increased risk for cardiovascular disease—another Alzheimer's risk factor. If you don't feel rested when you wake up, talk to your doctor about your sleep quality.

What I do: I often take a 10-minute nap during the day. Brief naps (especially between 2 pm and 4 pm, which syncs with most people's circadian rhythms) can be restorative.

STEP 4: Don't be a loner. Having regular social interaction is strongly associated with healthy aging.

Scientific evidence: Older adults who frequently spend time with others—for example, sharing meals and volunteering—have about a 70% lower rate of cognitive decline than those who don't socialize much.

What I do: To stay socially active, I regularly Skype, attend conferences and stay in touch with other scientists and postdoc students.

If you're lonely, any form of social interaction is better than none. One study found that people who used computers regularly—to write e-mails, for example—were less lonely than those who didn't. If you can't connect in person, do a video chat or Facebook update at least once a day.

Also helpful: Having a pet. Pets are sometimes better listeners than spouses!

STEP 5: Stay calm. People who are often stressed are more likely to experience brain shrinkage.

Scientific evidence: In a three-year study of people with mild cognitive impairment (a condition that often precedes Alzheimer's), those with severe anxiety had a 135% increased risk for Alzheimer's, compared with those who were calmer.

What I do: I go for long walks.

Other great stress reducers: Having a positive mental attitude, deep breathing, yoga, tai chi, meditation—and even watching funny movies. Practice what works for you.

STEP 6: Push yourself intellectually. So-called "brain workouts" help prevent Alzheimer's—perhaps by increasing cognitive reserve (the stored memories/cognitive skills that you can draw on later in life)…and possibly by accelerating the growth of new brain cells.

Scientific evidence: In an important study, older adults (including those with a genetic risk factor for Alzheimer's) who frequently read, played board games or engaged in other mental activities were able to postpone the development of the disease by almost a decade.

But don't fool yourself—if you're an accomplished pianist, then banging out a tune won't help much even though a nonmusician is likely to benefit from learning to play. Push your mental abilities—do math problems in your head, memorize a poem, become a tutor, etc.

What I do: To challenge myself intellectually, I read novels and practice my foreign language skills—I do research in Latin America, so I work on my Spanish.

The Diet That Cuts Your Alzheimer's Risk in Half

Martha Clare Morris, ScD, professor and director of the Section of Nutrition and Nutritional Epidemiology at Rush University, Chicago, where she is assistant provost for community research. She specializes in dietary and other preventable risk factors in the development of Alzheimer's disease and other chronic diseases in older adults.

Some of the same diets that are good for cardiovascular health also are good for the brain. But there's a new diet—combining the best aspects of other diets—that is so effective it reduces the risk for Alzheimer's disease even in those who don't give the diet their best effort.

The MIND diet blends components from DASH (a blood pressure–lowering diet) and the popular Mediterranean diet, with an extra emphasis on berries, leafy greens and a few other brain-healthy foods.

How good is it? People who carefully followed the diet were about 53% less likely to develop Alzheimer's disease in subsequent years. Those who approached it more casually didn't do quite as well but still reduced their risk considerably, by about 35%.

BLENDED BENEFITS

The MIND diet was developed by researchers at Rush University who examined years of studies to identify specific foods and nutrients that seemed to be particularly good—or bad—for long-term brain health. The MIND (it stands for Mediterranean-DASH Intervention for Neurodegenerative Delay) diet is a hybrid plan that incorporates the "best of the best."

In a study in the journal *Alzheimer's & Dementia*, the researchers followed more than 900 participants. None had dementia when the study started. The participants filled out food questionnaires and had repeated neurological tests over a period averaging more than four years.

Some participants followed the MIND diet. Others followed the older DASH diet or the Mediterranean diet. All three diets reduced the risk for Alzheimer's disease. But only the MIND diet did so even when the participants followed the plan only "moderately well."

This is an important distinction because few people are perfect about sticking to diets. Most cheat now and then and eat more unhealthy foods than they should.

The MIND diet specifies "brain-healthy" food groups and five groups that need to be limited, either eaten in moderation or preferably not at all.

WHAT TO EAT

•**More leafy greens.** Kale really is a superfood for the brain. So are spinach, chard, beet greens and other dark, leafy greens. The Mediterranean and DASH diets advise people to eat more vegetables, but they don't specify which ones.

The MIND diet specifically recommends one serving of greens a day, in addition to one other vegetable. Previous research has shown that a vegetable-rich diet can help prevent cognitive decline, but two of the larger studies found that leafy greens were singularly protective.

•**Lots of nuts.** The diet calls for eating nuts five times a week. Nuts are high in vitamin E and monounsaturated and polyunsaturated fats—all good for brain health.

The study didn't look at which nuts were more likely to be beneficial. Eating a variety is probably a good idea because you'll get a varied mix of protective nutrients and antioxidants. Raw or roasted nuts are fine (as long as they're not roasted in fat and highly salted). If you are allergic to nuts, seeds such as sunflower and pumpkin seeds are good sources of these nutrients as well.

•**Berries.** These are the only fruits that are specifically included in the MIND diet. Other fruits are undoubtedly good for you, but none has been shown in studies to promote cognitive health. Berries, on the other hand, have been shown to slow age-related cognitive decline. In laboratory studies, a berry-rich diet improves memory and protects against abnormal changes in the brain. Blueberries seem to be particularly potent. Eat berries at least twice a week.

•**Beans and whole grains.** These fiber-rich and folate-rich foods provide high levels of protein with much less saturated fat than you would get from an equivalent helping of meat. The MIND diet calls for three daily servings of whole grains and three weekly servings of beans.

•**Include fish and poultry—but you don't need to go overboard.** Seafood is a key component of the Mediterranean diet, and some proponents recommend eating it four times a week or more. The MIND diet calls for only one weekly serving, although more is OK. A once-a-week fish meal is enough for brain health.

There is no data to specify the number of poultry servings needed for brain health, but we recommend two servings a week.

•**A glass of wine.** People who drink no wine—or those who drink too much—are more likely to suffer cognitive declines than those who drink just a little.

Recommended: One glass a day. Red wine, in particular, is high in flavonoids and polyphenols that may be protective for the brain.

FOODS TO LIMIT

•**Limit red meat, cheese, butter and margarine—along with fast food, fried food and pastries and other sweets.** The usual suspects, in other words.

All of these food groups increase the risk for Alzheimer's disease, probably because of their high levels of saturated fat (or, in the case of some margarines, trans fats). Saturated fat has been linked to higher cholesterol, more systemic inflammation and possibly a disruption of the blood-brain barrier that may allow harmful substances into the brain.

However, most nutritionists acknowlege the importance of letting people enjoy some treats and not being so restrictive that they give up eating healthfully altogether.

Try to follow these recommendations...

Red meat: No more than three servings a week.

Butter and margarine: Less than one tablespoon daily. Cook with olive oil instead.

Cheese: Less than one serving a week.

Pastries and sweets: Yes, you can enjoy some treats, but limit yourself to five servings or fewer a week.

Fried or fast food: Less than one serving a week.

---

7 Natural Ways to Boost Your Brain's Alzheimer's Defense

Study titled "Higher brain BDNF gene expression is associated with slower cognitive decline in older adults" by researchers at Rush University Medical Center, Chicago, Brigham and Women's Hospital, Boston, Harvard Medical School, Boston, Broad Institute, Cambridge, Massachusetts, published in *Neurology*.

Andrew Rubman, ND, medical director, Southbury Clinic for Traditional Medicines, Southbury, Connecticut. SouthburyClinic.com

---

There's a protein in your brain that protects you from Alzheimer's disease.

It's called brain-derived neurotrophic factor (BDNF), and it promotes the survival of neurons in the brain.

Here's the latest research that is establishing the importance of this natural protective protein—including seven simple, practical ways to boost your levels.

A NATURAL MEMORY PROTECTOR—EVEN IF YOU GET ALZHEIMER'S DISEASE

While there is growing evidence in both animals and humans that BDNF plays a key role in the brain's ability to repair itself from dementia, until now the evidence has been largely indirect. Low blood levels of BDNF in people, for example, are statistically associated with an increased risk for Alzheimer's. But blood levels don't always track well with brain levels.

A new study is more definitive. Researchers at Rush University Medical Center in Chicago studied the cognitive function of 535 older men and women—some with Alzheimer's and some not—for an average of six years, and, when they died, autopsied their brains.

Results: The amount of BDNF proteins in their brains was directly related to the documented rate of cognitive decline that those men and women experienced in the years before they died. *Findings...*

• **Study participants with the most BDNF protein** (top 10%) in their brains had 50% slower cognitive decline than those with the least (lowest 10%).

• **Even among those with Alzheimer's disease,** higher levels of BDNF were associated with less severe cognitive effects.

Even this new study doesn't prove that BDNF protects against Alzheimer's, but it strengthens the case considerably. The good news is that there are straightforward ways to boost your levels.

7 WAYS TO BOOST BDNF

The research on how to boost BDNF levels in the brain isn't quite as definitive. After all, scientists can't exactly put people on treadmills and then look inside their brains. But studies in animals and humans point to some very practical healthy habits that can boost BDNF. *Here's what we know...*

1. Exercise—moderately and frequently. Several studies have found that exercise increases blood levels of BDNF. The good news is that regular moderate- and even low-intensity exercise appears to be effective. In one study of healthy men and women (55 to 80 years old), moderate-intensity walking for just 40 minutes increased blood BDNF and maintained cognitive performance—with the oldest people seeing the biggest boost—more than stretch/toning exercises did for the control group. Another study found that over a six-month period, regular low-intensity exercise (less than an hour of stretching with rubber tubing three times a week) led to increased BDNF levels in people

---

Side Sleepers Might Have Better Brains

Sleeping position may be linked to Alzheimer's risk. Research using rats found that when the animals slept on their sides, their brains cleared waste products more efficiently than when they slept on their stomachs or backs. Among the waste products removed are amyloid beta and tau proteins, which are associated with cognitive impairment.

Helene D. Benveniste, MD, PhD, professor, departments of anesthesiology and radiology, Stony Brook University School of Medicine, Stony Brook, New York, and leader of a study published in *The Journal of Neuroscience*.

---

who were previously inactive compared with participants who continued to be inactive.

2. Eat less. Animals on a calorically restricted diet have higher brain levels of BDNF compared with those that are allowed to eat as much as they want. While there are no comparable studies in people, there is evidence that avoiding overeating is beneficial. In a study of older adults (70 to 92 years old), those who consumed the most calories (more than 2,143 daily) had almost twice the risk for mild cognitive impairment as adults who consumed the least (fewer than 1,525 daily calories).

3. Eat better. Animal studies find that a diet that's very high in fat and sugar leads to lower brain BDNF. But carefully conducted clinical studies report that when it comes to preventing Alzheimer's, the quality of dietary fat is particularly important. The Mediterranean diet, which is low in sugar but includes plenty of healthy fats (olive oil, fatty fish, nuts), is protective, for example. So is the MIND diet, which is also low in sugar but high in healthy fats. Researchers believe that boosting BDNF may be a key way that these diets protect the brain—and they will be testing that hypothesis in an upcoming clinical trial.

4. Consider intermittent fasting. It's not for everyone, but eating just 500 or 600 nutritious calories on one or two days a week, while eating a normal amount on the other days, may boost BDNF.

The theory: Skipping meals stresses your neurons, and your body boosts BDNF to buttress neurons while you're undernourished. Several animal studies show that fasting increases BDNF. In one study, rats fed every other day for six months had nearly five times more BDNF than rats fed every day. Human studies that involve fasting are not easy to come by, but one small study of people who didn't eat at all during daylight hours showed increased blood BDNF.

5. Get spicy. Curcumin, a major component of the spice turmeric that's found in curries, appears to protect the brain—possibly by boosting BDNF. In India, people who consume the most curry have the lowest risk for Alzheimer's. In mice, curcumin protects against brain damage caused by an animal version of Alzheimer's, and a lab-made form of curcumin has been shown to boost BDNF in mice. Clearly we need to learn more, but we already know that turmeric's curcumin is powerfully anti-inflammatory—with other proven benefits. "It's effective at lowering cholesterol and reducing osteoarthritis pain," says naturopathic physician Andrew Rubman, ND, Health Insider's medical contributing editor. "It reduces aches and pains and inflammation throughout the body." Since curcumin is only about 2% of turmeric, you'll have to eat a lot of curry to get much curcumin—but fortunately curcumin supplements have a good safety profile. If you want to supplement, Dr. Rubman recommends taking 500 mg of a curcumin extract three or four times a day.

6. Stay social. Animal studies have shown that social isolation, compared with communal living, leads to reduced BDNF in the brain. One study in older humans also showed that social support is linked to increased blood levels of BDNF.

7. Catch rays. BDNF levels are higher in the spring and summer months than they are in fall and winter, according to a study of more than 2,800 men and women, with a direct relationship between the number of hours of sunshine per day and higher BDNF. Whether it's vitamin D (which, of course, is higher when you get sun exposure) that elevates BDNF isn't clear—one human study found that daily supplementation with 2,000 IU of vitamin D, a modest amount, didn't increase BDNF. So get some sun—in moderation, of course.

There is clearly much more we need to learn about BDNF, and there is already research toward creating a drug that boosts it. But you already have the power to create more of this protective natural brain compound yourself—every day.

Crafty Brain Boosters

Rosebud Roberts, MB, ChB, professor of epidemiology and neurology, Mayo Clinic, Rochester, Minnesota.

Sculpting, painting, woodworking and quilting aren't just enjoyable pastimes—such activities may also help protect against mild cognitive impairment (MCI). A recent study of 256 people found that those who did arts and crafts, socialized with others and/or used a computer to play online games, shop or do online searches were up to 73% less likely to develop MCI.

Why: Engaging the brain in these ways may stimulate existing neurons and/or produce new neurons that help maintain cognitive ability.

Stop Memory Loss

Pamela Wartian Smith, MD, MPH, codirector of the master's program in medical sciences at Morsani College of Medicine at University of South Florida and owner and director of the Michigan-based Center for Personalized Medicine. She is author of *What You Must Know About Memory Loss & How You Can Stop It*. CFHLL.com

Do you have trouble remembering names and phone numbers? How about where you put things? Do you sometimes struggle to come up with the right word?

Mild forgetfulness, known as age-related memory impairment, is a natural part of getting older. By age 75, a person's memory has declined, on average, by about 43%. After age 75, the hippocampus, the part of the brain most closely associated with memory, will eventually atrophy at the rate of 1% to 2% each year.

But you can improve memory with over-the-counter supplements—if you choose the right ones. Here are the supplements I find most effective with my patients. You can take several of these if you choose. You could start with phosphatidylserine and add others depending on your personal needs. For example, if you're taking a medication that depletes CoQ10, you might want to take that supplement. Or if you're under stress, add ashwagandha root. Of course, always check with your doctor before starting any new supplement. To find a practitioner trained in this field, go to *Metabolic-Anti-Aging Specialist.com.*

•**Phosphatidylserine (PS).** Most people haven't heard of it, but PS is one of my first choices for mild memory loss. It's a naturally occurring phospholipid (a molecule that contains two fatty acids) that increases the body's production of acetylcholine and other neurotransmitters. It improves cell-to-cell communication and "nourishes" the brain by improving glucose metabolism.

Studies have shown that healthy people who take PS are more likely to maintain their ability to remember things. For those who have already experienced age-related memory loss, PS can improve memory. It's also thought to improve symptoms caused by some forms of dementia.

Typical dose: 300 mg daily. You're unlikely to notice any side effects.

•**Co-enzyme Q10 (CoQ10).** This is another naturally occurring substance found in many foods (such as fatty fish, meats, nuts, fruits and vegetables) and in nearly all of your body's tissues. CoQ10 increases the production of adenosine triphosphate, a molecule that enhances energy production within cells. It's also a potent antioxidant that reduces cell-damaging inflammation in the brain and other parts of the body.

People with degenerative brain disorders, such as Alzheimer's, tend to have lower levels of CoQ10. Studies suggest that supplemental CoQ10 improves memory by protecting brain cells from oxidative damage.

Important: If you're taking a medication that depletes CoQ10—examples include statins (for lowering cholesterol)…metformin (for diabetes)…and beta-blockers (for heart disease and other conditions)—you'll definitely want to take a supplement. I often recommend it for people age 50 and older because the body's production of CoQ10 declines with age. Hard exercise also depletes it.

Typical dose: Between 30 mg and 360 mg daily. Ask your health-care professional how much you need—it will depend on medication use and other factors. Side effects are rare but may include insomnia, agitation and digestive problems such as diarrhea and heartburn.

•**Acetyl-L-carnitine.** A study that looked at people with mild cognitive impairment (an intermediate stage between age-related memory impairment and dementia) found that acetyl-L-carnitine improved memory, attention and even verbal fluency.

Acetyl-L-carnitine (it is derived from an amino acid) is a versatile molecule. It's used by the body to produce acetylcholine, the main neurotransmitter involved in memory. It slows the rate of neurotransmitter decay, increases oxygen availability and helps convert body fat into energy.

Typical dose: 1,000 mg to 2,000 mg daily. Check with your health-care professional before starting acetyl-L-carnitine to see what dose is best for you. If your kidneys are not functioning perfectly, you may need a lower dose. Some people may notice a slight fishy body odor. In my experience, you can prevent this by taking 50 mg to 100 mg of vitamin B-2 at the same time you take acetyl-L-carnitine.

•**Ashwagandha root.** This is an herb that improves the repair and regeneration of brain cells (neurons) and inhibits the body's production of acetylcholinesterase, an enzyme that degrades acetylcholine. It also improves the ability to deal with both physical and emotional stress—both of which have been linked to impaired memory and cognitive decline.

Typical dose: 500 mg to 2,000 mg daily. Start with the lower dose. If after a month you don't notice that your memory and focus have improved, take a little more. GI disturbances are possible but not common.

Warning: Don't take this supplement if you're also taking a prescription medication that has cholinesterase-inhibiting effects, such as *donepezil* (Aricept) or *galantamine* (Razadyne). Ask your health-care professional whether any of your medications have this effect.

•**Ginkgo biloba.** Among the most studied herbal supplements, ginkgo is an antioxidant that protects the hippocampus from age-related atrophy. It's a vasodilator that helps prevent blood clots, improves brain circulation and reduces the risk for vascular dementia, a type of dementia associated with impaired blood flow to the brain. It also increases the effects of serotonin, a neurotransmitter that's involved in mood and learning.

Bonus: In animal studies, ginkgo appears to block the formation of amyloid, the protein that has been linked to Alzheimer's disease. There's strong evidence that ginkgo can stabilize and possibly improve memory.

Typical dose: 60 mg to 120 mg daily. Most people won't have side effects, but ginkgo is a blood thinner that can react with other anticoagulants. If you're taking warfarin or another blood thinner (including aspirin and fish oil), be sure to check with your health-care professional before taking ginkgo.

•**Fish oil.** Much of the brain consists of DHA (docosahexaenoic acid), one of the main omega-3 fatty acids. It is essential for brain health. People who take fish-oil supplements have improved brain circulation and a faster transmission of nerve signals.

Studies have found that people who eat a lot of fatty fish have a lower risk for mild cognitive impairment than people who tend to eat little or no fatty fish. One study found that people with age-related memory impairment achieved better scores on memory tests when they took daily DHA supplements.

Typical dose: 2,000 mg daily if you're age 50 or older. Look for a combination supplement that includes equal amounts of DHA and EPA (another omega-3). Fish-oil supplements can increase the effects of blood-thinning medications such as aspirin and warfarin if the dose is above 3,000 mg a day.

•**Huperzine A.** Extracted from a Chinese moss, this is a cholinesterase inhibitor that increases brain levels of acetylcholine. It also protects brain cells from too-high levels of glutamate, another neurotransmitter.

Huperzine A may improve memory and could even help delay symptoms of Alzheimer's disease. A study conducted by the National Institute of Aging found that patients with mild-to-moderate Alzheimer's who took huperzine A had improvements in cognitive functions.

Recommended dose: 400 mcg daily. Don't take it if you're already taking a prescription cholinesterase inhibitor (as discussed in the "Ashwagandha root" section).

Does Fish Protect the Brain—or Poison It With Mercury?

Study titled "Association of Seafood Consumption, Brain Mercury Level, and APOE ε4 Status with Brain Neuropathology in Older Adults" by researchers at Rush University Medical Center, Chicago, Missouri University Research Reactor, Columbia, and Wageningen University, the Netherlands, published in *JAMA*.

When it comes to preventing dementia, eating seafood is a double-edged sword. On the one hand, it's high in mercury, a neurotoxin. Bad for the brain. On the other hand, it's high in omega-3 fatty acids, which support nerve functioning. Good for the brain.

So what happens to people who eat seafood regularly, compared with those who eat little or none? They're less likely to get dementia. All those omega-3s protect the brain even with the extra mercury.

This is something of a breakthrough finding. While earlier population studies had suggested that the cardiovascular and other benefits of eating seafood outweighed the risks of consuming contaminants, doubts remained. In a new study, researchers at Rush University Medical Center in Chicago looked at what you might call hard evidence—autopsies of 286 men and women (average age 90). They had already been studying these people when they were alive, so they knew how much seafood they were eating, and now they could look directly at their body tissues and inside their brains to see if there was accumulation of mercury—and neurological evidence of Alzheimer's disease.

The surprise answer was that while the seafood eaters did have higher levels of mercury, there was no increased incidence of Alzheimer's. That's true even for those who had the highest levels of mercury.

While mercury didn't harm, however, seafood protected those at the highest risk. These are the estimated about one-quarter of the population who carry a gene variant (apolipoprotein E4) that triples Alzheimer's risk. Seafood didn't protect everyone, but in this group, those who ate seafood regularly, compared with those who rarely or never ate it, were 47% less likely to show the brain pathology that defines Alzheimer's disease.

Bottom line: By all means, choose seafood lowest in mercury—good choices include catfish, clams, flounder, salmon, sardines, scallops, shrimp, squid and light (not albacore) tuna. But don't let worry about mercury stop you from getting the brain-protective benefits of seafood.

For a Sharper Brain, Eat These 4 Foods

Drew Ramsey, MD, an assistant clinical professor of psychiatry at Columbia University College of Physicians and Surgeons in New York City. Dr. Ramsey is also co-author of *The Happiness Diet: A Nutritional Prescription for a Sharp Brain, Balanced Mood, and Lean, Energized Body* and *Fifty Shades of Kale: 50 Fresh and Satisfying Recipes That Are Bound to Please.*

We all know that a strong cup of coffee can give us that extra mental boost we may need to complete a brain-draining project or meet a tight deadline.

What works even better: Strategic eating is a healthful and reliable way to improve your ability to concentrate for the long haul—not just for a few hours at a time when you're hyped-up on caffeine.

There's no single food that will suddenly have you speed-reading a book in one sitting, but you can improve your overall powers of

concentration by including the following foods in your diet…

•**Eggs.** When it comes to mental focus, it doesn't get much better than eggs! They're a leading source of a nutrient called choline, a precursor to the neurotransmitter acetylcholine—a key molecule of learning.

Eggs (including the yolks) also contain a variety of B vitamins, most of which have been stripped from the refined carbs that are so ubiquitous in the typical American diet. In particular, eggs are rich in vitamins B-6 and B-12, which are crucial for carrying out most cognitive functions (three large eggs will give you about half of your daily B-12 requirement)…and vitamin B-9 (also known as folate).

For optimal brain health, include up to 12 eggs in your diet each week. While cholesterol in one's diet has only a minimal effect on blood levels of cholesterol, consult your doctor for advice on appropriate intake of eggs if cholesterol is a concern.

•**Mussels.** Three ounces of mussels—which is a modest serving—contain 20 micrograms (mcg) of vitamin B-12 (that's nearly 10 times your daily requirement). Even a mild deficiency of this crucial brain-boosting vitamin can impair concentration and lead to fuzzy thinking.

But that's not all. Three ounces of mussels will also give you 430 mg of docosahexaenoic acid (DHA)—the equivalent of two to three typical fish oil supplement capsules. DHA is a type of omega-3 fatty acid needed for healthy brain function. Mussels are also loaded with zinc, a nutritional workhorse involved in more than 100 chemical reactions in the brain. Enjoy mussels twice a month.

Don't like mussels? Other smart brain-boosting seafood selections include oysters (six oysters deliver three to four times your daily zinc needs)…anchovies, which have more omega-3s than tuna…and clams, which are an excellent source of vitamin B-12.

Tasty choices: Caesar salad with anchovies…clam chowder…or pasta alle vongole (with clams).

•**Beef.** You've probably heard that eating too much red meat is linked to heart disease and even some types of cancer. However, you can minimize these risks and maximize your brainpower with a few small servings per week.

Here's why: Beef is a potent source of heme iron (the most absorbable form), which is needed to transport oxygen through the blood and to the brain.

What I recommend: Opt for grass-fed beef. It has fewer calories, less fat and more nutrients (such as vitamin E) than conventional beef. Meat from grass-fed animals has two to three times more conjugated linoleic acid (CLA) than meat from grain-fed animals. CLA helps protect the brain by counteracting the effects of harmful stress hormones.

Try to have grass-fed beef once or twice a week—but give it a supporting role instead of making it the star of your meal. Think grass-fed vegetable beef stew instead of a large steak.

Note: Even though grass-fed beef is more expensive than conventional beef, you can save by opting for nontraditional cuts, such as beef shank, stew meats and roasts. If you are a vegetarian or vegan, black beans are an excellent substitute.

• **Cruciferous vegetables.** Take your pick—the list includes brussels sprouts, kale, arugula, bok choy, cauliflower and collard greens. As members of the Brassica plant family, these veggies contain sulfur-based anti-inflammatory compounds that help protect the brain. One of these compounds, sulforaphane, has even been shown to improve memory and learning after brain injury.

Aim for at least two cups of cruciferous vegetables daily—I put that much in my kale-blueberry smoothie every morning!

Sing for a Super Brain!

Singing can improve brain function. After 10 weeks of coaching by a singing teacher, patients under age 80 with mild dementia showed improvements in memory, thinking skills, mood and the ability to find their way around.

Teppo Särkämö, PhD, is a researcher in the Cognitive Brain Research Unit, University of Helsinki, Finland, and leader of a study published in *Journal of Alzheimer's Disease*.

Note: Consult your doctor before changing the amount of leafy greens you eat if you take warfarin, a blood thinner, since vitamin K–rich foods may interact.

Other good choices: Add purple cabbage to a stir-fry...or mash cauliflower instead of potatoes and season with brain-boosting turmeric and black pepper (to increase the absorption of turmeric).

Best Workouts to Keep Your Brain "Buff"

Cynthia R. Green, PhD, a practicing clinical psychologist and the founder and president of Memory Arts, LLC, a brain-health and memory fitness consulting service in Montclair, New Jersey, TotalBrainHealth.com. Her most recent book is *Your Best Brain Ever: A Complete Guide & Workout.*

We all want to keep our brains in top shape. But are crossword puzzles, online classes and the other such activities that we've been hearing about for years the best ways to do that? Not really.

Now: To improve memory and preserve overall cognitive function, the latest research reveals that it takes more than quiet puzzle-solving and streaming lectures.

Even more intriguing: Some activities that we once thought were time wasters may actually help build intellectual capacity and other cognitive functions.

To learn more about the most effective ways to keep your brain "buff," we talked to Dr. Cynthia R. Green, a psychologist and a leading brain trainer.

A HEALTHY BRAIN

The most important steps to keep your brain performing at optimal levels are lifestyle choices...

• **Getting aerobic exercise (at least 150 minutes per week).**

• **Maintaining a healthy body weight.**

• **Not smoking.**

• **Eating a diet that emphasizes fruits and vegetables and is low in refined sugar**

and white flour—two of the biggest dietary threats to brain health that have recently been identified by researchers.

Additional benefits are possible with regular brain workouts. In the past, experts thought that nearly any game or activity that challenges you to think would improve your general brain functioning.

What research now tells us: An increasing body of evidence shows that improved memory requires something more—you need to work against a clock. Games with a time limit force you to think quickly and with agility. These are the factors that lead to improved memory and mental focus. *Among Dr. Green's favorite brain workouts—aim for at least 30 minutes daily of any combination of the activities below…*

BRAINY COMPUTER GAMES

Specialized brain-training computer programs (such as Lumosity, Fit Brains and CogniFit) are no longer the darlings of the health community. Formerly marketed as a fun way to reduce one's risk for dementia, recent evidence has not supported that claim.

These programs do provide, however, a variety of activities that may help improve intellectual performance, attention, memory and mental flexibility. Lumosity and other programs are a good option for people who enjoy a regimented brain workout, including such activities as remembering sequences and ignoring distractions. Monthly prices range from $4.99 to $19.95.

Other options to consider trying…

•**Action video games.** These games were once considered "brain-numbing" activities that kept players from developing intellectual and social skills. Recent research, however, shows that action video games can promote mental focus, flexible thinking, and decision-making and problem-solving skills. Because these games are timed, they also require quick responses from the players.

Good choices: World of Warcraft, The Elder Scrolls and Guild Wars, all of which involve role-playing by assuming the identity of various characters to battle foes and complete quests, often with other virtual players. These games

are available in DVD format for Mac or PC and with an online subscription for virtual play.

Caveat: An hour or two can be a brain booster, but don't overdo it. Too much role-playing takes you away from real-life interactions.

•**Free brain-boosting computer game for a cause.** At *FreeRice.com*, you can answer fun and challenging questions in such subjects as English vocabulary, foreign languages, math and humanities. With each correct answer, the United Nations World Food Programme donates 10 grains of rice to a Third World country. To date, players have "earned" a total of nearly 100 billion grains of rice—enough to create more than 10 million meals.

To increase the challenge: Set a timer so that you must work against the clock.

APPS FOR YOUR BRAIN

If you'd prefer to use an "app"—a software application that you can use on a smartphone or similar electronic device—there are several good options. *Among the best fun/challenging apps (free on Android and Apple)…*

•**Words with Friends.** This ever-popular game allows you to play a Scrabble-like game against your friends who have also downloaded the app on an electronic device. The game provides even more benefits if it's used with the time-clock feature.

•**Word Streak with Friends** (formerly Scramble with Friends) is a timed find-a-word game. You can play on your own or with friends.

•**Elevate** was named Apple's Best App of 2014. It provides a structured game environment that feels more like a test, focusing on reading, writing and math skills, than a game. Still, this timed app will give Apple users a good brain challenge.

TECH-FREE OPTIONS

If you'd rather not stare at the screen of a computer or some other electronic device for your brain workout, here are some good options…

•**Tech-free games.** SET is a fast-paced card game that tests your visual perception skills. Players race to find a set of three matching cards (based on color, shape, number or shading) from an array of cards placed on a table.

Bonus: This game can be played by one player or as many people as can fit around the table. The winner of dozens of "Best Game" awards, including the high-IQ group Mensa's Select award, SET is fun for kids and adults alike.

Another good choice: Boggle, which challenges you to create words from a given set of letter cubes within a three-minute period. It can be played by two or more people.

•**Drumming.** Playing any musical instrument requires attention and a keen sense of timing. Basic drumming is a great activity for beginner musicians (especially if you don't have the finger dexterity for piano or guitar).

Even better: Join a drumming circle, which provides the extra challenge of matching your timing and rhythm to the rest of the drummers, along with opportunities for socialization.

Bonus: Research has demonstrated that some forms, such as African djembe drumming, count as a low- to moderate-intensity activity that may reduce blood pressure, which helps protect the brain from blood vessel damage.

•**Meditation.** This practice improves cognitive function and sensory processing and promotes mental focus. Meditating for about 30 minutes daily has also been linked to greater blood flow to the brain and increased gray matter (associated with positive emotions, memory and decision-making). The benefits have even been seen among some people with early-stage neurodegenerative diseases, such as Alzheimer's disease.

A good way to get started: Begin with a simple "mindful eating" exercise—spend the first five minutes of each meal really focusing on what you're eating. Don't talk, read the paper or watch TV...just savor the food. Eventually, you'll want to expand this level of attention to other parts of your day. Such mindfulness habits are a good complement to a regular meditation practice.

•**Coloring.** If you have kids or grandkids, don't just send them off with their crayons. Color with them.

Even better: Get one of the new breed of coloring books with complex designs for adults. While there hasn't been specific research addressing the brain benefits of coloring, this form of play has been shown to reduce stress in children, and it is thought to boost creativity and have a meditative quality. You can find coloring books made for adults at bookstores and art-supply stores.

New Hope for Parkinson's Patients

Plymouth University

A cholesterol-lowering drug has been shown to affect the protein clumping that occurs in Parkinson's patients. A multicenter clinical trial to test the effects of *simvastatin* (Zocor) in Parkinson's patients is now under way.

Brain Implant for Parkinson's

William Maisel, MPH, acting director, Office of Device Evaluation, Center for Devices and Radiological Health, US Food and Drug Administration, Silver Spring, Maryland.

Brain implant may help Parkinson's symptoms. The Food and Drug Administration recently approved the Brio Neurostimulation System, an implantable device that helps reduce the symptoms of Parkinson's disease and the movement disorder called essential tremor. The conditions are not curable, but the implanted device may help patients who have difficulty walking and with balance problems, as well as patients for whom medication alone is not effective. The device includes a small battery-powered electrical-pulse generator implanted under the skin of the upper chest, along with wire leads that are attached to electrodes placed within the brain. It is the second device of this type to be approved by the FDA.

Dementia Clue

Study by researchers at University College London, UK, published in *Journal of Alzheimer's Disease*.

Change in sense of humor may signal dementia. People who develop frontotemporal dementia tend to have behavior and personality changes—not memory troubles—in the years before the condition is diagnosed. One such change involves laughing at things that people don't usually find funny, such as a badly parked car. Friends and relatives of people with this form of dementia report noticing changes at least nine years before dementia symptoms appear. These changes are not associated with Alzheimer's disease—but people with both frontotemporal dementia and Alzheimer's tend to prefer slapstick humor to humor that is satirical or absurdist.

Aquariums Whet Appetites

Study of 70 patients, ages 59 to 99, at three residential facilities by researchers at Purdue University, West Lafayette, Indiana, published in *Alzheimer Disease & Associated Disorders*.

Fish tanks can boost appetites of patients with neurocognitive disorders. When aquariums containing eight large, colorful fish were rolled into the dining area during the evening meal every day for 10 weeks, people who were insti-tutionalized with advanced dementia—who are at risk for excessive weight loss—ate enough food to gain more than two pounds.

Possible reason: The fish tanks may have had a calming effect, allowing patients to focus on eating.

When Certain Noises Make You Nuts

Pawel J. Jastreboff, PhD, ScD, professor of otolaryngology, Emory University School of Medicine, Atlanta.

Repetitive sounds, such as gum chewing or throat clearing, are classic triggers for a condition known as *misophonia*. People with misophonia (also known as selective sound sensitivity syndrome) become anxious or angry when they hear a specific sound that would not cause a similar reaction in most other people. Sometimes just the sight of someone putting a stick of gum in his/her mouth, for example, is enough to make the misophonia sufferer angry.

Researchers don't know what causes misophonia but believe that it's a disorder in the way the brain processes sound. Sound waves are transformed into electrical signals that go into certain areas of the brain that control emotions. In people with misophonia, the brain cannot filter past negative associations with certain sounds. In some cases, the condition is linked to obsessive-compulsive disorder. Many people with tinnitus (a ringing in the ears) also have misophonia.

A treatment method called tinnitus retraining therapy has been shown to improve symptoms significantly in 85% of misophonia patients. They listen to a recording of enjoyable sounds (such as favorite music) mixed with the offensive sound set at a very low level. Over a period of three months (sometimes longer), the enjoyable sound is gradually decreased so the listener can develop a tolerance for the sound that triggers negative reactions. Cognitive behavioral therapy can also help change negative thoughts about the sound.

Write Longhand for a Memory Boost

Handwriting boosts learning and memory. Physically drawing letters activates a distinct neural pathway that improves reading comprehension and memory of language.

Claudia Aguirre, PhD, neuroscientist and mind-body expert based in the Los Angeles area, writing at *Huffington Post.com*.

Finally...Real Relief for Tinnitus

Murray Grossan, MD, an ear, nose and throat specialist in private practice in Los Angeles with more than 30 years of experience in treating tinnitus and hearing loss. He is the author of *The Whole Person Tinnitus Relief Program*, an e-book available at DrGrossanTinnitus.com.

It's estimated that about one in 10 Americans hears noise—ringing, buzzing, roaring, hissing, whooshing or clicking sounds—when no external sound is present. This condition, known as tinnitus, can be a minor annoyance, or the sound can be loud enough or persistent enough to make concentration, sleep and communication impossible. The torment even drives some sufferers to suicide.

About 20% of people with tinnitus seek medical help. But far too many are told there's nothing that can be done and they should "learn to live with it"—a hopeless prognosis that only compounds their suffering.

Recent development: A panel of leading experts from the American Academy of Otolaryngology—Head and Neck Surgery Foundation has developed new diagnostic and treatment guidelines, which will help tinnitus sufferers get much better care. What you need to know...

DETERMINING THE CAUSE

When you see a doctor for tinnitus, he/she should start with a physical examination and detailed medical history to determine if it's caused by a treatable condition, such as...

•**Ménière's disease.** Intense vertigo is the most dramatic symptom of this condition, but hearing loss and tinnitus can be symptoms as well. Diuretics or steroids, taken as needed, may help the disease and relieve the tinnitus.

•**Cochlear hydrops.** This condition, caused by increased fluid pressure in the inner ear, is like Ménière's disease but without the vertigo. It can often be cured by reduced intake of salt and use of a diuretic, taken as needed, to eliminate fluid, which in turn alleviates the tinnitus.

•**Temporomandibular joint (TMJ) syndrome,** whiplash or head or shoulder muscle injury. These issues can activate nerve signals that the brain interprets as sound. Physical therapy, chiropractic treatment and/or orthodontia may help these problems and the tinnitus.

•**High blood pressure.** Elevated blood pressure alters the inner ear chemistry to cause tinnitus in some people. Effective treatment of hypertension may stop the tinnitus.

•**Anxiety and depression.** Tinnitus aggravated by anxiety and depression may be alleviated by therapy for these conditions.

•**Excessive earwax.** Removal of the wax stops the tinnitus.

•**Medications.** Most commonly, nonsteroidal anti-inflammatory drugs (NSAIDs), such as aspirin, *ibuprofen* (Advil, Motrin) or *naproxen* (Aleve), can cause tinnitus and should be stopped if suspected.

Note: Low-dose aspirin (81 mg), often used for heart health, is not known to cause tinnitus.

What a physical exam should include: A hearing test (audiometry). Hearing loss is common with tinnitus, and a hearing aid sometimes makes it better (see "Sound therapy" below).

More advanced tests like magnetic resonance imaging (MRI) are usually not required. But when tinnitus and hearing loss are limited to one side, such tests may be needed to rule out a benign tumor on the acoustic nerve—a rare condition known as acoustic neuroma.

Many tinnitus cases, however, are "idiopathic"—there's no identifiable underlying disease.

TREATMENTS THAT HELP

The expert panel approved the following two therapies for idiopathic tinnitus. *Patients can try both at the same time or do them individually...*

•**Cognitive behavioral therapy (CBT).** This type of therapy aims to alter negative thinking about tinnitus and its effects on your life. When the patient understands tinnitus better (for example, "It's not my fault"), it takes away some of the mystery and reduces associated distress. To find a CBT therapist, go to the website of the American Tinnitus Association, *ATA.org*.

•**Sound therapy.** Just as the ticking of a clock in a quiet room becomes inaudible when there's traffic in the street outside, background sound can reduce or relieve tinnitus. This masking effect is the simplest form of sound therapy. To mask the tinnitus sound, the patient wears earbuds that deliver white noise, nature sounds or low-volume music. In other forms of sound therapy, enjoyable sounds or music is mixed with the sound that mimics a patient's tinnitus.

Simply getting a hearing aid to correct hearing loss is also a type of sound therapy—restoring normal perception of external sound often makes the phantom noise much less noticeable.

According to recent sound therapy research, such treatments reduce tinnitus over time, possibly by retraining the brain circuits that generate the perceived sound.

You can develop your own sound therapy program by using apps such as Nix Tinnitus Ear Amp at *Bxtel.com* ($1.99, iOS)…and Tinnitus Balance at *Phonak.com* (free, iOS and Android).

Important: Stress does not cause tinnitus, but sufferers will tell you that it can worsen it. Do all you can to keep stress levels in check.

Helpful: Counting breaths.

What to do: As you inhale slowly, count from one to four. Then, as you exhale, count from one to six. The longer exhale makes this exercise particularly relaxing. Repeat these breaths for about a minute, every waking hour for several weeks, to establish the habit. Then you can use these exercises any time you need to de-stress.

WORTH TRYING?

The evidence is limited or mixed for the following treatments, and the recent guidelines advise against most of them. *But some people report that these approaches help, so you may want to consider trying them…*

•**Supplements.** Numerous studies suggest possible benefits of supplements for tinnitus. For example, magnesium may improve hearing loss, and alpha-lipoic acid may protect the ears against damage from loud noise or drug toxicity. Also, some research has shown an association between tinnitus and low levels of B vitamins or other nutrients. In practice, some clinicians report improvements in patients who take the supplements described above as well as coenzyme Q10, zinc, selenium and/or other antioxidants that are important for hearing chemistry.

•**Alternative and experimental approaches.** Acupuncture has been used for tinnitus since the fifth century BC, but scientific reviews have found no conclusive evidence that it works (the panel made no recommendation for or against this treatment). Repetitive transcranial magnetic stimulation (rTMS), in which external magnetic fields are applied in an attempt to change brain function, is now being offered for tinnitus in some clinics, but the FDA has not approved the treatment for this condition and research has not yet shown evidence that it offers long-term benefit.

Resveratrol for Alzheimer's Treatment: Time to Celebrate?

Study titled "A randomized, double-blind, placebo-controlled trial of resveratrol for Alzheimer disease" by researchers at Georgetown University, Washington, DC, et al., published in *Neurology*.

You'd have to drink 1,000 bottles of red wine to get the amount of the antiaging compound resveratrol that's used in a recent Alzheimer's study. Scratch that idea. But it may be worth uncorking a bottle to celebrate the positive findings of the longest and largest human resveratrol study to date.

Researchers gave 119 people with mild-to-moderate Alzheimer's super-concentrated synthetic resveratrol supplements for a year. It was safe. It got into their brains. It arrested "biomarkers" that indicate the disease is progressing. And there was a modest improvement in the ability to do daily tasks. Next stop on this clinical train—a larger study specifically designed to study effectiveness.

The researchers say it's too early to recommend supplements yet for Alzheimer's patients. Certainly anyone being treated for the disease should discuss any supplement with his/her doctor first.

Want to Boost Short-Term Memory? Watch a Funny Video

Gurinder Singh Bains, MD, PhD, assistant professor and primary research coordinator, Loma Linda University School of Allied Health Professions, Loma Linda, California. His study was published in *Alternative Therapies*.

You forget that thing that someone told you…this morning. You misplace your keys. You walk into the kitchen to do something…but once you get there, you forget what it is.

What you're experiencing is a decline in short-term memory. It starts to go down as early as your 40s…and it's perfectly normal. (Forgetting where you live or what your keys are for, that's a different story.)

But wouldn't it be great if there were something simple and easy that you could do to improve it?

There is. In fact it's so simple, it's funny.

HOW RED SKELTON ENHANCES BRAIN POWER

Watching a humorous video for 20 minutes may be all it takes to improve your ability to remember things you've just heard or read, found researchers at Loma Linda University in California. They showed 20 older men and women (average age 70) either a video of Red Skelton (the former clown who had a popular TV comedy show in the 1950s, '60s and early '70s)…or a montage from America's Funniest Home Videos.

None of the participants had any cognitive impairment. However, half of them (10) had diabetes, which is known to contribute to short-term memory loss. An additional 10 participants, who did not have diabetes nor cognitive impairment and were of the same age, were the control group. They did not watch the videos but instead were asked to sit silently in a quiet room.

Before and after watching funny videos…or sitting in silence…the participants took three components of a short-term-memory test. First, a researcher read aloud 15 words, and participants were then asked to say from memory as many as they could remember…a test of learning. The test was repeated five times. The same test was then given with a different list, and then participants were asked to remember what had been on the first list…a test of recall. Finally, participants were given a piece of paper with 50 words on it and asked to circle words that had been on the first list…a test of visual recognition. Finally, a little saliva was swabbed at five different points, including before and after—you'll see why in a moment.

Result? Laughter worked. After watching the humorous videos, the healthy adults did 39% better on the learning test, 44% better on the recall test and 13% better on the visual recognition test. Those with diabetes also saw significant improvements—a 33% boost in learning, a 48% jump in recall and a 17% gain in visual recognition. Sitting silently also seemed to benefit the control group but not nearly as much. Their gains were 24%, 20% and 8%, respectively.

How can a little mirth improve memory? That's where the saliva comes in.

THE STRESS CONNECTION

Saliva contains cortisol, a stress hormone. All of the participants who watched the funny videos experienced a significant decrease in salivary cortisol levels. Stress, as the researchers already knew, suppresses the function of the brain's hippocampus, where short-term memory is pulled together. (Over time, chronic stress can even damage…and shrink…the hippocampus.) Feeling less stress and producing fewer stress hormones, the researchers speculate, is what led to better learning and memory in the video watchers.

This wonderfully simple experiment suggests a wonderfully simple way that we could all boost our short-term memory—watch humorous videos. *There are literally thousands that are easily found online…but here are three good (and free) ones…*

•**The hilarious well-known scene from the *I Love Lucy* TV show**—when Lucy and Ethel get jobs at a candy factory.

•**Comedienne Carol Burnett's spoof on *Gone With the Wind*.**

•**Frasier,** from the TV comedy series Frasier, sings "Buttons and Bows."

If you want to stretch out the experience, try these funny full-length movies—*Blazing Saddles*

(1974), *Airplane!* (1980), *Raising Arizona* (1987), *A Fish Called Wanda* (1988), *Liar Liar* (1997), *There's Something About Mary* (1998), *Little Miss Sunshine* (2006), *Death at a Funeral* (2007) and *Bridesmaids* (2011). For more choices, see "Classic Comedies to Make You Laugh Out Loud" at BottomLineInc.com.

Of course, you don't have to watch a video to relax and laugh. Although it wasn't studied, it's a reasonable speculation that anything that lowers stress levels may enhance short-term memory. While this is the first research to show memory improvement, other research has shown that humor and laughter stimulate the immune system, make pain more tolerable, improve mood and even reduce markers of inflammation. That's fun with benefits.

Is It a Migraine, Low Blood Sugar, a Seizure…or a Stroke?

Edward Jauch, MD, professor and director, division of emergency medicine, professor, department of neurosciences, comprehensive stroke program, and director, acute stroke trials, Medical University of South Carolina, Charleston.

They're called stroke mimics. The symptoms are similar to a stroke—slurred speech, a weakness on one side of your body and confusion—but what you're experiencing is actually low blood sugar, a migraine or another condition. If you know you have diabetes, suffer from migraines, have a seizure disorder or other conditions, you may be tempted to ignore possible stroke symptoms.

That's a big mistake.

Reason: When you're having a stroke, minutes—even seconds—count. Getting emergency treatment with blood clot–dissolving medications—typically tissue plasminogen activator (tPA)—or other therapies can mean the difference between life and death and can dramatically affect recovery. To learn more about stroke mimics, we spoke with Edward Jauch, MD, director of the division of emergency medicine at the Medical University of South Carolina.

MIMIC #1: LOW BLOOD SUGAR (HYPOGLYCEMIA)

When blood sugar dips too low, a common problem for people who take medication for diabetes, the symptoms mimic a stroke—confusion, feeling dizzy or light-headed, slurred speech and/or muscle weakness.

Clues that it may be hypoglycemia, not stroke: Symptoms may build up slowly, rather than occur suddenly, as they do with a stroke. If you do a finger prick and discover your blood sugar is low, and if symptoms resolve after eating a glucose tablet or drinking a half cup of fruit juice, it's likely not a stroke.

But if you have any doubts, call 911. Be sure to tell the EMS professionals that the patient is a diabetic so they can rule out hypoglycemia with a finger-prick test—and maybe save a trip to the ER. It's actually standard practice to test everyone's glucose right away, whether or not they have diabetes, but it's not always followed, says Dr. Jauch.

MIMIC #2: HEMIPLEGIC MIGRAINE

You may remember when the newscaster Serene Branson frighteningly lost her speech during a live broadcast, and everyone thought she had had a stroke. Well, it turned out to be a hemiplegic migraine. This type of migraine can cause loss of speech, weakness and other strokelike symptoms.

Clues that it may be a migraine, not a stroke…

•**You know you get migraines,** the pain is familiar, and an aura precedes the symptoms.

•**The headache comes on gradually,** over several minutes or longer, intensifies to a peak and tends to be throbbing or a dull ache.

•**You have known triggers such as stress,** caffeine, foods, weather changes, etc.

•**You have visual disturbances such as seeing flashing lights or wavy lines.**

Signs that it may be a stroke, not a migraine…

•**You're older than 50, and you've never had a migraine.** Migraines don't tend to develop after age 50.

•**The headache comes on suddenly** and is the worst headache of your life.

•**You have visual disturbances that involve loss of part of your visual field**—you may bump into things because you don't see them, for example.

As always, when in doubt, call 911. It's particularly important for people who get migraines frequently to pay attention to possible stroke symptoms. "There's a small increased risk for stroke in people who have migraines, but we are still researching if treatment of a migraine reduces stroke risk," says Dr. Jauch.

MIMIC #3: A SEIZURE

Some seizures leave people with neurological symptoms such as difficulty speaking or a weakness in one or more limbs often on one side of the body, known as Todd's paralysis. "When you have a seizure, your brain turns off, just like when you shut down a computer," Dr. Jauch explains. "When you turn the computer back on, it takes a while to boot up. Your brain, too, may take some time to get back to normal."

Clues that it may be a seizure…

•**The patient has a history of seizures, a bite mark on the side of the tongue**—or confusion that gradually improves.

•**Typically symptoms subside with time**…from a few minutes to a few hours.

Clues that it may be a stroke: If there is confusion, it is persistent and doesn't improve.

If you're concerned that it's a stroke, time isn't on your side. EMS guidelines state that the ER team should consider stroke if someone has a seizure and has symptoms of neurological deficits, such as weakness, numbness or language issues, particularly if the patient doesn't have a history of seizures. Sometimes, seizures are symptoms of a stroke.

MIMIC #4: BELL'S PALSY

Bell's palsy causes facial drooping, but it's not because of a stroke. It's typically caused by a viral infection such as shingles or the flu or Lyme disease that leads to an inflammation or infection in the facial nerve (called the seventh cranial nerve). It can also cause your eyelid to droop, drooling, dryness of the eye or mouth or excessive tearing in one eye. Though this is easy for the pros to diagnose, patients often confuse it with a stroke.

Clues that it may be Bell's palsy…

•**It typically causes significant facial distortion including the forehead.** Facial symptoms are your only symptoms.

Clues that it may be a stroke…

•**You're older than 60,** when Bell's palsy becomes less common.

•**You have other stroke symptoms, not just facial droop.**

Not sure? You know what to do—call 911.

MIMIC #5: A BRAIN TUMOR

Brain tumors can also cause symptoms that mimic stroke, such as headache, confusion, nausea, weakness and disturbance in the way you walk.

Clues that it's a brain tumor rather than a stroke: Symptoms are headaches that are worse in the morning, when coughing, exercising or changing position.

Both are serious ailments, of course, so these symptoms, whatever the cause, require immediate attention. For any of these unexplained symptoms, you would likely be given a CT scan, which would pick up the tumor versus signs of a stroke.

WHAT HAPPENS IF I THINK IT'S A STROKE AND IT'S NOT?

Stroke mimics confuse even health-care professionals. In one study, about 20% of the time when neurologists thought patients were having a stroke, the cause was a different condition. The result can be getting a CT scan and treatment when it's not needed, with all the anxiety that entails. But the risk for harm is much lower than having a stroke and not getting it promptly treated.

Here's what you can do: Help health-care professionals by giving them the right information. Let them know if the symptoms came on suddenly (common in strokes) or more gradually (uncommon), and let them know when the symptoms began or when the person was last known to be normal. If the patient has diabetes or is subject to frequent migraines or has a seizure disorder, tell the EMS professionals right away. Also let them know if the person takes any form of regular medications. It'll help them sort things out quicker.

HOW TO SPEED UP STROKE TREATMENT

Everyone should know the classic signs of a stroke, made easy to remember with the acronym, FAST…

•**Face drooping.** One side of the face may droop or become numb. Ask the person to smile, and check to see if the smile is uneven.

•**Arm weakness.** One arm only may be weak or numb. Ask the person to raise both arms, and check to see if one arm drifts downward.

•**Speech problems.** Speech may be slurred, or the person may have trouble speaking or being understood. Ask the person to repeat a simple sentence, such as "The sun is shining."

•**Time,** as in, act quickly! If you think you or someone you're with is having a stroke, call 911 immediately. "We know that if you use the ambulance, you will get to the hospital faster, you see a doctor faster, you get a CT scan faster, you're more likely to get tPA, and you're more likely to get it faster." After calling 911, check the time so that the first responders know when symptoms started. When the ambulance arrives—and again when you get to the ER—say the word stroke if you think that's what you or the patient is having. Don't just say, "my arm is numb" or "I'm dizzy." Says Dr. Jauch, "The sooner someone says, 'I think I'm having a stroke,' the sooner health-care providers can start the proven system called the "Stroke Chain of Survival."

Scientists Uncover Clues to Origins of Schizophrenia

Steven McCarroll, PhD, director, genetics, Broad Institute's Stanley Center for Psychiatric Research, and associate professor, genetics, Harvard Medical School, Boston. Vishwajit Nimgaonkar, MD, PhD, professor, psychiatry and human genetics, University of Pittsburgh. *Nature*, online.

Individuals might develop schizophrenia when a normal process of brain development goes haywire in adolescence and early adulthood, Harvard researchers report.

Everyone undergoes what is called "synaptic pruning" as they move into adulthood, explained study author Steven McCarroll, PhD, director of genetics for the Broad Institute's Stanley Center for Psychiatric Research and an associate professor of genetics at Harvard Medical School in Boston.

It's how extra brain cells and synapses (the junctions where nerve signals cross from one brain cell to the next) are eliminated in the cerebral cortex, to increase the efficiency of function, he said.

But a gene that contributes to synaptic pruning may increase a person's risk of schizophrenia if certain mutations cause things to go wrong, Dr. McCarroll and his colleagues explained.

"Somehow, this biological process becomes miscalibrated and removes too many synapses," Dr. McCarroll said. "Something about this process of maturation, if it goes awry, results in brain wiring that can no longer perform some of the basic functions that it used to be able to perform."

The findings were published online in the journal *Nature*.

BACKGROUND ON SCHIZOPHRENIA

About 1% of U.S. adults have schizophrenia, and about seven or eight people out of every 1,000 will have schizophrenia in their lifetime, according to the U.S. National Institute of Mental Health (NIMH).

People with schizophrenia may hear voices or see things that aren't there, or develop irrational delusions of grandeur or persecution, according to NIMH. Patients might also display disorganized thinking, agitated body movements or emotional withdrawal. Symptoms most frequently appear in patients when they are teenagers or young adults.

The gene implicated in this study, C4, normally acts as a regulator of the immune system, Dr. McCarroll said. The gene helps target debris, viruses and other pathogens for destruction by immune cells.

Earlier research had linked the C4 gene to schizophrenia, leading some to believe the mental disorder might be caused by some sort of virus or infection, he said.

STUDY DETAILS

However, the research team learned that the C4 gene also "moonlights" in synaptic pruning, playing a role in the process by tagging synapses for elimination, Dr. McCarroll said.

His team's analysis of genetic data for more than 65,000 people revealed that patients who had particular forms of the C4 gene showed a higher expression of that gene and, in turn, had a higher risk of developing schizophrenia.

"This is a promising model because it addresses what has been two of the central mysteries of schizophrenia—the age of onset, in adolescence, and genetic results that have seemed to point to immune molecules as having some role in the illness," Dr. McCarroll said.

Synaptic pruning is particularly active during adolescence, which is the typical period of onset for schizophrenia symptoms. And brains of schizophrenic patients tend to show fewer connections between neurons (brain cells), the researchers said.

And "when we got to the bottom of this genetic effect, yes, it's an immune molecule, but it's an immune molecule with a different job in the brain," Dr. McCarroll said. "It's important when we got to the bottom of this genetic effect, it's not pointing to a virus or infection, it's pointing to brain wiring."

IMPLICATIONS OF STUDY

Schizophrenia currently is treated mainly through the use of antipsychotic medications, according to NIMH. Patients might also need therapy and rehabilitation to help them lead a normal life, once medication has stabilized their condition.

The new discovery by Dr. McCarroll and his team could lead to new medicines for the treatment, and possible prevention, of schizophrenia in people who carry this genetic risk, he said.

"I get emails every day" from drug companies interested in exploring possible treatments based on this research, Dr. McCarroll said, although he warned that "it takes many, many years to go from biological discovery to a new medicine."

EXPERT COMMENT

Vishwajit Nimgaonkar, MD, PhD, a professor of psychiatry and human genetics at the University of Pittsburgh, praised the new study as "very sophisticated and fairly comprehensive."

However, Dr. Nimgaonkar added that the findings really are just a first step along a promising new line of research.

"I don't think they've proved conclusively this is one of the mechanisms that causes schizophrenia, but they've certainly got a lot of minds thinking," he said. "This might lead to new drugs for treating schizophrenia, but we really need to figure out the mechanism properly first, and then figure out a way to treat the problem."

info For more on schizophrenia, visit the U.S. National Institute of Mental Health at *Nimh.nih.gov.*

Why Learning a Second Language Is Easier for Some

Society for Neuroscience, news release.

New research helps explain why learning a second language is easier for some adults than others.

Language learning success or failure has to do with differences in the strength of connections between certain areas of the brain, according to the study published in the *Journal of Neuroscience.*

Even when you're resting and not doing any specific tasks, the different regions of your brain are communicating with each other, the Canadian researchers explained.

The strength of these connections varies between people, and previous research has linked these differences to variations in language ability.

STUDY DETAILS

In this study, researchers at McGill University in Montreal scanned the brains of 15 adult English speakers before they began an intensive 12-week French course. The participants' language abilities were tested in speaking and reading tests before and after the course.

Those with greater improvement in speaking French by the end of the course had stronger connections between the left anterior insula/frontal operculum—which plays a role in verbal fluency—and the left superior temporal gyrus, an important part of the language network, the researchers found.

Participants with greater improvement in reading speed had stronger connections between the visual word form area and a different region of the left superior temporal gyrus language area, the study authors said.

"These findings have implications for predicting language learning success and failure," study co-leader Xiaoqian Chai said in a news release from the Society for Neuroscience.

EXPERT COMMENT

According to Arturo Hernandez, a neuroscientist at the University of Houston, "The most interesting part of this finding is that the connectivity between the different areas was observed before learning," he said in the news release.

"This shows that some individuals may have a particular neuronal activity pattern that may lend itself to better learning of a second language," added Hernandez, who studies second-language learning and was not involved in the new study.

But Chai said that the findings don't mean that brain wiring is the only factor that affects a person's ability to learn a second language, because the brain can be shaped by learning and experience.

The study is "a first step to understanding individual differences in second language learning," and "might help us to develop better methods for helping people to learn better," Chai concluded.

info Learn more about how the brain works at Harvard Medical School's Whole Brain Atlas, *http://www.med.harvard.edu/aan lib/home.html*

CHAPTER 4

Cancer Care and Breakthroughs

Best of Integrative Cancer Care

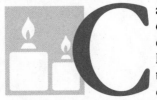

Cancer is a complex disease—elusive and difficult to control, let alone cure. To get the best possible outcome, you want to have all hands on deck.

More than the conventional approach: While modern oncology has given us powerful weapons to fight cancer—drugs, surgery and radiation that attack tumors head on—the most effective integrative cancer therapies focus on the cancer patient, bolstering his/her natural defenses to help suppress tumor growth. Combining these approaches not only fills in gaps but also creates a powerful synergy.

BUILD YOUR DEFENSES

While there are a multitude of integrative approaches now available for cancer patients, ranging from acupuncture and massage to aro-matherapy and music therapy, it's crucial to fortify your body's defenses to fight the inflammation associated with cancer. *Here's how…*

•**Diet.** Strive for a plant-based diet (especially cruciferous vegetables and berries—both are extremely rich in cancer-fighting nutrients) with plenty of whole grains, nuts and omega-3–rich fatty fish (omega-3s have been linked to reduced cancer risk). Cut back on animal proteins and sugar—these foods are associated with cancer-promoting inflammation.

•**Exercise.** Try to get 150 minutes weekly of moderately vigorous exercise (such as brisk walking) to help optimize your body's own cancer-fighting abilities. An ideal regimen could include some aerobic activity (such as cycling)… some stretching (such as yoga or tai chi)…and some strength training (with hand weights or resistance bands).

Dwight McKee, MD, a medical oncologist based in Aptos, California, who is also board-certified in nutrition and integrative and holistic medicine. Dr. McKee is coauthor of *After Cancer Care: The Definitive Self-Care Guide to Getting and Staying Well for Patients After Cancer.*

•**Stress reduction.** The first weeks after diagnosis are likely to be the most stressful of your life.

There are a myriad of ways to control stress, including meditation, hypnosis, yoga and tai chi, but one method that seems particularly effective is progressive muscle relaxation, which involves systematically relaxing all the muscle groups in the body, one after another. Twenty minutes daily has been shown to provide major benefits to people with cancer.

For a free video demonstrating progressive muscle relaxation, go to: *CMHC. utexas.edu* (search "progressive muscle relaxation video").

•**Herbs and supplements.** While adopting the inflammation-fighting lifestyle practices described earlier, anti-inflammatory herbs, such as curcumin and boswellia, can be powerful aids.

In addition, a typical herb-and-supplement regimen for a colon cancer patient, for example, may include some combination of the following: Vitamin D, green tea extract, resveratrol, grape seed extract, probiotics and omega-3 fatty acids.

Important: For specific advice on herbs and supplements, work with a skilled, experienced complementary/alternative doctor or herbalist.

GETTING RID OF THE TUMOR

While conventional methods, such as surgery, radiation and chemotherapy, can be quite effective, they have important downsides, too. For example, chemotherapy and radiation not only have harsh side effects, including nausea and hair loss, but they also suppress the immune system at a time when it should be working overtime to fight the cancer.

Newer alternatives: The immune-suppressing effects of chemo and radiation can be avoided with thermal ablation. With this approach, doctors insert a needle into the tumor, often guided by computed tomography (CT) imaging, to kill the cancer cells with heat (radiofrequency or microwave ablation) or freezing (cryoablation). Irreversible electroporation (the NanoKnife) uses electrical pulses to kill cancer cells by disrupting their cell membranes. These methods are also much less invasive and traumatic than surgery.

Right now, ablation is mainly used for tumors that can't be treated with conventional surgery, due to their location or number, and for isolated metastases in the lung and liver. But ablation and electroporation have the potential to replace a considerable amount of surgery.

IMMUNOTHERAPY

Scientists are actively developing new medications that help undo the tumor's ability to produce chemicals that inactivate the body's cancer-fighting immune cells.

Examples: *Ipilimumab* (Yervoy) and *pembrolizumab* (Keytruda) have been approved for the treatment of melanoma. Clinical trials to investigate their use against a wider range of malignancies, including certain kinds of lung cancer, and bladder, colon and metastatic prostate cancer, are also under way. For details on clinical trials using these drugs, check ClinicalTrials.gov.

Because these drugs target molecular mechanisms driving cancer, they are far less toxic than conventional chemotherapy. The drugs are, however, extremely expensive (costing up to $150,000 a year). If insurance won't cover the drug and a clinical trial is not available, sometimes the pharmaceutical manufacturer will donate it to a patient without the financial resources to purchase it so that it can be administered by his/her oncologist.

GETTING THE HELP YOU NEED

It's risky for cancer patients to try to treat themselves with integrative approaches. Some therapies, including certain herbs, such as St. John's wort, may even interfere with conventional treatment. But finding oncologists, herbalists and other health-care professionals who are knowledgeable about the latest approaches in integrative cancer care is also challenging.

To find a health-care professional who specializes in integrative oncology: Ask your doctor for a referral or consult the Society for Integrative Oncology, IntegrativeOnc. org. When you find an experienced integrative professional, ask him/her to work with your primary oncologist in coordinating your care.

Breakthrough Cancer Treatment That Saved Jimmy Carter

Louis Weiner, MD, director, Lombardi Comprehensive Cancer Center, Georgetown University, Washington, DC. He is an internationally recognized medical oncologist specializing in the treatment of gastrointestinal cancers. His lab researches novel immunotherapy treatments.

A new way of fighting cancer uses the body's own immune system to wage war on cancer cells. Many leading cancer experts believe this approach, known as cancer immunotherapy, could revolutionize how we treat many forms of cancer.

When it comes to certain cancers, the revolution has already begun. In fact, former President Jimmy Carter, in his early nineties, is now said to be "cancer free" (based on MRI scans) after using one of these drugs for the melanoma that spread to his brain.

The new treatments aren't about enhancing immunity in general. Instead, this is an intriguing approach that can prevent cancerous tumors from hijacking our own immune defenses—so that our amazing immune system can do its job.

6 THINGS YOU NEED TO KNOW

Here are the details on this latest form of cancer immunotherapy...

1. It treats the body's immune system so the immune system can fight the cancer. T cells are the immune system's main line of defense, but they're not always effective against cancer cells. In the 1990s, cancer researchers identified a class of molecules in the body that are known as immune checkpoints. These molecules keep T cells from attacking normal cells, but cancer cells can hijack them for their own purposes. Cancer cells employ immune "checkpoints" to turn off killer T cells that would otherwise recognize and destroy a cancer that was growing in a person's body. Drugs that block these checkpoints so T cells can do their job are game changers called immune checkpoint inhibitors.

2. It still has side effects, but early results suggest a less toxic experience. All of us would love to see a day when very toxic chemotherapy agents that cause hair loss, low blood counts, fatigue, etc., are no longer the backbone of therapy for cancer. With checkpoint inhibitors, there will potentially be fewer side effects and certainly different ones. So far, the most common side effects caused by checkpoint inhibitors already in use include fatigue, cough, nausea, skin rash and itching. But more serious side effects including severe diarrhea, colitis and intestinal inflammation (even perforation) have also been reported.

3. It can be very effective and long-lasting. Consider the effects of checkpoint inhibitors against end-stage Hodgkin's disease, where patients had already received every imaginable therapy and were running out of hope. More than 90% of these patients went into remissions, many of them complete. When checkpoint inhibitors are combined against metastatic melanoma—the most deadly form of skin cancer—more than half of those cancers are eliminated or controlled, with benefits that have lasted for many years in some cases.

4. It works against many forms of cancer. In a viewpoint recently published in *JAMA*, James Allison, PhD, who pioneered the use of immune checkpoint inhibitors against cancer, wrote: "The therapy does not target the tumor cell but rather engages a target on the patient's immune system. Thus, there is no inherent reason that it would not be successful against a wide variety of tumors."

At this time, checkpoint inhibitors are FDA approved for treating only certain types of melanoma and lung cancer. But studies show that they also work against no fewer than 20 different cancers, including certain forms of kidney cancer, triple negative breast cancer, stomach cancer, Hodgkin's disease, bladder cancer and head and neck cancer.

5. It is very expensive. It can cost tens of thousands of dollars or more to have a course of therapy with these drugs, especially if you start combining them with other expensive cancer therapies.

6. It is still evolving. One promising innovation in cancer immunotherapy that is currently being researched is chimeric antigen receptor (CAR) T-cell therapy. In this case, a patient's T cells are genetically engineered to produce antibodies against a specific type of cancer. When these T cells proliferate, they pass their cancer-killing modifications along.

So far, this experimental treatment has had outstanding results against a hard-to-treat and deadly form of leukemia called acute lymphocytic leukemia.

WHAT'S AVAILABLE NOW

While many checkpoint inhibitors are in development, currently only three have been approved by the FDA...

•**Nivolumab (Opdivo) and *pembrolizumab* (Keytruda) are approved for advanced-stage non-small cell lung cancer** that has spread and that is not responding to conventional platinum-based chemotherapy... and for advanced melanoma.

•***Ipilimumab* (Yervoy) is approved for melanoma that has spread within the body (metastasized) or that cannot be removed by surgery.**

Until new drugs for different cancers make it through the FDA approval process—or the existing approved ones get future approvals for different cancers—these are the only three of this type of cancer treatment that insurance companies or Medicare are likely to cover. If you have the financial wherewithal, you may be able to have your doctor prescribe the approved drugs off-label and pay for them yourself.

For everyone else, however, there is another potential option. If there is an immunotherapy cancer drug in development for a cancer that you are being treated for, ask your oncologist whether there is a clinical trial that you can join. You can also check the website *ClinicalTrials.gov.*

4 Secret Cancer Fighters

The late Mitchell Gaynor, MD, founder of Gaynor Integrative Oncology in New York City and author of The Gene Therapy Plan: Taking Control of Your Genetic Destiny with Diet and Lifestyle. *GaynorWellness.com*

The new science of epigenetics shows that it is possible to "upregulate" (trigger) the "expression" (activity) of powerful anticancer genes using a whole-foods diet, regular exercise, restful sleep, stress reduction—and concentrated nutritional and herbal compounds.

These natural compounds can activate genes that tell the body to turbocharge the immune system so that it can locate cancer cells...kill those cells...douse chronic, low-grade inflammation, which generates "growth factors" that fuel cancer...decrease the liver's production of insulin-like growth factor one (IGF), the most deadly "tumor promoter"...reduce a tumor's cancer-spreading blood supply...and even improve the effectiveness of chemotherapy.

In addition to taking vitamin D daily, I recommend these four powerful anticancer supplements for preventing or controlling cancer or stopping its recurrence. Take one, two or all four. At the dosages recommended, they are very safe. Of course, always check with your doctor before taking any new supplement.

MAGNOLIA EXTRACT

This herbal supplement from the bark of a magnolia tree contains honokiol, which has anticancer functions—it is anti-inflammatory and anti-angiogenic (limiting blood supply to tumors), and it targets many biochemical compounds that "signal" cancer to start and to grow, such as nuclear factor-kappaB and epidermal growth factor receptor.

Scientific research: More than 200 studies show that honokiol (and magnolol, another compound in magnolia bark) can fight cancer. In a recent cellular study, published in *International Journal of Oncology*, honokiol activated a gene that "suppressed" the spread of kidney cancer and deactivated two genes that allow kidney cancer cells to invade and colonize the surrounding tissue (metastasize).

Typical dosage: 200 mg, daily.

Suggested product: Magnolia Extract from NutriCology.

ARTICHOKE EXTRACT

This extract from artichoke leaves contains rutin, quercetin, gallic acid and chlorogenic acid—all of which have been shown in laboratory studies to kill a variety of cancer cells, including colon, breast and liver cancers, and leukemia. Artichoke extract also contains cynarin, which decreases inflammation. Plus, the extract has been shown in people to improve insulin sensitivity, the body's ability to utilize the glucose-regulating hormone insulin. When insulin is used efficiently, the body makes less insulin—and less cancer-sparking IGF.

Recent study: A cellular study published in *Asian Pacific Journal of Cancer Prevention* showed that artichoke extract triggered tumor suppressor genes.

Typical dosage: 320 milligrams (mg), once daily.

Suggested product: Artichoke Extract from Enzymatic Therapy.

BLACK CUMIN SEED OIL

Many years ago, a patient of mine with prostate cancer started taking black cumin seed oil (Nigella sativa) with honey, three times a day, on the recommendation of a naturopathic physician. His Gleason score (a measure of the severity of prostate cancer) went from nine on a scale of one to 10 (an aggressive, invasive cancer with poor prognosis) to six—essentially, a precancerous lesion. Amazed, I started investigating this compound, which has been used in Turkish cooking for millennia—and started taking it myself, adding the seed to blended shakes and the oil to foods as seasoning. I recommend that patients use the oil—rich in thymoquinone, which is found in few other foods—either in their diets or as a supplement.

Compelling research: Researchers at Barbara Ann Karmanos Cancer Institute at Wayne State University School of Medicine in Detroit reviewed hundreds of cellular and animal studies on thymoquinone and cancer and concluded that the compound is anti-inflammatory...stops cancer cells from dividing and spreading by triggering their death...limits the formation of blood vessels that nourish the tumor (angiogenesis)...and "sensitizes" cells to chemotherapy.

Example: In a recent animal study, published in *Archives of Medical Science*, researchers found that thymoquinone "decreased the expression" of both BRCA1 and BRCA2 genes—genes that increase the risk for breast cancer three- to five-fold and the risk for ovarian cancer as much as 30-fold.

Typical dosage: 500 mg, twice daily.

Suggested product: Black Cumin Seed Oil from Amazing Herbs.

BEE PROPOLIS, BEE POLLEN AND ROYAL JELLY

Bee propolis (a waxlike material used by bees to repair holes in hives) is rich in caffeic acid phenethyl ester (CAPE), chrysin and cinnamic acid, compounds that affect cancer genes. Studies show they are immune-strengthening, anti-inflammatory and anti-angiogenic and can reduce the growth of many cancers, including colon, prostate and kidney. Bee propolis also has been used clinically to reduce mouth sores caused by chemotherapy and radiation.

Recent study: In a cellular study on prostate cancer from the University of Texas Medical Branch, researchers found that CAPE boosted the cancer-killing power of chemotherapeutic drugs.

Another cellular study shows that bee pollen can inhibit vascular endothelial growth factor (VEGF), which helps create blood supply to tumors.

Royal jelly (a milky secretion produced by worker bees) contains several epigenetic factors. It has been shown to suppress the blood supply to tumors.

Typical dosage: 500 mg, once daily.

Suggested product: Triple Bee Complex from Y.S. Organic Bee Farms, which contains bee propolis, bee pollen and royal jelly.

Caution: People who are allergic to bee stings should not take bee products.

Itching After a Shower and Other Surprising Cancer Symptoms

Eugene Ahn, MD, hematologist and oncologist at Cancer Treatment Centers of America (CTCA) and medical director for clinical research in integrative oncology at CTCA at Midwestern Regional Medical Center in Zion, Illinois. CancerCenter.com

Certain cancer symptoms almost always prompt a visit to the doctor. A breast lump. A mole that changes in size, shape or color. Blood in the stool.

But there are other symptoms that most people ignore.

Startling new finding: In a study published in *British Journal of General Practice*, nearly half of people with a warning sign of cancer decided not to see a doctor about it, often because they thought the symptom was insignificant.

For the following symptoms, your first step is to visit your primary care physician who can perform the appropriate tests and/or refer you to a specialist.

If you have any one of these symptoms in isolation, the likelihood of you having cancer is less than 1%. That doesn't mean you should dismiss the symptom. But it does mean that you shouldn't panic if it shows up.

HEARTBURN

Most likely cause: Gastroesophageal reflux disease (GERD).

But it could be a sign of: Esophagus or stomach cancer. Symptoms of heartburn can include burning pain or discomfort in the stomach, upper abdomen, chest and/or throat... and/or excessive burping, bloating or nausea after eating. If those symptoms are chronic, it's time to see a doctor for a workup. You might have Barrett's esophagus, a precancerous condition that is triggered by chronic inflammation and increases the risk for esophageal cancer. Or you might have H. pylori, a bacterial infection of the stomach that increases your risk for stomach cancer (and ulcers)—but is easily treatable with a two-week treatment that includes antibiotics and possibly a proton-pump inhibitor.

What to do: Ask your doctor if you need an esophagogastroduodenoscopy (EGD), in which an endoscope is used to explore your esophagus, stomach and duodenum (the first section of the small intestine). A biopsy can be taken during the procedure if there is suspicious-looking tissue.

ITCHING AFTER A HOT SHOWER

Most likely cause: Dry skin or a contact allergy to a cleansing product.

But it could be a sign of: Polycythemia vera, a common myeloproliferative disorder, a type of blood cancer. In the early stages of this cancer, histamine-containing mast cells (cells behind allergic reactions) become hypersensitive, causing the skin to react to hot water.

What to do: If you're over age 40 (when this cancer most commonly occurs), ask your doctor for a complete blood count (CBC), which will detect an elevation of red blood cells, a feature of polycythemia vera.

EATING ICE

Likely cause: Iron deficiency.

But it could be a sign of: Gastrointestinal cancers, bladder cancer or any cancer that leads to blood loss. Called pica, this phenomenon—a compulsion to eat ice, sand, soil, clay, paper or chalk or to chew on something metallic—usually occurs during pregnancy and can be a sign of iron deficiency. But iron deficiency also can signal chronic internal blood loss, sometimes from cancer.

What to do: Ask your doctor about a blood test for iron deficiency. If you have an iron deficiency, work with your doctor to determine the cause.

UNBEARABLE PAIN IN A BONE WHEN TOUCHED

Most likely causes: Trauma, rheumatological disease or infection.

But it could be a sign of: Bone metastases (the spread of an original, primary tumor into the bone). This symptom is a hallmark of bone cancer.

What to do: If you have unexplained pain that tends to increase over a month—particularly if it's sensitive to the touch—talk to your doctor about imaging studies, such as a CT scan, a bone scan, an X-ray or an MRI.

DIARRHEA PLUS FACIAL FLUSHING

Likely cause: Irritable bowel syndrome (IBS).

But it could be a sign of: Neuro-endocrine tumor, metastasized to the liver. Diarrhea alone rarely leads to a diagnosis of cancer, but diarrhea and flushing of the face are a unique pair of symptoms that could indicate a neuroendocrine tumor—a type of cancer arising from the hormone-producing cells in the body.

What to do: Talk to your doctor about possible imaging (CT, PET or MRI) to potentially detect liver metastases and primary tumor.

REDDENED SKIN ON THE BREAST

Likely cause: Skin infection.

But it could be a sign of: Breast cancer. A lump is not the only warning sign of breast cancer. Redness of the breast—particularly if the skin also is thickened, with the texture of an orange peel—is a sign of inflammatory breast cancer, a rare and aggressive form of the disease that can be missed by a mammogram, an ultrasound or an MRI.

What to do: Ask your doctor about a breast biopsy, the best way to detect this type of cancer.

Important: If the doctor diagnoses the redness as an infection and treats it with antibiotics, and the redness doesn't resolve or worsens, return quickly for a follow-up examination.

BLOOD CLOT

Likely causes: Leg or arm injury, such as a sprained ankle…recent hospitalization or surgery…a long period of inactivity, such as a plane ride.

But it could be a sign of: Breast, pancreatic, ovarian and many other cancers. A blood clot (a symptom of deep vein thrombosis, or DVT) is a common problem, affecting 900,000 Americans yearly. But DVT is not commonly understood as a potential early warning sign of cancer and so is often overlooked as a cancer symptom, even though as many as one in 10 patients with an unexplained blood clot may have some type of cancer.

What to do: If you have a blood clot (typically signaled by a sudden, painful swelling of an arm or a leg) without any of the common triggers, talk to your doctor about a workup for cancer. This is an early warning sign that often is missed.

BLOATING

Likely cause: Eating too much or too fast.

But it could be a sign of: Ovarian cancer. Bloating is a common symptom that is rarely a sign of cancer. But persistent bloating can be a sign of cancer in the peritoneal cavity, a common feature of advanced ovarian cancer, particularly if accompanied by a persistent, dull ache in the abdomen and unexplained weight loss (a symptom of advanced cancer).

What to do: Your doctor may recommend a CT scan or a transvaginal ultrasound. If the results are negative, ask about getting a laparoscopy, in which a thin, lighted tube is put through an incision in the belly to look at the abdominal and reproductive organs. A CT scan or a transvaginal ultrasound can easily miss ovarian cancer.

QUITTING SMOKING EASILY

Likely cause: You decided to quit, and you succeeded.

But it could be a sign of: Lung cancer. A chronic smoker who suddenly finds it unusually easy to quit may be experiencing a strange physiological symptom of lung cancer—inexplicably losing the desire to smoke. Usually, non-small-cell lung cancer is diagnosed three to four years after a chronic smoker easily quits, and small-cell lung cancer (a more aggressive type) is diagnosed about six months after quitting.

What to do: If you have been a lifelong smoker who suddenly finds it easy to quit, talk to your doctor about having a chest CT scan for lung cancer. You also would benefit from routine annual surveillance even if the scan is negative.

Cancer-Fighting Purple Potatoes

Study titled "Anthocyanin-containing purple-fleshed potatoes suppress colon tumorigenesis via elimination of colon cancer stem cells" by researchers at Penn State University, University Park, Pennsylvania, published in *The Journal of Nutritional Biochemistry*.

Maybe you've seen them at the farmers market or in your regular market—purple potatoes. They go by names such as Purple Peruvian, Peru Purple, Purple Fiesta, Purple Majesty and Purple Passion. You get the idea. Purple. The first time you cut into one, you may be pleasantly surprised to find that they are a pretty shade of purple all the way through.

Here's an even better surprise—anthocyanins, the compounds that turn these spuds purple, may protect you from colon cancer. In the latest study, researchers induced colon cancer in mice and gave one group a baked purple potato extract and a control group a standard painkiller.

Results: In the mice given purple potato extract, colon cancer stem cells, which spread the disease, were suppressed—and colon cancer cells were more likely to die. Other studies have linked anthocyanins to prevention of other cancers (and heart disease). Purple potatoes are particularly rich in anthocyanins, which are also found in berries, red and purple grapes, red wine, cherries, eggplant and red cabbage.

COOKING WITH PURPLE POTATOES

Purple potatoes are just as versatile as the bag of russets or red potatoes in your pantry, and they'll add a pop of color to your meal. With a medium starch level and thin, tender skins, purple potatoes resemble white-skinned potatoes with their creamy, dense texture, but they have a slightly earthier taste. Whether you roast, steam or sauté them, they'll hold their texture after cooking. Boiled, they'll mash to velvety perfection. They'll make your next potato salad a colorful affair, turn a puréed potato soup a lovely pastel color and liven up a potato gratin.

Fear of Heights: The Cancer Link

Take that, Randy Newman. Shorter people may be less likely to get cancer. When Swedish researchers tracked health records of more than five million people over more than 50 years, they found that for each four inches of adult height, men were 11% and women 18% more likely to develop cancer. Other studies have also reported the association.

Study by researchers at the Karolinska Institute, Stockholm, Sweden, presented at the annual meeting of the European Society for Paediatric Endocrinology.

Secrets to Getting the Best Colonoscopy

Douglas K. Rex, MD, director of endoscopy at Indiana University Hospital in Indianapolis. He is coauthor of the colorectal cancer screening recommendations of the American College of Gastroenterology. Douglas KRex.com

If you're age 50 or older, chances are you've had a colonoscopy—and maybe more than one. If so, you've taken a crucial step in protecting your health.

Why this test is so important: It's estimated that if every person age 50 and older had a colonoscopy, 64% of people with colorectal cancer would have never developed the disease.

But since you are going to the trouble to get this test (and we all know the bowel-cleansing prep is no picnic), then it also makes sense to make sure you're getting the best possible screening. *How to ensure that you get the maximum cancer protection from your colonoscopy...*

HOW GOOD IS YOUR DOCTOR?

One of the most important aspects of a colonoscopy is the doctor's ability to detect a type of polyp called an adenoma—the doctor's so-called "adenoma detection rate" (ADR). This varies widely depending on the doctor's skill.

If your doctor has a low ADR, you're more likely to get colon cancer before your next colonoscopy. Gastroenterologists are more likely to have good ADRs than primary care physicians and general surgeons who might perform colonoscopies, but there's a wide range of performance within each group.

Precisely defined, a doctor's ADR is the percentage of screening colonoscopies in patients age 50 or older during which he/she detects one or more adenomas.

My advice: Look for a doctor with an ADR of 20% or higher in women and 30% or higher in men (who have more adenomas)…or a "mixed-gender" rate of 25% or higher—in other words, the doctor detects at least one adenoma in 25% of the screening colonoscopies he conducts.

Startling recent finding: A 10-year study published in *The New England Journal of Medicine* evaluated more than 300,000 colonoscopies conducted by 136 gastroenterologists—and found that for every 1% increase in ADR, there was a 3% reduction in the risk of developing colorectal cancer before the next colonoscopy. This means that having your colonoscopy performed by a doctor with a high ADR (as described earlier) is a must for optimal screening. But how does a patient ask about his doctor's ADR without seeming to question the physician's competence?

My advice: Ask about your doctor's ADR on the phone, during the colonoscopy scheduling process, when you are talking to an administrator or a nurse. If that person doesn't know, request that someone get back to you with the number. That will make your query less confrontational.

However: Even your doctor may not know his own ADR. Monitoring of ADRs is endorsed by several professional medical societies, such as the American Society for Gastrointestinal Endoscopy and the American College of Gastroenterology, but there is no law mandating that doctors must track it. Or your doctor may refuse to disclose his ADR—a response you should find concerning. If you don't get the information you need from your doctor, it's probably a good idea to find a new one.

Also important: Make sure your colonoscopy is being performed with a high-definition colonoscope, the current state-of-the-art in colonoscopy. Inquire about this when you ask about a doctor's ADR.

A BETTER BOWEL PREP

Another key to a truly preventive colonoscopy is the preparation. Before the procedure, a patient drinks a defecation-inducing liquid (prep) that cleanses the rectum and colon of stool so that the doctor can clearly see the lining. In some patients, a four-liter prep (about one gallon), or even more, is best for optimal cleansing. If you don't have a condition associated with slow bowel motility, such as chronic constipation, or use constipating medications such as opioids, you may be eligible for one of the regimens that requires only two or three liters of fluid. (A pill preparation is also available, but it is seldom used because it can cause kidney damage.) Ask your doctor what regimen will give you the best combination of excellent cleansing and tolerability.

A common mistake: Many people think that they can drink the prep one to two days before the procedure and then drink nothing but clear fluids (such as Gatorade, apple juice or water) until the day of the colonoscopy.

But even during the prep, the small intestine (the section of bowel after the stomach and before the colon) continues to produce chyme, a thick, mucousy secretion that sticks to the walls of the ascending colon—so that seven to eight hours after drinking the prep the colon is no longer completely clean.

Best: A split prep, with half the prep ingested the day before the procedure and half ingested four to five hours before (the middle of the night when the colonoscopy is scheduled for the morning…or the morning when the colonoscopy is scheduled for the afternoon).

Scientific evidence: Split preparation improves ADR by 26%, according to a study in *Gastrointestinal Endoscopy.*

Also helpful: Drinking the prep can be difficult, even nauseating. *How to make it more palatable…*

Chill the liquid thoroughly, and drink it with a straw. Follow each swallow with ginger ale or another good-tasting clear liquid. Suck on a clear menthol lozenge after you drink the prep. And if you throw up the prep, wait 30 minutes (until you feel less nauseated) and then continue drinking the prep as instructed—it can still work.

Several recent studies have found that eating a fiber-free diet all or part of the day prior to colonoscopy allows for better cleansing of the colon. Some doctors advise avoiding high-fiber foods such as corn, seeds and nuts for about a week before a colonoscopy. Ask your doctor what he advises for you.

Six Ways to Reduce Your Risk of Colon Cancer

Alice Bender, RDN, head of nutrition programs, American Institute for Cancer Research, Washington, DC.
American Institute for Cancer Research, news release.

Half of the colon cancer cases in the United States could be prevented if people followed six proven steps to reduce their risk, a cancer and nutrition expert says.

Colon cancer is the second leading cause of cancer death, and the third most common type of cancer in the United States. In 2016, there will be over 134,000 cases of colon cancer, the U.S. National Cancer Institute estimates.

"Research now suggests that 50% of colorectal cancers in the United States are preventable each year through diet, weight and physical activity. That's about 67,200 cases every year," Alice Bender, RDN, head of nutrition programs at the American Institute for Cancer Research, said in an institute news release.

Bender outlined six evidence-based measures you can take to try to lower your risk of developing colon cancer...

•**Maintain a healthy weight and control belly fat,** which has been linked to increased risk of colon cancer, regardless of body weight.

•**Get regular moderate physical activity,** which can range from house cleaning to running.

•**Eat plenty of high-fiber foods.** For every 10 grams of fiber (a bit less than a cup of beans) in your daily diet, your risk of colon cancer falls by 10%, Bender said.

•**Reduce red meat consumption and avoid processed meats,** such as hot dogs, bacon, sausage and deli meats. Ounce for ounce, processed meats boost the risk of colon cancer twice as much as red meat.

•**Avoid alcohol or limit your intake to no more than two standard drinks a day for men and one for women,** Bender advised.

•**Go heavy on the garlic.** Evidence suggests that a diet rich in garlic reduces the risk of colon cancer, Bender said.

The American Cancer Society recommends that people age 50 or older talk with a doctor about colon cancer screening. Screening can detect the cancer before symptoms develop, when it's easier to treat and survival rates are more favorable.

info The American Cancer Society has more on colon cancer at *cancer.org*

Elderly with Advanced Colon Cancer Often Get Costly, Dubious Treatments

Cathy Bradley, PhD, associate director, population science research, University of Colorado Cancer Center, and professor, Colorado School of Public Health, Aurora.
Alfred Neugut, MD, PhD, oncologist and epidemiologist, professor, Columbia University Medical Center, and co-director, Cancer Prevention Program, New York-Presbyterian Hospital, New York City.
Medical Care, online

Expensive drugs are being given far more often to elderly patients with advanced colon cancer, but they offer almost no benefit, a new study suggests.

"This research found that there is a trend for elderly late-stage colorectal cancer patients to receive newer, more expensive drugs," said lead author Cathy Bradley, PhD, associate director for population science research at the University of Colorado Cancer Center. "However, in spite of their receiving more drugs, no [significant] survival benefit was observed."

STUDY DETAILS

In the study, published recently in the journal *Medical Care*, Dr. Bradley and her colleagues analyzed data on more than 16,000 Medicare patients with advanced, or metastatic, colon cancer and 4,000 patients with advanced rectal cancer. (Metastatic means the cancer has spread from the original tumor to other parts of the body.)

They discovered that among patients aged 75 and over, the percentage receiving three or more drugs to treat the disease rose from 2% to 53% over a 10-year period.

These agents included new drugs such as ox*aliplatin* (Eloxatin), *cetuximab* (Erbitux), and *panitunumab* (Vectibix), as well as *bevacizumab* (Avastin), which works by starving tumors.

These drugs have been shown to be more effective in younger people or those with less advanced disease, the researchers said in background notes.

For patients aged 65 to 74 who took these newer therapies, overall survival increased by about eight months. But those over 75 who took these medications improved their median survival rate by only one month.

NEW THERAPIES ARE COSTLY AND DANGEROUS

The study authors stressed that these new therapies can also be expensive. Treatment costs for colon cancer patients taking these anticancer drugs in the first year following diagnosis increased 32% over the study period. These same costs rose by 20% for rectal cancer patients.

Patients and their families often have to cover a significant portion of these costs, the authors noted. These patients paid approximately $16,000 in out-of-pocket costs for care in 2009, compared with $11,000 in 2000, according to the research.

To illustrate the higher costs of newer drugs compared to older ones, investigators noted the average cost for oxaliplatin in 2006 was $11,593, while the older 5-FU/leucovorin treatment only cost an average of $1,028.

Dr. Bradley said newer therapies not only cost more than older ones, but they're tied to worse side effects.

"Common toxicities associated with newer therapies include diarrhea, dehydration, bowel wall injury, hemorrhage, wound-healing complications and GI [gastrointestinal tract] perforation," Dr. Bradley said. "The main concern is that these toxicities will be incurred without any survival benefit, potentially worsening the patient's health status. These toxicities would seem to have a negative impact on quality of life."

To cope with these side effects, patients may also need to take supportive medications, which can push costs even higher.

EXPERT COMMENT

Alfred Neugut, MD, PhD, co-director of the Cancer Prevention Program at New York-Presbyterian Hospital in New York City, said that despite the soaring costs, side effects and no real survival benefits, patients may still pursue these newer therapies when standard treatments do not work.

"Patients and their doctors often do not want to give up," he said. "The patients have to ask themselves, do they live out life now the best way possible or do they keep trying new treatment even if it impairs quality of life. Physicians usually encourage a non-passive approach. And the presence of insurance removes the patient and doctor's inhibitions regarding cost."

ALTERNATIVE FOR OLDER PATIENTS

Dr. Bradley added that palliative care could be a good option for the elderly. This approach aims to relieve the symptoms and mental stress of a serious illness without curing the disease.

"Only the patients and their physician can decide what is best for the situation," said Dr. Bradley. "However, palliative care may offer some symptom relief without inflicting additional toxicities."

info There's more on colon cancer treatment at the U.S. National Cancer Institute website, *cancer.gov* (search "colon cancer treatment")

Drink This to Prevent Colon Cancer

Study titled "Coffee Consumption and the Risk of Colorectal Cancer" by researchers at University of Southern California, Los Angeles, Carmel Medical Center, Clalit Health Services National Cancer Control Center, Technion-Israel Institute of Technology, all in Haifa, Israel, published in *Cancer Epidemiology, Biomarkers & Prevention.*

The good news about coffee keeps getting better. The latest—a few cups a day might avert colon cancer, the third most common kind of cancer, which kills 50,000 Americans a year.

Although bioactive compounds in coffee have been thought to be protective against this common cancer, evidence has been lacking—until now. A new study of 9,000 men and women compared those who had recently been diagnosed with colorectal cancer with healthy controls. *Results…*

Those who drank one or two cups of coffee per day were 26% less likely to have colon cancer.

Those who drank 2.5 or more cups a day had 50% lower risk.

It didn't matter what kind of coffee—the benefit was equal for espresso, instant, filtered and even decaffeinated. So if you can't take the caffeine jolt of regular coffee, you can still get the benefits with decaf.

Sunscreen Myths Debunked

Barney Kenet, MD, a board-certified dermatologist and dermatologic surgeon at New York-Presbyterian/Weill Cornell Medical Center and in private practice, both in New York City. He specializes in cosmetic dermatology and in the diagnosis of melanoma and other skin cancers. He is the author of *Saving Your Skin.*

Even though dermatologists have cautioned for years that burned—or even suntanned—skin can lead to skin cancer, far too many people are failing to heed that warning. In fact, only about 20% of men and 43% of women use sunscreen regularly, according to a new survey by the Centers for Disease Control and Prevention.

Why do so few of us take advantage of this basic form of skin protection? Part of the problem is that there are so many misconceptions about sunscreens and skin cancer.

Among the most common myths…

MYTH #1: If you wear sunscreen, you'll develop vitamin D deficiency.

Truth: Our skin needs to be exposed to sunlight in order for our bodies to manufacture vitamin D. Deficiencies of this crucial vitamin are now being linked to everything from bone loss and multiple sclerosis to heart disease and dementia.

It's true that if you were perfectly covered in sunscreen every minute of every day, then you could, theoretically, develop a vitamin D deficiency. This, however, isn't a reality for most people.

Dr. Kenet's take: To produce sufficient vitamin D, you need only about 10 to 15 minutes of sun exposure three times a week on your arms or face (without sunscreen). If you are worried because you live in an area where you get limited sun exposure, ask your doctor for a blood test to measure your vitamin D level. If your level is low, you may need to take a vitamin D supplement.

MYTH #2: Only fair-skinned people develop skin cancer.

Truth: While it is true that fair-skinned people are at highest risk for melanoma, the deadliest form of skin cancer, olive-skinned and dark-skinned people are also at risk. Among African-Americans, for example, melanomas mainly occur on parts of the body that are not pigmented, such as the palms of the hands, the soles of the feet and the skin beneath the nails.

Dr. Kenet's take: No matter what your skin tone, use sunscreen to help protect against skin cancer. Be sure to cover areas that frequently get overlooked—the back, behind the ears and the backs of the legs.

If you have dark skin, you might not need to wear sunscreen on a daily basis, but I advise using it when you are spending time outdoors in intense sunlight.

MYTH #3: Sunscreen is all you need to avoid skin cancer.

Truth: Sunscreen is just one tool in skin cancer prevention.

Dr. Kenet's take: When it comes to skin protection, think "belt and suspenders"—that is, no single approach will guarantee safe skin, so do as much as possible.

Reduce your exposure to ultraviolet (UV) radiation by avoiding outdoor activities during the peak UV-risk hours of 10 am to 4 pm.

Hide your skin from the sun by seeking shady areas…using a wide-brimmed hat that shades your face and ears…and wearing a tight-weave, long-sleeved shirt. Also, consider wearing clothing made with UV-protective fabric. Check Coolibar.com…and SunPrecautions.com.

Important: Don't forget sunglasses—ocular melanoma is a real risk, especially for people with light (blue or green) eyes. One in four Americans rarely or never wears sunglasses, according to a new survey. Be sure your sunglasses block out 99% to 100% of both UVA and UVB rays.

Important: Skin cancer can develop on the lips, too, so use a lip balm that includes sun protection factor (SPF). It doesn't have to be anything fancy—ChapStick Ultra Lip Balm with SPF 30 works great.

MYTH #4: When it comes to SPF, the higher the better.

Truth: Sunscreens with SPF 15 filter out 93% of UVB rays (the primary cause of sunburn)…SPF 30 filters 97%…and SPF 50 filters 98%. There is very little difference between the protection offered by SPF 30 and SPF 50+.

People often mistakenly assume that a high-SPF product that blocks sunburn is adequate, not realizing that it may not protect them from the effects of UVA exposure, which is more closely associated with skin cancer. "Broad-spectrum" products provide protection against both UVB and UVA exposure.

Dr. Kenet's take: For maximum sun protection, purchase a broad-spectrum sunscreen with at least SPF 15, then be sure to reapply it every two hours (use a golf ball–size dollop—

roughly one ounce). And yes, that means you'll go through a bottle of sunscreen very quickly!

Note: People who have lupus or a family history of skin cancer should use an SPF of at least 30.

It is a good idea to wear sunscreen year-round. Apply it before you get dressed (this helps reduce the chance that you'll miss a spot).

MYTH #5: It's fine to choose any form of sunscreen, as long as it's broad-spectrum and has an SPF of at least 15.

Truth: That's true in theory, but the form of the sunscreen can make a big difference in whether you actually use it.

Dr. Kenet's take: Spray-on sunscreens can be practical for people playing golf or tennis, for example, who need to reapply quickly and often. Because concerns have been raised about potential dangers due to inhaling spray-on sunscreens, these products shouldn't be sprayed on the face. Instead, spray the sunscreen on your hands and then apply it to your face.

Gel sunscreens are water-based and easy on the skin for people who are prone to acne. However, gel sunscreens are not good if you plan to spend a lot of time in the water or tend to get very sweaty. For these people, sunscreens containing titanium dioxide and/or zinc oxide work well (they do leave a white coating on the skin).

DR. KENET'S TOP SUNSCREEN PICKS

As a dermatologist and skin cancer expert, Barney Kenet, MD, recommends the following sunscreen products for his patients…

•**Olay Complete All Day Moisture Cream with Sunscreen.** Broad-spectrum, SPF 15. This product is designed for people with sensitive skin and good for daily use. It is also available in SPF 30.

•**Neutrogena Ultra Sheer Dry-Touch Sunscreen.** Broad-spectrum, SPF 30. This sunscreen, which is not oily, is great for people who resist sunscreens because of the "greasy" feel. For babies, try Neutrogena Pure & Free Baby Sunscreen Lotion.

•**Avène Mineral Ultra-Light Hydrating Sunscreen Lotion (Face).** Broad-spectrum, SPF 50+. This sunscreen is lightweight and free of parabens (chemicals used as preservatives). It's more expensive than many other sunscreens (about $22 for a 1.3-ounce bottle) but provides good protection with a luxurious feel to the skin.

Should You Be Screened For Melanoma? Check Your Arm

Study titled "Prediction of high naevus count in a healthy UK population to estimate melanoma risk" by researchers at King's College London published in *British Journal of Dermatology*.

If you have more than 11 moles on your right arm, you're at increased risk for melanoma, the deadliest form of skin cancer, according to a recent study. It means that you likely have more than 100 moles over your entire body, a known risk factor.

The arm check is a quick way to see if you need further screening. If your count is high, schedule regular full-body exams with a dermatologist. Early detection is a lifesaver when it comes to melanoma.

Got fewer moles? You're not off the hook! Not all melanomas emerge from existing moles. It's important to know what's normal for your skin and to let your doctor know if you see any change in the size, shape, color or feel of a mole—or any other patch of skin.

New Tests May Help Combat Melanoma

American Academy of Dermatology, news release

Genetic and molecular tests can be valuable in helping to diagnose and treat deadly melanoma skin cancer.

The tests are widely available in the United States, and many are covered by insurance or offered at no extra cost, said Emily Chu, MD, PhD. She is an assistant professor of dermatology and pathology and laboratory medicine at the University of Pennsylvania, in Philadelphia.

Melanoma rates in the United States have doubled over the past three decades, according to the U.S. Centers for Disease Control and Prevention. Tissue biopsy is typically used to diagnose skin cancer, but biopsy results aren't always definitive. In such cases, genetic and molecular tests can help determine if a patient has skin cancer, Dr. Chu said.

She added that such tests may also help identify the most effective treatments for patients with advanced melanoma.

Continuing research into specific melanoma mutations and targeted treatments could lead to more effective therapies in the future, the researcher said.

Not Safe from the Sun

Neal Schultz, MD, dermatologist in private practice, New York City, and host of DermTV.com.

Car windows do not protect skin from sun damage. While glass does block burning UVB rays, it still allows 60% of damaging UVA rays through.

Daily Low-Dose Aspirin Linked to Reduced Risk of Certain Cancers

Andrew Chan, MD, MPH, Massachusetts General Hospital, Boston.
Ernest Hawk, MD, MPH, vice president, division of cancer prevention and population sciences, University of Texas MD Anderson Cancer Center, Houston.
Eric Jacobs, PhD, strategic director, pharmacoepidemiology, American Cancer Society.
JAMA Oncology, online

Taking low-dose aspirin every day may lower the overall risk of cancer by 3%, mostly due to a 15% lower risk for gastrointestinal cancers and a 19% lower risk for cancers of the colon and rectum, the recent findings showed.

But the benefit was only seen after six years of taking aspirin almost daily, the study authors said.

"That makes sense, because cancers don't typically develop overnight. They take years to develop, so you would have to take aspirin for a long time to prevent cancer," said senior researcher Andrew Chan, MD, MPH, from Massachusetts General Hospital in Boston.

"There is scientific evidence that aspirin has an effect on certain biological pathways that can result in cancer," he said. And it also reduces inflammation and the amount of some cancer-causing proteins.

STUDY DETAILS

For the study, Dr. Chan and colleagues looked at the link between aspirin and cancer among more than 130,000 women and men who took part in the long-term Nurses' Health Study and the Health Professionals Follow-up Study.

During more than 30 years of follow-up, there were more than 20,000 cancers among more than 88,000 women, and more than 7,500 cancers among nearly 48,000 men, the study found.

Aspirin, however, was not associated with a lower risk for other major cancers, such as breast, prostate or lung cancer, the investigators found.

Taking aspirin regularly might prevent 17% of colon cancers among those who are not screened with colonoscopy and 8.5% of colon cancers among those who are, the research indicated.

EXPERT COMMENTARY

"Aspirin may serve as a relatively low-cost primary prevention for gastrointestinal and colon cancers, with reductions in cancers complementing recommended cancer screening," Ernest Hawk, MD, MPH, vice president of cancer prevention and population sciences at the University of Texas MD Anderson Cancer Center in Houston.

Although the evidence is mounting that aspirin may reduce the risk of colon and other cancers, the American Cancer Society does not currently have recommendations for or against aspirin use, said Eric Jacobs, PhD, the cancer society's strategic director for pharmacoepidemiology.

People who have had a heart attack or stroke are usually prescribed aspirin unless there is a good reason not to, such as a recent history of stomach ulcers, Dr. Jacobs said.

RECOMMENDATIONS

"People who have not had a heart attack or stroke need to consider the overall balance of risks and benefits, including lower risk of heart disease and colon cancer, but higher risk of serious stomach bleeding," he said. "This makes more sense than thinking about taking aspirin just for prevention of cancer."

People who are wondering if they should start taking aspirin should first talk to their physician. The doctor will be able to take into account the patient's risk for heart disease, as well as reasons why regular aspirin use might not be right for them, Dr. Jacobs said.

Aspirin is not a substitute for getting screened for colon cancer, he said. "All Americans 50 or older should talk to their doctor about getting tested for colon cancer so that polyps can be detected and removed before they get a chance to develop into cancer," Dr. Jacobs explained.

Lung Cancer Is on the Rise Among Nonsmokers

Timothy Burns, MD, PhD, assistant professor of medicine in the department of medicine, division of hematology/oncology, at the University of Pittsburgh Cancer Institute, where his laboratory focuses on discovering targeted therapies for lung cancer.

People who have never smoked often assume that they'll never get lung cancer. But they can—and the prevalence of these cases is increasing at a troubling rate.

Update: Two important recent studies show that rates of lung cancer among so-called "never-smokers" (less than 100 cigarettes smoked in a lifetime) are mysteriously skyrocketing—in one study, from 9% to 20% of all such malignancies.

But it's not all bad news.

The recent discovery of genetic mutations called "oncogenes" that drive lung cancer in never-smokers has fueled the development of powerful medications that are often more effective and have fewer side effects than conventional chemotherapy.

Bonus: These new drugs are taken orally rather than intravenously, as is more common with conventional chemotherapy.

TESTING FOR MUTATIONS

If you're one of the roughly 24,000 never-smokers diagnosed with lung cancer each year in the US, it's crucial for you (as well as current and former smokers) to be tested for a genetic mutation that might be driving your disease.

Shockingly, many of these patients are not tested despite the recommendations of national cancer organizations. This is due, in part, to the lack of awareness of many community oncologists in the US.

The most accurate test uses a tissue biopsy to screen for a handful of critical mutations that predict a more than 70% chance of responding to FDA-approved drugs. If the size and location of the tumor make a biopsy impossible, the oncologist should order a blood or urine test to check for mutations.

Important: If possible, get your genetic testing at one of the 45 medical institutions designated by the National Cancer Institute (NCI) as a "Comprehensive Cancer Center" (check *Cancer.gov/research/nci-role/cancer-centers/find*). You will get the most accurate testing at one of these centers and the most reliably up-to-date information on the latest cutting-edge medicine and clinical trials. A medical oncologist near you can administer the treatment. If you're not able to travel to an NCI-designated center, a tissue sample from a biopsy performed at your local medical facility can be sent to certain institutions (such as the Mayo Clinic and Johns Hopkins) that offer molecular testing.

KEY GENETIC MUTATIONS

If you have a genetic mutation, a targeted medication can be used to treat the lung cancer. (Patients who do not test positive for a mutation receive standard cancer care, including conventional chemotherapy and/or radiation.)

Genetic mutations may include…

•**Epidermal growth factor receptor (EGFR).** This is the most common mutation in never-smokers with lung cancer, occurring in about 40% of these patients. Several FDA-approved drugs called EGFR-inhibitors can counter this mutation, including *gefitinib* (Iressa)…*erlotinib* (Tarceva)…and *afatinib* (Gilotrif). Additionally, *icotinib* (Conmana) is in clinical trials.

•**Anaplastic lymphoma kinase (ALK).** About 5% to 8% of lung cancer patients (most of these never-smokers) have this genetic mutation. The FDA-approved drug is *crizotinib* (Xalkori) for ALK-positive patients who have never received lung cancer treatment.

TIME FOR A DIFFERENT DRUG

Even when a genetic mutation is identified, eventually a new mutation is generated and the tumor starts growing again—a phenomenon called acquired resistance. This typically occurs after about a year of treatment. Therefore, patients on these therapies undergo regular CT scans at two- to three-month intervals to make sure their disease is not growing.

Best approach: When your tumor develops acquired resistance, it's important to have another biopsy so that your doctor can determine which drug is right for you. Two months after starting a second-line drug, the patient will undergo a new CT scan to make sure it is shrinking the tumor.

Important: The patient should alert the physician if he/she is taking any over-the-counter supplements—some can have life-threatening interactions with the targeted therapies.

EARLY DETECTION

The cause of lung cancer in never-smokers is unknown, but it is believed that up to 50% of cases are due to exposure to radon, a naturally occurring radioactive gas, and/or secondhand smoke. A distant third is indoor air pollution, such as particles from wood-burning stoves and cooking fumes from stir-, deep- or pan-frying. *Main risks…*

•**Radon.** Get your home tested. If levels are high (4 pCi/L or above), hire a state-licensed "radon mitigation contractor" to reduce levels to 2 pCi/L or below by installing a pipe that vents the gas outdoors.

•**Secondhand smoke.** Avoid it whenever possible.

•**Indoor air pollution.** If you have a wood stove, get a high-efficiency particulate arresting (HEPA) air filter...if you fry food, vent the fumes—they may contain harmful carcinogens.

Important: If you are a never-smoker who has one or more of the symptoms of lung cancer—a persistent cough, chest pain, shortness of breath and/or sudden weight loss...or if you've had pneumonia that's persisted for months in spite of several rounds of antibiotics—ask your doctor to test for lung cancer.

Unfortunately, never-smoker lung cancer often has no (or only vague) symptoms that doctors may not immediately suspect as a malignancy. For this reason, it is usually diagnosed when the cancer has spread to the bone, brain, liver and/or other organs. At that point, the most that can be done is to control the disease, giving the patient as much as three to five or more extra years of life if the disease is treated. As new therapies continue to emerge, the goal is to make never-smoker lung cancer a chronic disease and to someday provide a cure.

Better Lung Cancer Follow-Up

Niels-Chr. G. Hansen, MD, pulmonologist, Odense University Hospital, Denmark.

In a new finding, a CT scan follow-up program after surgery for lung cancer significantly increases survival rates.

Details: About 400 patients who received CT scans of the thorax (chest) and upper abdomen every three months for two years and then every six months for three more years had a survival rate during the study of 67.8% versus a survival rate of 55.7% for those who did not receive CT scans.

If you have had surgery for lung cancer: Ask your doctor about getting regular CT scans.

Pancreatic Cancer? Only 1 in 5 Patients Gets This Critical Test

Only one in five gets the widely available CA 19-9 blood test, which assesses levels of a particular tumor marker, according to a new study of 97,000 pancreatic cancer patients. Results of this test can help determine the best treatment. Pancreatic cancer patients with elevated CA 19-9 levels may get better results by having chemotherapy before surgery.

The study's senior author is Mark Truty, MD, gastrointestinal surgical oncologist, Mayo Clinic, Rochester, Minnesota.

How to Get Into a Cancer Clinical Trial...

Toni Kay Mangskau, a social worker and clinical trials referral coordinator at the Mayo Clinic Cancer Center in Rochester, Minnesota. She counsels cancer patients, helps determine their eligibility for clinical studies and provides logistical support for study participants.

About 20% of newly diagnosed adult cancer patients in the US are eligible for clinical trials, studies for which people volunteer to test new drugs or other treatments. Yet only about 3% to 5% actually participate.

Why? Most people assume that clinical studies are an option for only the sickest patients for whom there are no effective treatments. Not true! The only requirement for many studies is having a specific type of cancer or being in a certain age group or other demographic category. Also, many people assume that one group in a study receives a placebo. The fact is that a placebo is not used in the vast majority of studies. In treatment studies, some patients are given the drug/procedure under investigation...others are given the best available standard treatment.

Here's what else you need to know about clinical trials...

WHAT'S AVAILABLE?

At any given time, thousands of clinical trials are under way. The National Cancer Institute website alone lists more than 12,000 trials that are looking for participants. The studies that get the most attention are those that look at break-through cancer treatments, but that's just the tip of the iceberg. Other trials compare single drugs with combination treatments…find new uses for old drugs…study new surgical techniques or radiation treatments, etc.

For some studies, all you have to do is give researchers permission to review your medical records.

Example: Researchers at the Mayo Clinic Cancer Center learned from chart review studies that patients with chronic lymphocytic leukemia responded better to treatments when they had normal blood levels of vitamin D.

RANDOM SELECTION

Typically, a computer will assign a participant to a group in a clinical trial. One group will be given the new drug/treatment. The control group will be given a standard treatment.

If you're randomly assigned to the control group, you'll still get the same treatment that you likely would have gotten if you hadn't joined the study. Those in the "active" group will get something that's expected to be at least as good—and possibly better.

THE RISKS

New drugs/procedures can have side effects or other complications that the researchers didn't anticipate. Should you take the risk?

It's a valid concern, particularly if it's an early-phase study, with a lot of unknowns. But most treatment studies already have a long history. Cancer drugs typically have been studied for at least six years in the laboratory before they make it to clinical trials with humans. It may take another eight years before drugs are approved—or not—by the FDA.

Researchers may not know everything about the drug/treatment, but they know a lot by the time these studies begin. It's always possible that the therapy being researched in the clinical trial is going to be less effective than the standard treatment. But typically study data is reviewed while the study is under way—and a study could be stopped because of side effects or because a treatment is not showing effectiveness.

My advice: If you are considering joining a particular study, ask the researchers how familiar they are with the treatment being researched. Some treatments have been used for other purposes for decades—they're unlikely to bring too many surprises. The diabetes drug metformin, for example, now is being studied as a treatment for breast and ovarian cancers. Doctors are knowledgeable about the drug and the probable side effects.

HOW TO PARTICIPATE

•**Talk to your oncologist.** In one poll, patients reported that 70% of their doctors never mentioned a clinical trial as an option. So ask. Even if your doctor isn't personally involved in a clinical trial, he/she can talk you through the issues—the pros and cons of participating…where to look for studies that involve your type of cancer…and what the studies are likely to involve.

Helpful: For a list of cancer clinical trials, go to *Cancer.gov/clinicaltrials*.

•**Make the decision early.** One of the first things you should ask your oncologist is how quickly you must make a decision about treatment options. Some studies accept only patients who haven't started other treatments.

Important: If you decide to participate in a study, you can change your mind later. Patients can quit a study at any time.

Is it practical? Even if you would like to participate, you may find that it's not a good fit.

Example: A study might require weekly tests at a medical center hundreds of miles away. That's not practical for most people. But other studies may involve monthly visits at a site closer to home. Or there may be times when routine blood work or imaging may be done at your local doctor's office and results sent to the study team.

Study participants typically get more face time with doctors—along with additional checkups, tests, etc.—than patients who don't participate in studies. One study found that 95% of those who participated in one clinical study said that they would consider doing so again.

Too Much Chemo Is Possible

Chemotherapy might hurt more than help end-stage cancer patients. Doctors often prescribe chemo to patients expected to live six months or less to shrink tumors and make them feel better—but side effects such as nausea and vomiting can make them feel worse. And if cancer has progressed despite two or more courses of chemotherapy, the chance that another regimen will work is very small.

Self-defense: Question your doctor on the pros and cons.

Holly G. Prigerson, PhD, is director of the Center for Research on End-of-Life Care, Weill Cornell Medical College, New York City.

• **Check the costs.** Many tests and treatments will be paid for by the study sponsor—but that doesn't mean all of your care is free. In most cases, you (or your insurer) still will be responsible for "routine" care costs—for example, routine blood work or scans. Travel expenses are rarely covered.

Under the Affordable Care Act, some health plans are required to cover the routine costs of study participants. Check with your insurance company, or contact your state's Health Insurance Commission.

THE 4 PHASES OF A STUDY

Before joining a clinical trial, ask about the study phase. This will give you some idea of how much is known about the treatment.

Phase 0 is the earliest stage. Small doses of a drug are tested in just a few people to find out if it reaches the tumor, how it's metabolized, etc. A participant won't benefit from a phase 0 study, but future patients might.

Phase 1 studies are used to determine the highest drug dose that can be given safely and identify possible side effects. Sometimes, these are referred to as "dosing" studies. Researchers also may make sure that the treatment has some benefit, such as slowing tumor growth.

Phase 2 trials involve slightly larger numbers of patients. The goal is to see if the treatment actually works—for example, if it causes a tumor to shrink. If enough patients benefit and side

effects aren't too much of a problem, the drug then may go on to the final stage.

Phase 3 studies look at anywhere from hundreds to thousands of patients. These are the treatment studies that most cancer patients join. If the drug is clearly effective, an application for approval is submitted to the FDA.

Take an Aspirin After Chemo...Live Longer

Study titled "Aspirin in the Treatment of Cancer: Reductions in Metastatic Spread and in Mortality: A Systematic Review and Meta-Analyses of Published Studies" by researchers at Cardiff University, Hywel Dda University Health Board, University of Cambridge, all in the UK, published in *PLOS ONE.*

Aspirin, already known to reduce risk of getting cancer, may soon become part of the regimen for patients who already have cancer.

Researchers at University of Cardiff conducted a meta-analysis of 47 studies—two randomized trials and 42 observational studies—of people with cancers of the breast, bowel and prostate, some of whom took low-dose aspirin in addition to their regular cancer treatment.

Results: For those who had aspirin therapy added at some point to their cancer treatments, their cancers were less likely to spread and, over the five-year period studied, they were 20% less likely to die.

Aspirin has been around for more than 100 years and is one of the most researched medicines in the world. It's easily available, cheap and relatively safe. But it's not risk-free. For one thing, taking aspirin regularly increases the chance for internal bleeding, although the researchers did report that no serious or life-threatening bleeding was reported in the studies that they analyzed.

For someone who is being treated for cancer, the best advice is to discuss with your doctor whether it makes sense to add low-dose aspirin to your treatment plan. Given the strength of the potential benefit, it's an essential conversation.

Anti-Nausea Chemo Drug Gets FDA Nod

Emmanuel Antonarakis, MD, associate professor of oncology, Johns Hopkins Sidney Kimmel Comprehensive Cancer Center, Baltimore.

Chemotherapy can trigger nausea and vomiting that may last for days.

Now: The FDA recently approved *rolapitant* (Varubi), a new drug that suppresses an enzyme needed to metabolize certain cancer drugs. Rolapitant was found to be effective in reducing vomiting and nausea in three different studies involving 2,800 patients taking chemo drugs known for causing sickness. Side effects included hiccups, dizziness and low white blood cell count.

Better Brain Cancer Treatment

Marina N. Nikiforova, MD, director, molecular & genomic pathology laboratory, University of Pittsburgh Medical Center.

In a recent study, a newly developed test called GlioSeq correctly identified all known genetic alterations in 54 adult and pediatric brain tumor samples, allowing physicians to tailor drug treatment for best response and possibly improved survival. The test may be covered by insurance.

Antioxidants Linked to Cancer

Sean Morrison, PhD, director of the Children's Medical Center Research Institute at UT Southwestern in Dallas. He led the team of scientists who conducted a recent study investigating the effect of antioxidants on melanoma cells.

Several studies have strongly suggested that antioxidants might significantly accelerate the spread of cancer among people who have the disease and increase the odds of getting cancer among people in high-risk groups. This might come as a shock to anyone used to reading about the health benefits of antioxidants such as vitamins C and E and beta-carotene. Research has suggested that antioxidants might protect our cells from certain types of damage, slowing the aging process and providing some defense against serious health problems, including heart disease.

Why would antioxidants also promote cancer? The most likely explanation is that they provide the same protection to cancer cells that they do to normal, healthy cells. In fact, cancer cells appear to benefit even more than normal cells. One study of more than 35,000 men over age 50 found that taking large doses of vitamin E increased their risk for prostate cancer by 17%...another study of more than 18,000 former smokers and workers exposed to asbestos found that taking large doses of beta-carotene and retinol (a form of vitamin A) increased their risk for lung cancer by 28%.

Bottom line: I would not take antioxidant supplements if I had been diagnosed with cancer...or was at high risk for cancer, perhaps because of family history or a long-term smoking habit. There is not enough evidence to state whether people who currently are healthy and not in a high-risk group are better or worse off if they take antioxidant supplements regularly. But everyone should continue to consume foods that contain antioxidants, such as berries, nuts and leafy green vegetables.

You Can Use Exercise to Fight Cancer

Study titled "Voluntary Running Suppresses Tumor Growth through Epinephrine- and IL-6-Dependent NK Cell Mobilization and Redistribution" by researchers at University of Copenhagen, Copenhagen University Hospital, et al.

The big news in cancer treatment these days is a new kind of high-tech immunotherapy that unleashes the body's own ability to target and kill tumor cells.

But new research has found that there may be something very similar that goes on in your body—any day you exercise a certain way—that unleashes the body's tumor-fighting response in a way that may both prevent and treat cancer. The research involved mice, but those results often transfer to humans. *Here's what was discovered…*

HOW EXERCISE PROTECTS

In a series of experiments, researchers trained one set of mice to run on treadmills while another group was more sedentary. They then injected the mice with tumor-producing carcinogens.

The exercising mice fought the tumors better. They had fewer tumors, and the tumors that they did develop were smaller and lighter, with fewer growth factors and less metastasis. Compared with couch-potato mice, their tumor burden was reduced by more than 60%.

The how was even more illuminating. Certain kinds of exercise stimulated a specific immunological response that sent the body's natural killer immune cells directly into tumors to destroy them—a kind of "immunological spark" that ignites other cells in the immune system to fight cancer, according to the study's authors.

The key was adrenalin, a "stress" hormone also known as epinephrine. When you exercise vigorously enough to get your heart really pumping, your body sends out more adrenalin—and it's that adrenalin surge, the researchers report, that stimulates natural killer cells to scour and destroy tumors.

Human studies will be needed to pinpoint exactly how intense exercise needs to be to optimize this immune response. But we already know that exercise that raises your heart rate significantly and makes you break a sweat causes the release of much more adrenalin than milder exercise. You don't have to be an Olympic athlete to reach those levels.

Of course, if you're not fit, you'll want to start slowly and safely. But becoming fit has its own separate reward—people who exercise regularly and are more fit tend to produce more adrenalin for the same level of exercise intensity compared to less fit people. In short, training boosts the adrenalin response.

If you're being treated for cancer, it's understandable if you don't have much energy for vigorous exercise. Do what you can, and talk with your doctor about ways to get more exercise. Even moderate exercise like walking has wonderful benefits for people undergoing cancer treatment, from reducing nausea to improving muscle tone to enhancing mood. But if you can work out hard, that adrenalin rush may be adding an immunological boost to your cancer fight, too. And once you've beaten the cancer, regular heart-pumping exercise may help prevent it from ever coming back.

Fish Oil and Chemo Can Clash

Emile Voest, MD, PhD, professor of medical oncology, Netherlands Cancer Institute, Amsterdam.

Fish oil could cause chemo resistance, we hear from Emile Voest, MD, PhD.

Recent research: In animal models, fatty acids in fish oil and fatty fish, such as herring or mackerel, were found to interfere with the metabolism of certain chemotherapy drugs. These resistance-inducing fatty acids are also found in human blood after consumption of fish oil and fatty fish.

If you're on chemotherapy: Ask your doctor if it's safe for you to take a fish oil supplement or eat fatty fish.

CHAPTER 5

Consumer Health Alerts

It's Not Your Imagination: Food Has Less Flavor

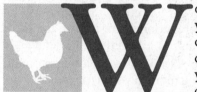

Wondering why you can't re-create the wonderful flavor of your mother's chicken recipe? It isn't your fault—it's the chicken's.

Most meats and vegetables and some fruits have significantly less flavor than they did decades ago. Chicken has become especially bland—it has almost no flavor now.

Agricultural companies and large-scale farms strive to produce as much food as possible as quickly and inexpensively as possible—even if that means sacrificing flavor. That has resulted in big savings for consumers—the typical five-pound supermarket chicken now costs around $7, for example, less than one-quarter of what it would have cost in 1948 after adjusting for inflation—but it also explains why today's food lacks flavor. *Modern chickens are...*

•**Fed inexpensive but bland feed.** Bland feed—typically a blend of seeds—produces bland meat.

•**Butchered very young.** Meat from young animals is less flavorful than meat from mature ones.

•**Bred to be plump, not tasty.** Today's chickens don't even look like the chickens of the past—their breasts are much larger.

The story is similar with other animals and crops. Pigs are 25% younger when slaughtered than they were in 1948, yet also 25% larger...beef cows are 50% younger but produce 60% more meat...hens lay twice as many eggs. All of the food from these animals is bland. Meanwhile, one acre of American farmland produces three times as much rice...four times as much corn... two-and-a-half times as much wheat...and five-and-a-half times as many strawberries.

Mark Schatzker, a food journalist whose work has appeared in *The New York Times* and *The Wall Street Journal*, among other publications. He is author of *The Dorito Effect: The Surprising New Truth About Food and Flavor.* He also is a radio columnist for the Canadian Broadcasting Corporation. MarkSchatzker.com

NOT AS HEALTHY

Eating bland food isn't just less enjoyable, it's also less healthful. There's a reason that nutritious meat, vegetables and fruits taste so good to us—our bodies are sending us the message that these foods contain beneficial vitamins, minerals and other nutrients. Today's foods don't taste as good largely because they contain fewer of these things.

Example: A study published in *Journal of the American College of Nutrition* in 2004 found that an assortment of 43 garden crops—39 vegetables, strawberries and three melons—contained 20% less vitamin A and 15% less vitamin C than the same crops grown in the 1950s.

The declining flavor and nutritional content of meats, vegetables and fruits are likely part of the reason why an increasing percentage of Americans are overweight. We must eat more of these foods to get the same nutritional content…we often cover these bland foods in high-fat and/or high-calorie sauces to give them flavor…and we resort to eating unhealthful processed foods that feature artificial flavors to find the flavor that's now missing from "real foods" such as meats, vegetables and fruits.

FINDING FOOD WITH FLAVOR

It is still possible to find healthful, flavorful foods. *Here's how…*

•**Buy meat from mature animals that ate natural diets.** Seek out grass-fed beef from cattle that lived to at least 22 months of age… pork, ham and bacon from pasture-raised pigs at least six to seven months old…and chicken from pasture-raised birds at least nine but preferably 12 to 18 months old. (If you live in an area where it is too cold to pasture-raise chickens during the winter, confirm that the birds are fed "green feed" during these months.)

The typical supermarket will not offer these meats, but some supermarkets now do. And a quality butcher shop, farmer's market, artisan farm or specialty poultry purveyor on the Internet is likely to (and can give you the ages of the animals).

Tip: The meat described above costs more than the meat typically sold in supermarkets. But I have found that when meat is more flavorful, smaller portions are satisfying. Or try buying relatively inexpensive braising cuts such as beef chuck, flank, brisket or round…and pork butt or shoulder roast. These have lots of flavor and are wonderful for stews, soups and roasts.

Sample savings: $15 per pound if you buy a chuck roast instead of a tenderloin roast.

•**Eat seafood.** Wild-caught seafood still tastes as good as it ever did. Farm-raised seafood might not be quite as flavorful as wild-caught fish, but the flavor dilution tends to be much less dramatic than it is with farm-raised meats. Farm-raised fish tend to consume diets closer to what they would have eaten in the wild.

Exception: Farm-raised tilapia often is fed corn. The result is an extremely bland fish—it's the chicken breast of the sea.

•**Buy produce at farmer's markets—or grow it yourself.** Farmers who sell at farmer's markets often prioritize flavor over crop yields. But sample before buying—just because something is sold at a farmer's market does not guarantee that it will be flavorful.

Tip: Buy green, leafy vegetables that have relatively dark leaves. These have more flavor than lighter-leafed varieties.

•**Or grow your own fruits and vegetables.** Prioritize garden crops that have lots of flavor. Ask other gardeners for tips on the most flavorful varieties, or search the Internet.

Example: A University of Florida program that is developing more flavorful tomato cultivars will send seed packets to anyone who donates $10 (*hos.ufl.edu/kleeweb/newcultivars.html*).

Also, heirloom varieties often feature smaller yields but pack incredible flavor.

If there are no farmer's markets in your area year-round, sample the produce available at high-end markets such as Whole Foods. In some cases, this will be more flavorful than the produce available at mainstream supermarkets. However, do not assume that food will be more flavorful simply because it costs more and is labeled "organic."

When you do purchase produce in supermarkets, favor relatively uncommon varieties. Less attention typically has been paid to increasing the yields of obscure crops than very popular ones, so the flavor might not have been degraded to the same degree.

Example: Arugula typically has much more flavor than iceberg lettuce…scallions have more flavor than the typical onion.

•**Limit your consumption of processed foods.** Regularly eating foods that feature lab-created flavors seems to reprogram the brain to crave these flavors and the often less nutritious foods to which they are added.

The Truth About Eggs: What 7 Tricky Terms Really Mean

Bonnie Taub-Dix, RDN, CDN, a registered dietitian and director and owner of BTD Nutrition Consultants, LLC, in Long Island and New York City. She is author of *Read It Before You Eat It*. Follow her on *Twitter@eat smartbd*. BonnieTaubDix.com

---

Now that research has settled the controversy about eggs—eating them does not affect cholesterol levels significantly in most people, as once believed—you may assume that the case is closed on these popular protein-rich foods.* Not so.

It's true that Americans are buying more and more eggs. The reasons are simple—eggs are inexpensive and can be prepared in minutes. But they're also great sources of key nutrients such as choline, a micronutrient that is vital for brain and liver health…and lutein and zeaxanthin, carotenoids that help prevent cataracts and other eye diseases.

The problem is, shopping for eggs now requires hefty label-decoding skills, thanks to new categories of "designer" eggs and often-confusing terms used to market them.

Before you spend extra money on those "cage-free," "vegetarian" or other specialized eggs, here is what commonly used terms on egg labels really mean…

---

*Most healthy people can eat seven eggs per week (but no more than two a day). Individuals with certain health conditions, such as heart disease or diabetes, should choose egg whites or limit whole-egg consumption to four times a week due to the cholesterol in egg yolks.

•**Brown.** Surprise! There is no reason to choose brown eggs over white, unless you find the hue more appealing. The shell color is usually a reflection of the feather color of the chicken—brown eggs come from chickens with brown feathers, and white eggs come from chickens with white feathers. Impact on nutrition? None. More humane? No.

•**Cage-free or free-range.** These eggs come from hens that are not confined to cages, but thousands of them may be crowded into a barn or warehouse. Free-range hens have access to the outdoors. However, there is no independent auditing of these practices unless the eggs are also certified organic (see next page). Impact on nutrition? None. More humane? Mildly.

•**Certified Humane.** If a carton bears an official-looking seal such as "Certified Humane," "Animal Welfare Approved" or "Food Alliance Certified," it means that the manufacturer's claim of "cage-free," "free-range" or "pasture-raised" has been verified by an independent third party. This labeling has everything to do with humane treatment and nothing to do with nutritional content.

There are multiple third-party certifiers, and each one has its own requirements—for example, a Certified Humane free-range hen has six hours of daily outdoor access and at least two square feet of outdoor space, while an American Humane Certified free-range hen gets 21.8 square feet of outdoor space but no minimum outdoor time. For a list of trustworthy certifiers, go to GreenerChoices.org/eco-labels, a website sponsored by *Consumer Reports*, and search "egg certifiers." Impact on nutrition? None. More humane? Yes—to varying degrees, depending on the certifier.

•**Omega-3–enriched.** These eggs come from hens that are fed a diet rich in algae, flaxseed, chia seeds and/or fish oil—all good sources of healthful omega-3s.

How does this diet affect the eggs? A conventional egg contains 37 mg of omega-3s…an omega-3–enriched egg has about 225 mg. To put those amounts in perspective, the American Heart Association recommends at least two 3.5-ounce servings of fatty fish per week for heart health, which is a total of about 3,500 mg of omega-3s.

Vegetarians who avoid fish may want to try omega-3–enriched eggs. Look for hens fed vegetarian diets (see below). They are also a good choice for people with fish allergies. However, if you eat fatty fish several times a week and/or take a daily omega-3 supplement, you might as well skip omega-3–enriched eggs and save yourself some money. Impact on nutrition? Yes. More humane? No.

•**Organic.** This label means that the USDA has certified that these eggs come from hens raised on feed that is free of pesticides, commercial fertilizers and animal by-products. Organic also means that the hens weren't given antibiotics and are cage-free with some amount of access to the outdoors. Eggs from hens treated with antibiotics cannot be labeled antibiotic-free even though the eggs do not contain antibiotic residue. Hormones are generally not used in any form of egg production.

If you're concerned about pesticides and fertilizers in your food, you might want to buy organic. But no research indicates that organic eggs are more healthful than conventional eggs.

The Cornucopia Institute, a nonprofit group that conducts research on sustainable and organic agriculture, has an organic egg scorecard that rates individual organic brands based on the amount of outdoor access and indoor space their birds receive, farming practices and other criteria. The scorecard is available at *Cornuco pia.org/organic-egg-scorecard*. Impact on nutrition? Possibly. More humane? Mildly.

•**Pastured/pasture-raised.** If you don't mind paying extra (about twice as much), these eggs could be the ideal choice for anyone seeking both enhanced nutrition and humane treatment. Pastured hens move about freely outdoors, have an organic diet and are allowed to eat grass, worms and bugs, all of which produce a deeper-colored yolk, creamier texture and richer flavor.

A study published in the journal *Renewable Agriculture and Food Systems* found that eggs produced by pasture-raised hens contained more than double the omega-3s and twice as much vitamin E as conventionally raised eggs. Impact on nutrition? Yes. More humane? Yes.

•**Vegetarian.** Eggs are considered vegetarian if the feed a chicken consumes doesn't contain animal by-products. But chickens are omnivores by nature, not vegetarians—wild chickens eat bugs and worms. If your eggs are labeled vegetarian and free-range, they might not be real "vegetarian" eggs, as roaming hens probably eat a bug or two. There is no nutritional difference between vegetarian and nonvegetarian eggs. Impact on nutrition? None. More humane? No.

Know Your GMO

The American Association for the Advancement of Science, *Environmental Sciences Europe*, *TIME* and other media.

I t's time for American consumers to know if the foods they are buying have GMO ingredients.

We're not saying that GMO foods are unsafe. So far, there hasn't been credible evidence that they pose health threats. But even scientists disagree about whether we really know enough yet to be sure. Some think the issue is settled and there's no health risk at all, while others argue that there's still no scientific consensus.

For many people, the issues go beyond health. To some, GMO food technology can help feed a world where many people might otherwise go hungry. To others, GMO food locks us more deeply into a farming system hooked on herbicides and pesticides and extends the control of mega-corporations over the food supply.

It's clear that Americans want to know what's in our foods—93% of Americans polled favor GMO labeling. As NYU nutrition professor and *Bottom Line* expert Marion Nestle, PhD, has written: "Labels, the FDA said, could mislead the public into thinking genetically modified foods differed from conventional foods. But GMOs can be considered different—DNA transfers sometimes come from completely different organisms—and the public wants that information."

Many of you are voting with your dollars— the supermarket chain Whole Foods has committed to GMO transparency and the restaurant chain Chipotle is banning GMO products from its menu. Meanwhile, the US Congress is debating federal transparency standards.

If you want to avoid GMO foods, the best bet right now is to buy organic foods, which by law cannot contain GMO ingredients. You can also search for non-GMO brands through the Non-GMO Project.

The Salmon Hoax

Karen Larson, editor of *Bottom Line/Personal*.

The Food and Drug Administration recently ruled that genetically engineered salmon can be sold in the US without any labels noting that its DNA has been altered. There is indeed strong scientific consensus that genetically modified foods are safe to consume. But safe or not, I believe I have a right to know what I'm eating. Label food for what it is, and let me decide for myself.

Thus I'm planning to buy my salmon at retailers such as Kroger, Safeway, Target, Trader Joe's and Whole Foods, which have announced that they will not stock the genetically modified fish.

But genetic modification isn't the only challenge for those of us who want to know what seafood we're consuming. When the nonprofit organization Oceana did DNA testing on the salmon sold in the US, it discovered that 43% of it wasn't what the seller claimed. Farmed Atlantic salmon often was sold as wild Pacific salmon. Oceana has found that other seafood has fishy labeling, too.

Here, advice from Oceana's Dr. Kimberly Warner...

•**Buy fish in supermarkets.** Oceana discovered that mislabeling is much less common in supermarkets—less than 20%—than in small markets, restaurants and especially sushi venues.

•**Eat fresh regional fish during its fishing season.** Misidentification is most common out of season, so lean toward buying regional seafood when you know it is in season.

Examples: Chesapeake blue crab is in season from April to December...Alaska wild salmon, in late spring through the fall.

•**Purchase whole fish when feasible.** Merchants are less likely to pass off one species as another when consumers can see the entire fish.

Five Food Health Myths the Industry Peddles... and That Consumers Believe

Andy Bellatti, MS, RD, is a Las Vegas–based nutritionist with a plant-centric and whole-food focus who takes an interest in food politics, deceptive food marketing, sustainability and social justice.

Coca-Cola recently came under fire for secretly funding the "Global Energy Balance Network," which blames society's growing weight problem primarily on our lack of exercise—rather than our food choices such as...soda. New York University nutrition professor Marion Nestle, PhD, neatly summed up the issue in a column entitled "Coca-Cola Says Its Drinks Don't Cause Obesity. Science Says Otherwise." *The New York Times* exposed Coke's cynical campaign of lies based on a tip from obesity doctor and blogger Yoni Freedhoff, MD and also ran a cartoon sarcastically featuring "The Sugar Water Workout."

That got us thinking—what other health myths stoked by the food industry are people swallowing? We spoke with registered dietitian Andy Bellatti, who works within his profession to minimize the negative effects of Big Food influence. Says Bellatti, "Every day I have to re-educate clients based on inaccuracies that have been set by the food industry."

Here are the myths—and the truth...

MYTH #1: Exercise is more important than diet when it comes to weight.

The truth: We could dub this one the "Coca-Cola myth" (see above). While sedentary lifestyles may play a role, the body of scientific research shows that poor dietary choices are far more to blame for the obesity epidemic. The contrast is even clearer when it comes to losing weight. After all, it takes three miles of walking to burn off the 140 calories in just one 12-ounce can of Coke. Exercise is essential for a healthy life, of course, but if you want to lose weight, start with what you eat and drink...especially sugar-laden beverages. As the saying goes, "You can't outrun a bad diet."

MYTH #2: Single nutrients make a food healthy.

The truth: Just because the package says a food is a "good source of [FILL IN THE BLANK NUTRIENT]!" doesn't mean it's actually a nutritious choice. Food companies use single nutrients to trump up the value of their unhealthy offerings. For example, "Most cereals are just whole-grain, low-fat cookies," says Bellati. That is, they are highly processed and stripped of many nutrients (that are later fortified back in), sugary and devoid of healthful fats. Even when they add in a little extra protein (or whatever) and tout it, they're just hoping we overlook all that added sugar.

Another "disaster" food Belatti recently spotted at a grocery store—a prepacked lunch containing a candy bar, a sugar-sweetened drink and corn chips with cheese dip. It was labeled as a good source of calcium! "It's a perfect example of the food industry's smoke and mirrors," Bellatti says. Look at the whole nutritional story when making choices.

MYTH #3: Taking out well-known "bad" ingredients makes a food "good" for you.

The truth: This is another Big Food sleight of hand trick.

Example: Foods that don't contain added white sugar but instead are "naturally sweetened" with honey, agave or maple syrup. "The term 'natural' on food labels is absolutely meaningless," Bellatti says. "From a caloric standpoint and from a health standpoint, sugar is sugar." Ditto for unhealthy foods with "good-for-you" attributes—a gluten-free donut is still, after all...a donut. The latest food industry bait-and-switch is removing artificial colorings and then crowing about it. It's a good step, to be sure. But beware of attempts to make these foods have a "health halo" that gives you permission to eat

more of them. No matter what is not in your food, what really matters is what is in it...and a donut is never going to be a peach.

MYTH #4: Low-fat or fat-free makes a food healthy.

The truth: Foods that are low in fat may claim that they're good for your heart for that reason, but that's not necessarily true. Fat is not the enemy of the heart—different fats have different effects on heart health. "There are lots of foods that are high in fat, such as nuts, seeds, avocado, cold-pressed extra-virgin olive oil and sardines, that are very heart healthy," Bellatti notes. Plus, we like fat because it makes food taste good, so when manufacturers cut fat from desserts, they typically add in more sugar to make them taste better. Meanwhile, there's growing evidence that diets that are high in added sugar are detrimental to heart health. Those low-fat cookies should be looking a lot less appealing to you now.

MYTH #5: It's fine to eat junk as long as you don't take in too many calories.

The truth: Quality matters, not just quantity. The food industry promotes the idea that as long as we're eating the right amount of daily calories, we're fine. But the number of calories we take in is not the only component of dietary health—the

Recent Food Guidelines Watered Down By Meat Industry

The industry, a powerful lobby, fights restrictions focused on reducing red-meat consumption. However, the health effects of meat are significant—eating more than one hot dog a week can reduce life expectancy by 25% to 35% over a 10-year period. Consume no more than a single hot dog or one bologna or salami sandwich per week—preferably less. For red meat that is not processed, eat a maximum of about two ounces a day.

Barry M. Popkin, PhD, is the W. R. Kenan, Jr. Distinguished Professor of Nutrition and an adjunct professor of economics at University of North Carolina, Chapel Hill.

quality of those calories is critical, too. "There's a huge difference between snacking on a Three Musketeers bar and eating the same amount of calories in almonds," Bellatti says. The candy bar will spike your blood sugar while providing almost no nutrients, but the almonds will give you protein, fiber, healthy fats, vitamin E, magnesium and much more. If weight is your concern, he adds, the more nutrient-dense choice is better for you even if it contains a bit more calories—especially if it has significant amounts of fiber and protein, which will help keep you fuller longer. It's also wise to remember that weight isn't the only marker of health. "You can lose weight but still be wrecking your arteries and having blood sugars fluctuate like crazy," Bellatti says. "The composition and quality of calories is very important for health, and the food industry tends to downplay that."

Don't Fall for These Myths About Meat Safety

Michael Doyle, PhD, food microbiologist, Regents Professor of Food Microbiology, director, Center for Food Safety, College of Agricultural and Environmental Sciences, The University of Georgia, Griffin. He has served as an adviser to the United Nation's World Health Organization.

You know that eating a rare hamburger can mean taking your life in your hands because of E. coli.

You're smart enough to cut raw chicken away from other foods because of Salmonella.

But when it comes to meat and food safety, are you still swallowing the following dangerous myths?

MYTH #1: Organic grass-fed beef has fewer bad bacteria.

Last year, a consumer organization released a report claiming that sustainably produced beef is safer than conventionally produced beef. The researchers found that conventional beef had higher levels of bacteria overall, as well as bacteria that were resistant to antibiotics. They recommended that consumers buy sustainably raised beef—from cattle that was raised, at a

minimum, without antibiotics and, ideally, by organic and grass-fed methods. The trouble with this report, however, is that the types of bacteria found most often during this testing process rarely cause foodborne illness. Of the bacteria types of greatest public concern, E. coli O157:H7 and Salmonella, only one of 300 beef samples had Salmonella and no E. coli O157:H7 were detected. There are good reasons to buy sustainably raised beef—nutritional, environmental and ethical—but avoiding foodborne illness is not one of them.

Bottom Line: In terms of foodborne illness, sustainably raised beef is no safer than conventionally raised beef.

MYTH #2: Halal beef is safer than other beef.

Halal is an Arabic word that means "permissible," and it's used to describe how animals should be raised and a process of slaughtering animals designed to minimize their pain. This makes the meat acceptable for devout Muslims to consume. Traditionally, the animal being slaughtered must be healthy, the animal must be facing Mecca at the time of slaughter, a very sharp knife must be used and the name of God must be said before slaughter. Today, in the US, most halal meat is produced in commercial slaughterhouses staffed with trained Muslim workers along with government inspectors. So while there is an extra layer of supervision, the focus is on spiritual purity and not science-based safety. Halal certification does not guarantee that the food is free from harmful pathogens.

Bottom Line: Halal meat is no safer than conventionally produced meat.

MYTH #3: Kosher chicken is safer than other chicken.

Like Halal meat, kosher meat is raised, slaughtered and prepared according to religious guidelines, in this case so that it's acceptable for consumption by devout Jews. One part of this process—salting the meat to draw out and remove any blood—has led some people to think this makes the meat safer because salting may help weaken harmful bacteria. But there is no scientific proof that it does. In addition, another kosher rule prohibits immersing the meat in scalding water, which can kill bacteria and is a common practice in the chicken industry. In fact, one study of more than 200 samples of raw kosher chicken purchased at 15 locations conducted at Northern Arizona University found that it harbored up to twice as much antibiotic-resistant E. coli as conventional poultry. While these E. coli bacteria were not E. coli O157:H7, because they are antibiotic-resistant they are still a public health concern. An Israeli study found that because kosher poultry is not scalded, the chickens have to remain longer in defeathering machines, which increases the risk for contamination with Listeria, one of the top five causes of death from foodborne illness, according to the CDC.

Bottom Line: Kosher meat is possibly less safe than conventionally produced meat.

THE FARMERS MARKET DELUSION

Now that we've burst your balloons about sustainable and religion-sanctioned meat, here's another bubble—farmers markets. The fast growth of farmers markets has been a boon to health-conscious people seeking in-season, locally grown and often organic food. It's important to support local agriculture. But these foods aren't necessarily safer. They're not always regulated, and the way food is handled and stored—from produce to meats to homemade dairy products and cider—varies greatly. Indeed, researchers at the University of Minnesota have found a statistically significant relationship between the presence of farmers markets in a community and a higher number of foodborne illness outbreaks. That's far from conclusive, to be sure. But it's also possible that there's an even stronger relationship because it's likely that these local outbreaks are small and go unreported—say a family gets sick after eating farm market products and chalks it up to a stomach bug—and the data are never recorded.

By all means, buy your meat—and produce—from farmers markets. Opt for grass-fed organic beef, not to mention organic chicken, if you can afford it, for the environmental and ethical benefits. Buy halal or kosher beef and chicken if you prefer their methods. Just don't labor under the impression that these virtuous buying habits will protect you from foodborne illness.

For that, you still need to follow the rules—wash your hands, cutting board and utensils after handling raw meat or poultry, and make sure it is fully cooked. The USDA recommends that steak be cooked to an internal temperature of 145°F, hamburger to 160°F and chicken to 165°F.

---

6 Things This Food-Safety Expert Won't Eat... and One Surprising Food He Will

Bill Marler, managing partner, Marler Clark, Seattle. Mr. Marler is a prominent foodborne-illness lawyer and a major force in food policy in the US and around the world. For the last 20 years, he has represented victims of nearly every large foodborne illness outbreak in the US. MarlerClark.com

---

Bill Marler is the most prominent food-safety lawyer in the US. He has represented victims in nearly every food-borne illness outbreak in the US in the last 20 years, including the recent ones at Costco and Chipotle. He knows just how scary these illnesses are. Shockingly, every year, foodborne bugs sicken 48 million Americans—sending 128,000 to the hospital and 3,000 to an early grave.

So we asked him if there are any foods that he never eats. He named six.

Then we asked him if there's a food that people avoid that is safe to eat. He named one that really surprised us.

6 FOODS BILL MARLER NEVER EATS

1. Unpasteurized ("raw") milk and packaged juices. Unpasteurized milk, sometimes called "raw" milk, can be contaminated with bacteria, viruses and parasites. Between 1998 and 2011, there were 148 food poisoning outbreaks linked to raw milk and raw milk products in the US—and keep in mind that comparatively few people in the country ever consume these products, so 148 outbreaks is nothing to ignore. As for unpasteurized packaged juices, one of Marler's earliest cases was the 1996 E. coli outbreak from unpasteurized Odwalla apple juice. As a result, he won't go near raw milk or juice. "There's no benefit big enough to take away the risk of drinking products that can be made safe by pasteurization," he says.

2. Raw sprouts. Uncooked and lightly cooked sprouts have been linked to more than 30 bacterial outbreaks (mostly of salmonella and E. coli) in the US since mid-1990s. As recently as 2014, salmonella from bean sprouts sent 19 people to the hospital. All types of sprouts—including alfalfa, mung bean, clover and radish sprouts—can spread infection, which is caused by bacterial contamination of their seeds. "There have been too many outbreaks to not pay attention to the risk of sprout contamination," Marler says. "Those are products that I just don't eat at all." He did add that he does eat them if they're cooked.

3. Meat that isn't well-done. Marler orders his burgers well-done. "The reason ground products are more problematic and need to be cooked more thoroughly is that any bacteria that's on the surface of the meat can be ground inside of it," Marler says. "If it's not cooked thoroughly to 160°F throughout, it can cause poisoning by E. coli and salmonella and other bacterial illnesses." As for steaks, needle tenderizing—a common restaurant practice in which the steak is pierced with needles or sliced with knives to break down the muscle fibers and make it more tender—can also transfer bugs from the surface to the interior of the meat. If a restaurant does this (Marler asks), he orders his steak well-done. If the restaurant doesn't, he'll opt for medium-well.

4. Prewashed or precut fruits and vegetables. "I avoid these like the plague," Marler says. Why? The more a food is handled and processed, the more likely it is to become tainted. "We've gotten so used to the convenience of mass-produced food—bagged salad and boxed salads and precut this and precut that," Marler says. "Convenience is great but sometimes I think it isn't worth the risk." He buys unwashed, uncut produce in small amounts and eats it within three to four days to reduce the risk for listeria, a deadly bug that grows at refrigerator temps.

5. Raw or undercooked eggs. You may remember the salmonella epidemic of the 1980s and early '90s that was linked mainly to eggs. If you swore off raw eggs back then, you might as well stick with it. The most recent salmonella outbreak from eggs, in 2010, caused roughly 2,000 reported cases of illness. "I think the risk of egg contamination is much lower today than it was 20 years ago for salmonella, but I still eat my eggs well-cooked," Marler says.

6. Raw oysters and other raw shellfish. Marler says that raw shellfish—especially oysters—have been causing more foodborne illness lately. He links this to warming waters, which produce more microbial growth. "Oysters are filter feeders, so they pick up everything that's in the water," he explains. "If there's bacteria in the water it'll get into their system, and if you eat it you could have trouble. I've seen a lot more of that over the last five years than I saw in the last 20 years. It's simply not worth the risk."

HERE'S ONE "DANGEROUS" FOOD YOU DON'T HAVE TO AVOID

It's sushi. You might be surprised that with all of his precautions, Marler is willing to dabble in raw fish. He says there have been only a handful of disease outbreaks caused by sushi, which is generally handled very carefully from the source to the sushi chef.

That doesn't mean he'll eat it from any purveyor, though—he won't touch the stuff sold at the grocery store or convenience store. "If you're going to eat sushi, spend the money and eat at a good sushi restaurant."

Many Food Cans Still Contain BPA

Study of 252 brands made by 119 companies between January and August 2014 by researchers at Environmental Working Group, an advocacy organization in Washington, DC.

The chemical bisphenol A often is used to line the inside of metal food cans to prevent food from touching the metal. It has been linked to health problems that affect the brain and the nervous system. While used less often than in the past, BPA still appears in about one-third of cans studied. Manufacturers are not required to identify cans with or without BPA. Among brands found to be BPA-free are Amy's, Earth's Best Organic, Health Valley, Seneca, Sprouts Farmers Market and Tyson. For more information on brands using BPA and those that are BPA-free, go to *EWG.org/research/bpa canned food.*

Arsenic Levels in Wine

Denise Wilson, PhD, is professor in the department of electrical engineering at University of Washington, Seattle, and leader of a study published in *Journal of Environmental Health.*

Arsenic levels in wine can be high. In a recent study, all but one of the domestic wines tested had arsenic levels higher than what is allowed in drinking water. This is not dangerous in itself, but a diet that includes significant amounts of wine plus foods that are also high in arsenic, such as apple juice, rice and rice syrup—or private well water—can be harmful. To prevent high consumption of arsenic, moderate-to-heavy wine drinkers should not rely on wine from a single region and should limit foods high in arsenic.

Lead: The Dangers No One Is Talking About

Hyla Cass, MD, a psychiatrist and integrative medicine practitioner located in Southern California. Dr. Cass is also the author of numerous articles and books, most recently *The Addicted Brain and How to Break Free.* CassMD.com

It started with Flint, Michigan, where outraged parents complained of toxic concentrations of lead in their drinking water. But anyone who reads newspapers, watches TV or goes online knows that lead continues to be a national problem.

Be Wary of Receipts

Be wary of handling receipts from cash registers, ATM machines and gas pumps, especially if your hands are wet from using hand sanitizer. These receipts typically are made of thermal paper—smooth paper coated with heat-activated printing developers, such as BPA. BPA is linked to obesity, type 2 diabetes, hypertension, heart attack, uterine disorders, sexual dysfunction and other conditions. Hands wet from hand sanitizer can absorb up to 100 times as much BPA as dry hands.

Frederick S. vom Saal, PhD, is curators' professor in the division of biological sciences, University of Missouri-Columbia.

A hidden danger: While attention has largely focused on the potential harms to children (including lasting damage to their developing brains and lowered IQs), adults are not immune to lead toxicity. *Here's how to protect yourself—and your family…*

HOW DAMAGE OCCURS

Lead poisons mitochondria (energy-producing structures within each cell), potentially harming your body in several ways. It blocks the production of glutathione, a naturally occurring antioxidant that keeps free radicals (implicated in a host of age-related chronic diseases) in check. The metal also interferes with the production of nitric oxide, a natural vasodilator that keeps blood flowing normally and blood pressure at proper levels.

As with children, high lead levels in adults can impair brain function, leading to memory problems, depression, anxiety, irritability and trouble concentrating. Headaches, insomnia and poor coordination are frequent, as are digestive difficulties such as constipation. Reduced sex drive in adults also can result.

When elevated lead levels persist over a period of years, high blood pressure can develop. Deaths due to cardiovascular disease become 50% more common as blood levels of lead rise, according to research published in the journal *Circulation.*

Even more concerning: The increased heart and stroke risks in this research occurred with blood lead concentrations of 2 micrograms per deciliter (mcg/dL)—less than half the level considered harmful by the CDC and EPA. Lead reaches or exceeds this level in almost 40% of American adults, according to data from the National Health and Nutrition Examination Survey.

SHOULD YOU BE TESTED?

Given the prevalence of lead toxicity, you might consider testing if you have one or more of the symptoms mentioned earlier. Age is a factor, too. As bones thin and break down with age, they release lead that may have been stored for decades in the skeleton.

Blood testing is simple and relatively inexpensive but won't tell the whole story—blood lead levels indicate exposures to the metal only during the past 35 days…and a low reading may mask high levels of lead stored in the bones.

Best test for lead: A "provocation test" in which you are given a dose of prescription medication to help release lead from tissues and bones. Then your body's lead level can be determined by checking for it in the urine collected in the next few hours.

No matter which test you use, the result can best be interpreted by an integrative medicine doctor, a doctor of osteopathy or a naturopathic doctor—all of whom are typically knowledgeable about lead toxicity. To find one near you, consult the American College for Advancement in Medicine…the American Academy of Environmental Medicine…or The Institute for Functional Medicine.

Many integrative practitioners are well versed in treatments, such as chelation therapy. This involves a series of IV injections of a chemical that binds to molecules of lead and other heavy metals for excretion in the urine. Since the body stores are generally so high, the course will likely need repeating as lead continues to be released. The treatment is generally not covered by insurance and costs about $75 to $125 per session.

Certain supplements can also be used to help fight lead toxicity, most of which boost glutathione, the body's master antioxidant. These include vitamin C, N-acetyl cysteine (NAC), quercetin, alpha-lipoic acid and cilantro. Discuss such therapy with your physicians first.

HOW TO PROTECT YOURSELF

Whether or not you already have elevated levels of lead in your body, we're all at risk and should try to limit exposure. *My advice…*

•**Test your water.** This is crucial if you live in a home built before 1986—but lead may also be found in newer homes. Until two years ago, the legal limit for "lead-free" pipes was up to 8% lead. If any questions have been raised about your municipal water supply, get an analysis from your water district. For your own home's supply, online kits are available or call a professional. The EPA supplies a list of certified labs in your area at *EPA.gov/dwlabcert.*

If there's any appreciable amount of lead (or other contaminants such as PCBs) in your water, get a kitchen filter (carbon or reverse osmosis) to remove them. You may also want to consider a whole-house filtration system. (For more information on lead pipes and testing water, see the following article "Rid Your Water of Lead.")

•**Limit lead dust.** If your home was built before 1978 (when lead paint was banned), have all air ducts thoroughly cleaned to remove lead dust. When stripping paint, use a respirator and protective clothing and scrupulously remove paint chips.

Best option: Hire a professional who is EPA-certified in lead paint removal.

To find such a professional, go to: EPA.gov/lead.

Lead can also be found in the soil, particularly if you live anywhere near a highway or busy street—particles may have settled there from the exhaust of cars using leaded gasoline, which was banned years ago. To avoid tracking lead-containing particulates into your home, remove your shoes before entering. Also test your soil before planting a vegetable garden.

•**Avoid lead-containing products.** Ceramic dishes and cookware should be made with lead-free glazes. Most US-manufactured items are safe, but there may be lead in imported products. When buying such items, you can check them by using the First Alert lead-testing kit that identifies the presence (not the amount) of lead

Watch Out for These Dangers to Your Teeth

Little-known dangers to teeth: Chlorine from swimming pool water can cause dental abrasion—so swim in saltwater whenever possible. Acidic beverages such as lemonade and sports drinks can weaken tooth enamel, so drink water instead—or at least have a glass of water after consuming one of these acidic drinks. White wine is more acidic than red wine and can erode tooth enamel, so drink water or eat bread between sips of wine. Berry juices and smoothies can discolor teeth—drink them with a straw to help liquid pass to the back of your mouth, avoiding your teeth.

EveryDayHealth.com.

on dishes, toys and other household items. It is available online and at home-improvement stores for about $17.

To confirm that lipstick and other cosmetics are free from lead and other toxins, consult the Environmental Working Group's database.

•**Watch your supplements.** Especially with herbs, which can be contaminated with lead, buy only from highly reputable manufacturers that can certify their purity. Look for brands that have been certified by NSF International or The US Pharmacopeia (USP).

Rid Your Water of Lead

Robert D. Morris, MD, PhD, an environmental epidemiologist based in Seattle and former professor at Tufts University School of Medicine, Boston. He is author of *The Blue Death*. EHTrust.org

If you are uncertain whether your home is connected to the water main by a lead pipe, check the home inspector's report conducted when you bought the property—if there's a lead pipe, this should be noted. Or find where your water supply enters your home—if this pipe is dull gray and can be easily scratched

with a sharp knife, it's probably lead. Or have a licensed plumber check for you ($45 to $150).

What to do: Install a water filter on your kitchen faucet or below your sink. Expect to pay $200 to $400 for an under-sink unit, plus a few hundred more to have it professionally installed. Faucet-mounted filters cost less than $100 and are easy to install but tend to slow water flow and don't fit every faucet. If you do not have a filter, run your tap for one to two minutes in the morning before using it (lead leaches into water as it sits in the pipes), and do not drink hot water from the tap (hot water absorbs more lead).

Not all water filters remove lead, so check the packaging or the manufacturer's website. Or use the independent-testing company NSF's online search tool to find lead-reduction filters (Info.NSF.org/certified/dwtu).

Surprising Dangers of Air Pollution

Neil Schachter, MD, medical director of the respiratory care department at Mount Sinai Hospital and the Maurice Hexter Professor of Pulmonary Medicine at the Icahn School of Medicine at Mount Sinai, both in New York City. He is the author of *The Good Doctor's Guide to Colds and Flu* and serves on the American Lung Association's Northeast Board of Directors.

More than 40% of Americans—nearly 140 million of us—breathe unhealthy air, according to a recent report by the American Lung Association.

Even when the sky appears crystal clear, you're inhaling exhaust fumes, ground-level ozone and microscopic particles—common pollutants that can increase your risk for health problems ranging from heart disease to asthma.

Small-town living helps but not completely. Even in the wide-open spaces of the American West, drought and high summer temperatures increase levels of dust and other airborne particles that can worsen conditions such as asthma and chronic obstructive pulmonary disease (COPD).

THE BIGGEST DANGERS

You would expect bad air to threaten lung health, but there's increasing evidence showing that the risk is far more pervasive. *Examples…*

•**Heart disease.** Air pollution is ranked ninth among the most important cardiovascular risk factors—making it more harmful than lack of exercise or elevated cholesterol, according to a report in the *European Heart Journal.*

What makes air pollution so hard on the heart? Airborne particles trigger inflammation in the lungs and blood vessels that can increase atherosclerosis and the risk for clots. Even brief exposures to PM2.5—common airborne particles that are about one-fifth the size of a speck of dust—may increase cardiovascular risks. You are likely inhaling these particles if you drive to work with your car windows open, walk past a construction site or light a fire in your fireplace. In areas where particle concentrations are persistently high, such as near busy roads, there's an 11% average increased risk of dying from heart attack, heart failure or stroke.

•**Stroke.** Even if you live in a rural, "wholesome" area, you will occasionally breathe high levels of carbon monoxide and other gaseous pollutants—when you're behind a truck, for example. Such limited exposures may seem harmless, but an analysis of more than 100 studies found that intermittent spikes in air pollution caused a corresponding increase in hospitalizations and deaths from stroke.

•**Heart-rate changes.** The varying intervals between heartbeats, known as heart-rate variability, are a sign of cardiovascular health. Bad air—even inside the home—can have a harmful effect. People who frequently use air fresheners are more likely to have reduced heart-rate variability, research has found. Many air fresheners contain terpenes, chemicals that can smell like pine or citrus. They interact with other chemicals in the air and form heart-damaging compounds.

WHAT CAN YOU DO?

To help protect your health…

•**Track the Air Quality Index (AQI).** The AQI is a rating based on daily levels of major pollutants—carbon monoxide, sulfur dioxide, particle pollution, etc. When the number rises above 100, it's wise to avoid outdoor activities—particularly if you have already been diagnosed with lung or heart disease or diabetes. For an up-to-date AQI, go to AirNow.gov.

•**Exercise away from major roads.** Levels of PM2.5 particles tend to be much higher in areas with heavy traffic. If you like to walk, jog or bike, do it as close to nature as possible—and away from busy streets. Pollution is usually highest within 50 feet of roads.

Also helpful: Avoid rush-hour traffic if you can…and drive with the windows closed (see below).

•**Use the AC.** It is nice to conserve power (and save money), but don't skimp on air-conditioning. It filters incoming air and traps large particles. In fact, a study in Taiwan found that people who used home air conditioners showed none of the "cardiovascular endpoints"—such as inflammation and heart rhythm disturbances—that were apparent when they kept windows open.

In the car: Be sure to use the "recirculate" setting. Research has found that recirculating air will keep out 80% of outside air pollution.

•**Filter the air.** Dust is a major irritant for people with asthma, COPD or other lung diseases, as well as for those with cardiovascular disease. And even if it's cleaned often, the average home has a lot of dust.

My advice: If you have any of the health issues mentioned above, invest in a HEPA air purifier for any room you spend a lot of time in. Many brands are available—most of which will remove up to 99% of suspended particles in a given room. They work more effectively than electrostatic air purifiers, and they don't produce the ozone (another lung irritant) that can result from electrostatic units. HEPA filtration is also available in central ventilation systems.

Also: To keep indoor air cleaner, install solid floors (such as wood or tile)—not wall-to-wall carpet…and avoid floor-to-ceiling curtains.

•**Use natural scents.** Commercial air fresheners may smell nice, but they all contain chemical compounds. Why take chances? Natural scents smell better—and cost less.

Examples: Spritz rosewater in the air…or simmer lemon or orange peels on the stove.

89

Organic Milk and Meat Have Higher Nutrient Levels

Carlo Leifert, PhD, research development professor for ecological agriculture, Newcastle University, UK. Newcastle University, news release.

New international research has good news for people who've been shelling out extra money to buy organic milk and meat—these products are healthier than conventional products in a number of ways.

"People choose organic milk and meat for three main reasons: improved animal welfare, the positive impacts of organic farming on the environment, and the perceived health benefits. But much less is known about impacts on nutritional quality, hence the need for this study," team leader Carlo Leifert, PhD, research development professor for ecological agriculture at Newcastle University in the United Kingdom.

"Several of these differences stem from organic livestock production and are brought about by differences in production intensity, with outdoor-reared, grass-fed animals producing milk and meat that is consistently higher in desirable fatty acids such as the omega-3s, and lower in fatty acids that can promote heart disease and other chronic diseases," he explained.

The researchers reviewed studies from around the world. The analysis included 196 studies on milk and 67 on meat. The investigators discovered that organic products provide higher levels of beneficial fatty acids, certain essential minerals and antioxidants.

For example, compared with conventional products, both organic milk and meat offer about 50% more healthy omega-3 fatty acids, the study found. Organic milk also provides 40% more conjugated linoleic acid. Organic milk also has slightly higher concentrations of iron, vitamin E and some carotenoids, the research revealed.

However, conventional milk has 74% more of the essential mineral iodine and slightly more selenium, the study authors pointed out.

Organic meat has slightly lower levels of two saturated fats that are associated with an increased risk of heart disease, the study found.

The results of the review suggest that switching to organic milk and meat would help increase people's intake of nutritionally important fatty acids, the researchers said.

The study was published in the *British Journal of Nutrition*.

The European Commission, the executive body of the European Union, and the Sheepdrove Trust, a British charity that supports organic farming research, paid for the analysis.

Don't Let Medical Bills Ruin You

Charles B. Inlander is a consumer advocate and health-care consultant based in Fogelsville, Pennsylvania. He was the founding president of the nonprofit People's Medical Society, a consumer advocacy organization credited with key improvements in the quality of US health care, and is the author or coauthor of more than 20 consumer-health books.

Even if you are fully insured, with either private insurance, Medicare and/or Medicaid, the cost of premiums, deductibles, co-payments and noncovered services could put your financial well-being at great risk…even leading to bankruptcy. In most cases, however, there are ways to get the health care you need—without going broke. *Here's how…**

•**Federally provided low-cost or free health care.** Let's say you need a checkup, dental care or a pricey prescription drug at little or no cost. You can get these services through a national network of health-care clinics administered by the federal Health Resources and Services Administration (HRSA), the prime agency responsible for helping uninsured, underinsured and medically vulnerable people with chronic and/or debilitating conditions get care based on their income.

*Financial eligibility criteria may vary by program.

To find a clinic near you: Go to HRSA.gov or call 877-464-4772.

•**Your local nonprofit hospital.** About 80% of US hospitals are nonprofit, and in order to retain their nonprofit status, they must provide a certain amount of charity care (the amount varies). That means nonprofit hospitals cannot deny you emergency room services or care for a serious illness if you cannot afford it. In addition, these hospitals have many free services such as nutrition counseling for diabetics and mental health counseling.

To learn what's available: Call hospitals in your area to find out which ones are nonprofit. Then check those hospitals' websites and/or call their social service departments and ask what they can do to meet your needs.

•**Free or low-cost medications.** Many new advanced medications that aren't available as generics can have monthly retail prices of up to $10,000 or more. Even with medication insurance, your co-pay may run up to 50% of that or more each month until you reach your insurance plan's out-of-pocket limits. What's more, many insurers don't include these high-cost drugs on their list of covered medications. Fortunately, most major pharmaceutical companies have patient-assistance programs that can help by discounting the drug if you can't afford it...or even providing the medication for free.

For additional information: Search online to find out what company manufactures the drug you need, and check its website or call the company for more details. Not all of these drug programs are based on income.

•**Other ways to get help.** You may also qualify for non-health-related programs that will help offset medical costs. For example, most states have programs that will help pay your utility bills, mortgage or rent. If you need cash for medical bills and have equity in your house, you may qualify for a reverse mortgage.

For more details: Contact your local Area Agency on Aging.

The Generic-Drug Rip-Off

David Belk, MD, a physician based in Alameda, California, specializing in internal medicine. He is founder of the True Cost of Healthcare blog, which provides information about health-care cost and billing issues. TrueCostofHealthCare.net

Using health insurance to fill a prescription for a generic drug could dramatically increase your out-of-pocket costs, particularly if you have not yet reached your policy's annual deductible. That's because people who use health insurance have to pay the price that the insurance company has set for the drug, and with generic drugs, these prices often are much higher than the prices you might pay when no insurance is used—sometimes hundreds of dollars higher for a 90-day supply.

Here's what happens behind the scenes: Many generic drugs cost pharmacies 10 cents a pill or less. A value-oriented pharmacy, such as those at Costco, Walmart and Kroger, or a reputable online pharmacy, such as *GoodRx.com* and *HealthWarehouse.com*, might charge as little as $4 for a 30-day supply or $10 for a 90-day supply—if you don't use insurance. What's more, even after you reach your deductible, many insurance policies require a co-pay that is higher than what these types of pharmacies charge for generic drugs.

Among the many widely used drugs that can be purchased without insurance as generics for as little as $10 for a 90-day supply are the blood pressure medications atenolol, carvedilol, clonidine and furosemide...blood-clot-prevention drug warfarin...diabetes drugs glimepiride, glipizide, glyburide and metformin...cholesterol medication lovastatin...antibiotic amoxicillin...and pain medication naproxen.

What to do: When filling a prescription for a generic drug, check whether it's cheaper to fill the prescription without using your coverage. Also, ask pharmacies whether they have a membership or rewards program that can further reduce the cost.

On the other hand, if you expect to spend a lot more than your deductible for medical costs in a given year, it might make sense to pay the higher prices so that you get past the deductible period more quickly. In some cases, depending on the specifics of your coverage, that might result in greater overall savings.

Talk to Your Doctor About Ways to Trim Health Care Costs

Peter Ubel, MD, professor, business, medicine and public policy, Duke University, Durham, North Carolina. Duke University, news release.

Discussing medical costs with your doctor could save you money without affecting your care, according to a recent study.

"Almost half the time that costs come up in conversation, either the doctor or the patient come up with some strategy to lower the patient's out-of-pocket cost. And it doesn't take long, usually less than a minute," study author Peter Ubel, MD, said in a news release from Duke University in Durham, North Carolina. Ubel is a professor in the schools of business, medicine and public policy at Duke.

He and his colleagues analyzed patient-doctor discussions from 1,755 outpatient visits across the United States. The patients had breast cancer, depression or rheumatoid arthritis, all of which have potentially high out-of-pocket costs. The doctors were oncologists, psychiatrists and rheumatologists.

Conversations about costs occurred in 30% of the visits, and nearly half of those included talking about how to reduce out-of-pocket costs. Doctors were as likely as patients to bring up the topic.

Money-saving ideas included: looking for a cheaper pharmacy, trying less expensive prescriptions, spacing medical visits further apart, and booking costly procedures after patients had met their deductibles.

"They're so simple and straightforward," Dr. Ubel said.

Dr. Ubel said many doctors are more aware now of the financial stress patients face and are suggesting ways to help patients get more affordable care.

"They're mentioning if a new medicine is expensive, or they're asking if something is covered by insurance. If more doctors adopted this approach, patients could really benefit," he said.

The study was published online recently in the journal *Medical Decision Making.*

Be Wary of Imported Supplements

U.S. Food and Drug Administration, news release.

You could be putting your health at risk if you buy imported dietary supplements and nonprescription drug products, the U.S. Food and Drug Administration warns.

Health fraud scammers often sell such products at ethnic or international stores, flea markets, swap meets or online, Cariny Nunez, MPH, a public health adviser in the FDA's Office of Minority Health, said in an agency news release. This may be because many people who shop at these places have poor English-language skills and limited access to health care services and information, she suggested.

"These scammers know that ethnic groups who may not speak or read English well, or who hold certain cultural beliefs, can be easy targets," she added.

For example, Native American, Hispanic, Asian and black people may have a long tradition of using herbal—or so-called "natural"—products, and many of these advertisers include the word "natural" on product labeling because they know it inspires trust in certain groups, Nunez said.

Gary Coody, RPh, the FDA's national health fraud coordinator, warned that just because a product is labeled "natural" doesn't mean that it's safe. These products may contain hidden drug ingredients or be contaminated with po-

Dangerous Athletic Wear

Shapewear can be dangerous, reports John Kuemmerle, MD. Shapewear and restrictive compression athletic tops and pants, worn to enhance the figure or improve athletic performance, put pressure on the abdomen. This can compress your stomach, intestines and colon—making acid reflux and heartburn worse. Shapewear also can worsen symptoms of irritable bowel syndrome and stress incontinence. And sweating in tight clothing can cause skin irritation and yeast infections.

John Kuemmerle, MD, is professor and chair, division of gastroenterology, hepatology and nutrition at Virginia Commonwealth University, Richmond.

tentially harmful chemicals, he said in the news release.

People should be suspicious about dietary supplements and nonprescription drug products that claim they are miracle cures, promise quick fixes or advertise that they can cure a wide range of diseases, the FDA officials said.

Before buying any unproven product or one with questionable claims, talk to a doctor or other health care professional, the experts said. In addition, consumers can check the FDA's website to find out if the agency has taken any action on the product.

"Remember, dietary supplements are not drugs," Coody said. "They are not substitutes for the drugs your health care professional prescribes. And you should let your health care professional know what supplements you are taking, because they may interact in a harmful way with prescribed medications or keep a prescribed drug from working."

If you or someone in your family has a bad reaction after using such a product, you can file a confidential report online at the FDA's MedWatch at *fda.gov/Safety/Med Watch/.*

Weight-Loss Supplements Might Not Be Worth the Risk

Joint study by researchers at the Food and Drug Administration, Silver Spring, Maryland, and Centers for Disease Control and Prevention, Atlanta, published in *The New England Journal of Medicine.*

Weight-loss supplements lead to about 23,000 ER visits a year. These include herbal pills, vitamins and minerals. The most common reasons for ER visits are allergic reactions, heart trouble, nausea and vomiting.

How to Pack Your Digital "Go Bag"

Joseph C. Kvedar, MD, vice president, Connected Health, Partners HealthCare, a Boston-based organization that uses information technology to improve health and wellness. A professor at Harvard Medical School, he is also the author of *The Internet of Healthy Things.*

We all know to keep water, ready-to-eat food and similar basic necessities packed in an emergency supply kit—aka a "go bag"—in case a natural disaster or some other crisis forces us to leave home at a moment's notice.

But these days, smartphones and other digital devices such as tablets offer several new options to help you and your loved ones stay safe. So-called "disaster apps" are game changers in the way that people can now find vital information, connect with one another and respond during a disaster.

PREPARE TO PREPARE

It's important to remember that smartphones still need to be charged to operate during a crisis, so it is wise to keep a small cell phone charger with you at all times—inexpensive ones (less than $10) can be found at electronics stores, discount stores and even drugstores.

Good to know: Data demands for text messages are smaller, so texts may go through even

93

if networks are overloaded during a disaster and cell phone calls can't be made.

5 PREPAREDNESS APPS

To stay safe, take some time—before you need them—to download the apps that are most appropriate for your family. Below are five excellent disaster apps that are free of charge and can be used on both Apple and Android phones and devices...

For convenience: Put several apps into a folder (named "disaster" or something similar).

The following apps require Wi-Fi or cell service...

•**American Red Cross** (*RedCross.org/mobile-apps/emergency-app*) is a good all-in-one app that offers 35 different alerts for severe weather (including hurricanes, winter storms and earthquakes) and a map to open Red Cross shelters. You receive text alerts when severe weather is predicted. With this app, you can monitor these conditions in your own area plus the locations of your loved ones.

Great feature: With "Family Safe," you can use this app to tell loved ones that an alert has been issued in their area and check to be sure they are safe.

•**Winter Survival Kit** (ag.*NDSU.edu/exten sion/apps/winter-survival-kit*). Developed by North Dakota State University, this app will help you find your location if you are stranded in severe winter weather, call 911 and notify your friends and family.

Great feature: The app's "gas calculator" estimates how long you can run your engine on your remaining fuel. The app also reminds you every 30 minutes to periodically turn off your engine to check your exhaust pipe for snow buildup—a crucial step in avoiding deadly carbon monoxide poisoning.

•**Outbreaks Near Me by HealthMap** (*HealthMap.org/outbreaksnearme*). This app shows all the current disease outbreaks in your community, including up-to-date tallies of flu cases in your area.

Great feature: You can set the app to alert you via text whenever an outbreak is occurring in your area.

•**ReUnite** (*lpf.nlm.nih.gov/PeopleLocator-Re Unite*) allows the public to report missing and/or found people after a large-scale disaster.

Great feature: This app allows you to upload photos and a physical description of a missing loved one to help disaster relief personnel find that person after an emergency.

•**Federal Emergency Management Agency** (*FEMA.gov/mobile-app*) gives tips on what to do before, during and after more than 20 types of disasters, as well as the locations of open shelters and disaster recovery centers in your area, which offer crucial services during floods, earthquakes and other natural disasters.

Great feature: This app's "Disaster Reporter" allows you to upload photos of damage and recovery efforts in your area.

Also helpful: In Case of Emergency (ICE) and flashlight apps—most reside on mobile devices and do not require Wi-Fi or cell service to operate. If you don't have a cell phone that will allow you to use an ICE app, be sure to create an emergency contact card that you carry with you at all times in your wallet or purse.

For a downloadable contact card that can be printed, go to: FEMA.gov/media-lib rary/assets/documents/108887.

Danger in New Clothes

Steven R. Feldman, MD, PhD, is professor of dermatology at Wake Forest University School of Medicine and director of the university's Center for Dermatology Research.

New clothes are not always unworn clothes—other shoppers might have tried them on in the store or even taken them home, then returned them. And that means these clothes can be infested with all sorts of things. Lice, scabies and bedbugs have been transferred this way. The likelihood is small, but possible, nevertheless, according to Steven R. Feldman, MD, PhD.

What's more, dyes and resins that manufacturers sometimes apply to new clothing to give it a wrinkle-free or crisp finish can cause allergic reactions, potentially producing an itchy rash wherever a garment comes in contact with the skin. Even if you have never exhibited these symptoms, that doesn't guarantee you never will—different clothing manufacturers use different chemicals and concentrations.

So always wash washable clothes. But what if the new clothes are dry-clean only, such as a wool jacket?

"Dry cleaning could get rid of infestations and some chemicals," said Dr. Feldman. "But it can introduce formaldehyde, another chemical that some people are allergic to." Even "organic" or "green" dry cleaners may be using chemicals that can cause allergic reactions. Put new clothes in a sealed plastic bag for two weeks. This won't get rid of chemicals, but it will kill bugs.

Are Electric Blankets Safe?

David O. Carpenter, MD, director of the Institute for Health and the Environment, University at Albany, New York.

You can stay cozy and safe under your electric blanket if you follow a few important guidelines. Electric blankets emit an extremely low frequency (ELF) level of radiation that has been linked to increased risk for certain types of cancer and Alzheimer's disease, although this link is still being debated. To be on the safe side, warm the bed before you get in and then turn the blanket off...or choose one with a timer that will automatically shut it off. And select a blanket with a UL logo on the label (this indicates it has met safety standards set by Underwriters Laboratories). Inspect it every month or so to make sure no wires are sticking out or the cord hasn't frayed, especially if your pet snuggles with you. A cat's or dog's paws can damage the wiring.

If you have diabetes or neuropathy, do not use an electric blanket. You may not sense when the blanket has become too hot and may end up with a burn.

Laminate Flooring Cancer Risk—Update

Jeffrey C. May, principal scientist with May Indoor Air Investigations LLC, Tyngsborough, Massachusetts. He is author of *My House Is Killing Me!* MayIndoorAir.com

In 2015, it was discovered that certain Chinese-made laminate flooring sold by the flooring company Lumber Liquidators released potentially cancer-causing levels of formaldehyde gas. Now the Centers for Disease Control and Prevention has essentially tripled its estimates of the danger. According to its revised projection, between six and 30 people per 100,000 exposed will develop cancer as a result of the flooring. This flooring could cause other health problems, too, including eye or throat irritation, difficulty breathing and other respiratory issues.

What to do: There is no need to avoid buying laminate flooring or to rip up any laminate flooring in your home. The majority of laminate flooring does not off-gas dangerous levels of formaldehyde, and Lumber Liquidators discontinued its sales of the unsafe flooring. Given the attention being paid to this problem, it is likely that retailers will pay close attention to laminate-flooring formaldehyde levels. What's more, even if your laminate floors initially did release dangerous levels of formaldehyde, they may not be doing so now if the floors were installed more than a year ago. *Still...*

•**If you want to be certain that new laminate floors are not dangerous,** unpackage the flooring and store it for two weeks or longer in your garage or some other dry location outside of your home's living area. Avoiding Chinese-made laminate flooring could reduce any risk of being exposed to high formaldehyde levels as well.

•**If you want to test installed laminate flooring for formaldehyde,** use Pure Air Control Services' test kit (*IndoorAirTest.com*, $97). Perform this test when relative humidity is above 60% and the temperature is above 70°F. If levels are high, find a pro who can help at the Indoor Air Quality Association (*IAQA.org*).

Flame-Retardant Furniture Is Bad for Your Health

RodaleNews.com.

Flame-retardant furniture is bad for your health. Chemicals used in the manufacture of flame retardants for foam furniture inserts have been linked to problems ranging from fertility issues to cancer. But a recent law passed in California is helping to phase out these dangerous chemicals. And companies that ship nationally will comply with the California law.

When shopping for furniture: Look for "TB 117-2013" on the label—that means the item may be flame-retardant–free, but confirm with the manufacturer. If the label says "TB 117," flame-retardant chemicals were used.

Brands that are eliminating flame retardants from sofas and armchairs: The Futon Shop, Ethan Allen, IKEA and La-Z-Boy.

CHAPTER 6

Diabetes Care

Check Your Risk for Diabetes

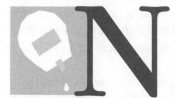**N**o one is excused from diabetes. That's the message behind a new public education campaign targeting the 86 million American adults with what's known as prediabetes.

More than one in three adults in the United States has prediabetes, a serious health condition that can lead to type 2 diabetes, heart attack and stroke, according to the U.S. Centers for Disease Control and Prevention.

If you have prediabetes, you have higher than normal blood sugar levels, but not high enough to be diagnosed with full-blown diabetes.

"Awareness is crucial in the effort to stop type 2 diabetes," David Marrero, PhD, director of the Diabetes Translation Research Center at Indiana University School of Medicine, said in a CDC news release.

To learn your risk, you can take a short online test at *DoIHavePrediabetes.org*. The test can also be taken through texts and interactive TV and radio announcements.

"This is a very simple and quick tool that will allow people to see if they are at risk for prediabetes or diabetes," said Mary Vouyiouklis Kellis, MD, an endocrinologist at Cleveland Clinic. "If they are at higher risk, this will hopefully prompt them to seek medical attention sooner."

The majority of people with prediabetes don't know they have it. Yet, if not treated, up to 30% of people with prediabetes will develop type 2 diabetes within five years, according to the news release.

"One of the problems with prediabetes and diabetes is that people sometimes don't feel sick until it's too late," Dr. Vouyiouklis Kellis said.

Some simple changes in activity and diet can prevent diabetes, however.

Mary Vouyiouklis Kellis, MD, endocrinologist, Cleveland Clinic, Cleveland, Ohio.

U.S. Centers for Disease Control and Prevention, news release.

"Losing 5 to 7% of body weight can significantly reduce your risk as well as making lifestyle changes, which include portion control, reducing foods with refined sugars and exercising regularly," she added. "Exercising just 30 minutes a day, five days a week, can also help reduce this risk."

Knowing you have prediabetes is just the first step in preventing type 2 diabetes, AMA President-Elect Andrew Gurman, MD, said in the CDC news release.

"As soon as someone discovers they may be at risk of prediabetes, they should talk with their physician about further testing to confirm their diagnosis and discuss the necessary lifestyle changes needed to help prevent type 2 diabetes," Dr. Gurman said.

Roughly 29 million people in the United States—more than 9% of the U.S. population—have diabetes, mostly type 2, according to the CDC.

info Here's where you can find the prediabetes risk test. *doihaveprediabetes.org/*

Alert: Doctors Are Not Treating Prediabetes

Arch Mainous III, PhD, chair, department of health services research, management and policy, College of Public Health and Health Professionals, University of Florida, Gainesville
University of Florida, news release

A large number of Americans with prediabetes aren't being treated for the condition, which suggests that doctors are missing opportunities to prevent diabetes, researchers report.

More than one-third of US adults have prediabetes, which means their blood sugar levels are higher than normal, but not high enough to be diagnosed with diabetes. People with prediabetes are at increased risk for circulatory problems, kidney disease, and nerve and retinal damage, the study authors said.

"We know that prediabetes is considered one of the biggest risk factors for the development of diabetes, with estimates ranging from 15 to 30% of people with prediabetes developing diabetes within five years," said lead investigator Arch Mainous III, PhD. Dr. Mainous is chair of the department of health services research, management and policy in the College of Public Health and Health Professions at the University of Florida.

"We also know that 90% of people who have prediabetes don't know they have it. So the question becomes, where is the doctor in all this? Is the doctor identifying people with prediabetes, telling them about it and providing treatment? That's what we wanted to find out," he said in a university news release.

Dr. Mainous and his colleagues analyzed 2012 federal government survey data on people aged 45 and older who had doctor-ordered blood tests within the past 90 days. About 34% of them had blood sugar levels that indicated prediabetes.

However, very few of those patients were told they had prediabetes and only 23% of them began treatment for the condition, such as lifestyle changes or drug therapy, according to the study. The findings were published in the *Journal of the American Board of Family Medicine*.

"Even with blood test results in front of them, physicians weren't detecting prediabetes in their patients in terms of making a diagnosis or providing some sort of management or treatment," Dr. Mainous said.

"Identifying people with prediabetes and getting them some sort of treatment has been shown to be effective for slowing the progression to diabetes or stopping it altogether, and that is the goal of prevention," he explained. "We don't want to manage half the population with diabetes. What we want to do is keep them from getting diabetes."

Dr. Mainous said he is now conducting a survey of thousands of family doctors to learn why so many patients with prediabetes aren't receiving treatment.

info The American Academy of Family Physicians has more about prediabetes at *familydoctor.org,* search "prediabetes."

How America's Top Diabetes Doctor Avoids Diabetes

George L. King, MD, chief scientific officer at the Boston-based Joslin Diabetes Center, one of the country's leading diabetes clinical care and research centers. He is also a professor of medicine at Harvard Medical School and the author, with Royce Flippin, of *The Diabetes Reset*.

You might think that a diabetes researcher would never develop the disease that he's dedicated his life to studying. But I can't count on it.

My family's story: My father was diagnosed with diabetes at age 72 and was promptly placed on three medications to control his insulin levels. What he did next made all the difference: Even though he began taking diabetes medication, he simultaneously went into action—walking an hour a day and going on the diet described below. A year and a half later, he no longer needed the prescriptions. He still had diabetes, but diet and exercise kept it under control.

As a diabetes researcher and physician whose own diabetes risk is increased by his family history, I've got a lot at stake in finding the absolute best ways to avoid and fight this disease.

Here are the steps I take to prevent diabetes—all of which can benefit you whether you want to avoid this disease or have already been diagnosed with it and are trying to control or even reverse it...

STEP 1: Follow a rural Asian diet (RAD). This diet includes the most healthful foods of a traditional Asian diet—it consists of 70% complex carbohydrates...15% fat...15% protein... and 15 g of fiber for every 1,000 calories. Don't worry too much about all these numbers—the diet is actually pretty simple to follow once you get the hang of it.

You might be surprised by "70% complex carbohydrates," since most doctors recommend lower daily intakes of carbohydrates. The difference is, I'm recommending high amounts of complex, unrefined (not processed) carbohydrates. This type of carb is highly desirable because it's found in foods—such as whole grains, legumes, vegetables and fruits—that are chock-full of fiber. If your goal is to reduce diabetes risk, fiber is the holy grail.

Why I do it: The RAD diet has been proven in research to promote weight loss...improve insulin sensitivity (a key factor in the development and treatment of diabetes) and glucose control...and decrease total cholesterol and LDL "bad" cholesterol levels.

To keep it simple, I advise patients to follow a 2-1-1 formula when creating meals—two portions of nonstarchy veggies (such as spinach, carrots or asparagus)...one portion of whole grains (such as brown rice or quinoa), legumes (such as lentils or chickpeas) or starchy veggies (such as sweet potatoes or winter squash)...and one portion of protein (such as salmon, lean beef, tofu or eggs). Have a piece of fruit (such as an apple or a pear) on the side. Portion size is also important. Portions fill a nine-inch-diameter plate, which is smaller than a typical 12-inch American dinner plate.

Helpful: I take my time when eating—I chew each bite at least 10 times before swallowing. Eating too quickly can cause glucose levels to peak higher than usual after a meal.

STEP 2: Fill up on dark green vegetables. I include dark, leafy greens in my diet every day. These leafy greens are one of the two portions of nonstarchy veggies in the 2-1-1 formula.

Why I do it: Dark green vegetables contain antioxidants and compounds that help your body fight insulin resistance (a main driver of diabetes).

My secret "power veggie": A Chinese vegetable called bitter melon. It is a good source of fiber and has been shown to lower blood sugar. True to its name, bitter melon tastes a little bitter but is delicious when used in soups and stir-fries. It is available at Asian groceries. Eat bitter melon as one of the two portions of nonstarchy veggies in the 2-1-1 formula.

STEP 3: Adopt an every-other-day workout routine. I try to not be sedentary and to walk as much as I can (by using a pedometer, I can tell whether I've reached my daily goal of 10,000 steps).

While this daily practice helps, it's not enough to significantly affect my diabetes risk. For that,

Lower Your Risk for Diabetes

●**Make up sleep for better insulin levels.** Sleep loss can play havoc with metabolism, increasing risk for diabetes.

New study: Insulin sensitivity declined 23% in men who got only 4.5 hours of sleep per night for four consecutive nights, but then recovered when they slept for 12 hours one night and 10 hours the next.

Takeaway: Whenever you lose sleep, try to then sleep in for a morning or two.

Josiane Broussard, PhD, assistant research professor of integrative physiology, University of Colorado Boulder.

●**Time your BP meds.** Taking blood pressure medication at bedtime (versus in the morning) cut the risk of developing diabetes by 57%, according to a recent study.

Why: ACE inhibitors, some beta-blockers and other such drugs block the effects of a hormone that narrows blood vessels, which can lead to increased blood pressure and decreased insulin sensitivity.

Important: Consult your doctor before changing the timing of your medication.

Ramon Hermida, PhD, professor of medicine, University of Vigo, Spain.

●**Reduce diabetes risk one serving at a time.** Start by substituting just one serving a day of water or unsweetened tea or coffee for one serving of a sugar-sweetened soft drink or dairy beverage.

Reason: Each daily serving of a sweetened soft drink or milk drink, such as a milk shake, raises diabetes risk by 14% to 27%. Each additional 5% of total calories from sweetened drinks raises the risk by 18%.

Study of data on diet and diabetes incidence in more than 25,000 British men and women, ages 40 to 79, by researchers at University of Cambridge, UK, published in *Diabetologia*.

●**Eat dark chocolate.** In a recent study, residents in the tiny country Luxembourg ate about 25 grams, on average—a little less than one ounce—of chocolate a day. When researchers studied those who ate the most chocolate and compared them with those who ate the least, the finding was sweet—the chocolate lovers had lower blood insulin levels and less insulin resistance, a measure of the body's ability to metabolize carbohydrates while keeping blood sugar low. In short, they had fewer risk factors for diabetes.

Study titled "Daily chocolate consumption is inversely associated with insulin resistance and liver enzymes in the Observation of Cardiovascular Risk Factors in Luxembourg study" by researchers at Luxembourg Institute of Health, Luxembourg, University of Maine, Orono, published in *British Journal of Nutrition*.

I have an every-other-day workout routine that consists of 30 minutes of jogging on the treadmill (fast enough so that I'm breathing hard but can still carry on a conversation)...followed by 30 minutes of strength training (using handheld weights, resistance bands or weight machines).

Why I do it: Working out temporarily reduces your insulin resistance and activates enzymes and proteins that help your muscles use glucose instead of allowing the body to accumulate fat—a beneficial effect that lasts for 48 hours (the reason for my every-other-day routine). Strength training is crucial—your muscles are what really kick your body's glucose-burning into high gear. A weekly game of tennis helps shake up my routine.

STEP 4: Keep the temperature chilly. At the courts where I play tennis, the temperature is naturally cool, but I wear a very thin T-shirt that leaves my neck exposed. This helps activate the "brown fat" in my body. Most people have this special type of body fat—mainly around the neck, collarbone and shoulders.

Why I do it: Brown fat burns calories at high rates when triggered by the cold. To help burn brown fat, exercise in temperatures of 64°F or lower...set your home's thermostat in the mid-60s...and dress as lightly as possible in cool weather. Walking for 50 or 60 minutes a day in cool weather also helps.

STEP 5: Get the "sleep cure." I make a point to sleep at least six hours a night during the week and seven hours nightly on weekends.

Why I do it: Lack of sleep has been proven to dramatically harm the body's ability to properly metabolize glucose—a problem that sets the stage for diabetes. Research shows that seven to eight hours a night are ideal. However, because of my work schedule, I'm not always able to get that much sleep on weekdays. That's why I sleep a bit longer on weekends.

Research now shows that the body has some capacity to "catch up" on lost sleep and reverse some—but not all—of the damage that occurs to one's insulin sensitivity when you're sleep deprived.

Antibiotics–Diabetes Link

Study by researchers at Center for Diabetes Research, Gentofte Hospital, and University of Copenhagen, both in Hellerup, Denmark, published in *The Journal of Clinical Endocrinology & Metabolism*.

Antibiotics are linked to an increased risk for type 2 diabetes. People with type 2 diabetes tend to take more antibiotics in the years before their diagnosis than people who don't develop diabetes. The association could mean that people have more illnesses requiring antibiotic treatment in the years before type 2 diabetes emerges…or that antibiotic use somehow contributes to the onset of diabetes.

A Surprising Health Benefit to (a Little) Hunger

Study titled "Let Hunger Be Your Guide? Being Hungry Before a Meal is Associated with Healthier Levels of Post-Meal Blood Glucose" by researchers at University of Illinois, Chicago, published in *Journal of the Association for Consumer Research*.

Anyone who aims for a healthy weight knows one key is to eat only when you are truly hungry. Eating for other reasons—you're bored or stressed or don't want to waste food—is a ticket to gaining weight.

But new research has discovered another reason to eat only when you're hungry. It's better for your body right away…every time you eat.

When you are moderately hungry before a meal, your blood sugar doesn't rise as high as it does when you're not really hungry but eat anyway, finds a new study. At University of Illinois in Chicago, 45 college students were asked to not eat for at least two hours, rate their hunger and then eat a dinner roll and a soda (a high-carb snack that tends to raise blood sugar). Afterward their blood sugar was tested. The study was repeated a week later to improve accuracy.

Results: Participants who said that they were pretty hungry had a lower level of post-snack blood sugar than those who said they weren't. That's a good thing, because postmeal blood sugar spikes damage cells, which, over time, can contribute to the risk of developing diabetes and cardiovascular disease.

What's going on? While human studies haven't teased out the physiology, animal research finds that cutting back on calories leads the hormone ghrelin to go up. It's a well-known hunger hormone in humans, too. But ghrelin does more than make us hungry—it improves the efficiency with which the body moves glucose (sugar) from the bloodstream into the muscles, where it's needed. In layman's terms, when you're hungry, your body is primed to digest a meal.

Getting ravenously hungry, however, may backfire. In that case, your body reacts by keeping blood sugar away from muscles to make sure there's enough sugar for essential organs, such as the brain. Indeed, in the study, those who were very hungry had higher blood sugar levels after the snack than the moderately hungry. They reacted more like those who weren't particularly hungry to start with.

It's the first such study, so more research is needed to confirm and expand the results. But we already know that getting in touch with your hunger is a good way to guard against mindless eating—and the weight that often follows.

The take-away: Eating when you are moderately hungry is not only best for weight management but may protect you from diabetes and heart disease, too. And there's no benefit to waiting until you could eat a horse.

To Prevent Diabetes, Say Hello to Your Kitchen

Study by researchers at Harvard T.H. Chan School of Public Health, Boston, and Montefiore Medical Center, New York City, presented at the annual meeting of the American Heart Association.

The path to diabetes prevention may lead to your stove, your oven and your pantry.

When researchers from Harvard's T.H. Chan School of Public Health analyzed data on nearly 100,000 men and women who were followed for up to 36 years, for each lunch eaten at home each week, the risk of developing diabetes went down 2%. For every weekly dinner, it dropped 4%. Those who ate 11 to 14 lunches or dinners at home each week compared with those who ate only six meals, for example, were 13% less likely to get diabetes.

Why? Many studies have found that home cooking tends to be lower in fat, sugar and calories than restaurant fare, especially fast food, so it's no surprise that the eat-at-home folks in the study weighed less than those who more frequently ate out. They also drank fewer sugar-sweetened beverages.

Beware This Diabetes Symptom

Xiang Gao, MD, PhD, director of nutritional epidemiology laboratory, The Pennsylvania State University, University Park.

A faster resting heart rate may be a sign of diabetes risk. In a recent study of 73,000 adults, those with a higher heart rate (above 80 beats per minute) were up to 70% more likely to develop diabetes within four years than those with lower heart rates (61 beats per minute).

Why: A faster heart rate may be a sign of increased nervous system activity, which can cause insulin resistance (a precursor to diabetes).

If your resting heart rate is above 80: Ask your doctor to test your blood sugar.

It's All About Blood Sugar

George L. King, MD, a professor of medicine at Harvard Medical School in Boston, chief scientific officer of Harvard's Joslin Diabetes Center, where he heads the vascular cell biology research section, and the author, with Royce Flippin, of *The Diabetes Reset*.

What's most frightening about diabetes is the fact that it increases one's risk for so many serious conditions such as heart disease and kidney disease.

How to fight back: People with diabetes who maintain a fasting blood sugar level of 70 mg/dL to 100 mg/dL—and a hemoglobin A1C (HbA1C) level, a measure of long-term glucose control, below 7%—are far less likely to suffer such diabetes complications.

THE LOWDOWN ON MEDICATION

In a perfect world, people with diabetes would be able to keep their glucose levels under control by eating a nutritious diet and getting adequate exercise. But the truth is, most people with diabetes need medication at some point. *My advice…*

•**Start with an insulin sensitizer.** *Metformin* (Glucophage), which reduces insulin resistance (in which the body becomes less responsive to insulin, increasing blood glucose levels), is widely used for type 2 diabetes. This medication helps prevent diabetes complications.

While metformin is among the least expensive yet most effective drugs for treating diabetes, new research suggests that it may have additional benefits.

Recent finding: There's some evidence that metformin and other such insulin sensitizers may reduce the risk for cancer and possibly heart disease and stroke—independently of their effects on insulin.

In most cases, metformin doesn't cause serious side effects. Some people may have diarrhea and/or nausea at first, but this usually goes away within a few weeks.

What helps: Taking it with meals.

•**Watch out for weight gain.** If metformin isn't enough to control glucose levels, it is often combined with synthetic insulin, a commonly used blood glucose–lowering drug.

Paradoxically, insulin and some of the other frequently prescribed diabetes drugs cause weight gain as a side effect—sometimes up to 10 pounds in the first year. Other diabetes medications that help with blood glucose control but can also cause weight gain include sulfonylureas, such as *glipizide* (Glucotrol)… and thiazolidinediones, such as *rosiglitazone* (Avandia).

Weight gain is particularly dangerous because 85% of adults with diabetes are already obese or overweight. Those who are carrying extra weight are more likely to have worse blood sugar control and higher cholesterol and blood pressure. They also tend to need larger doses of insulin or other medications.

Newer options: If your weight is a problem, in addition to adopting healthy lifestyle habits, switching to a newer form of insulin (such as Levemir) that minimizes weight gain may help. Other newer blood glucose–lowering medications that don't lead to weight gain include oral drugs called DPP-4 inhibitors, such as *sitagliptin* (Januvia)…and SGLT2 inhibitors, including *canagliflozin* (Invokana). New injectable drugs, such as *dulaglutide* (Trulicity), also do not promote weight gain. All drugs, however, may have some side effects. Ask your doctor for advice.

HABITS THAT REALLY HELP

It's entirely possible to go off diabetes medication if you are able to stabilize your glucose levels with diet and exercise. And even if you still do need medication, there's a good chance you can get by with lower or less frequent doses. *Here's how…*

•**Don't get caught up in finding the perfect diet.** There are many good diets to choose from.

My advice: Choose a diet that you can stick to! The best way to do this is to consult a dietitian who has experience working with people with diabetes to choose an eating plan that's both effective and enjoyable. This is usually covered by insurance if you have diabetes. Three to four sessions are recommended, with annual follow-ups. To find a qualified dietitian near you, check the Academy of Nutrition and Dietetics' Diabetes Care and Education website, *DCE.org/#2.*

•**Follow a two-pronged approach for exercise.** Aerobic exercise (such as biking, fast walking and swimming) helps with weight loss, improves cardiovascular health, increases bone density and even improves cognitive function. But that's not enough. If you've got diabetes, weight lifting and other forms of resistance training (such as exercising with elastic bands) are crucial. These workouts increase muscle mass—and muscle absorbs a large amount of glucose from the blood. Patients with type 2 diabetes who combine resistance workouts with aerobic exercise have a much lower risk for complications.

My advice: Get aerobic and resistance training, preferably for 30 to 45 minutes, most days of the week.

Diabetes Coach to the Rescue!

Lisa Foster-McNulty, RN, CDE, a registered nurse, certified diabetes educator and the director of patient care and education at Integrated Diabetes Services in Wynnewood, Pennsylvania, IntegratedDiabetes.com. She serves as co-chair of the Education Committee for the local affiliate of the American Association of Diabetes Educators.

If you've got diabetes, whether you're prescribed medication or not, your doctor may well give you a daunting to-do list with items such as "lose weight"…"cut back on carbs"…"lower your blood sugar"…and "get more exercise."

The challenging part is that you are on your own in reaching those goals! Most doctors don't have time to give patients the support they need in managing the self-care of their disease. But help is available.

Many people now depend on health coaches. A coach—ideally a "certified diabetes educator" (CDE), a health-care professional, such as a registered nurse, pharmacist or registered dietitian, with specialized training (see page 105)—can help people with diabetes navigate the intricate day-to-day details that determine how effectively they will control their disease.

HOW IT WORKS

With diabetes coaching, patients usually meet their coaches in person (the frequency and number of visits often depend on insurance coverage). The meetings can be private or in group settings at a doctor's office or medical center. In some cases, coaches also stay in touch with patients with phone calls, e-mail or Skype. What kind of help will you get? It depends entirely on what you need. *Examples...*

•**Exercise for nonexercisers.** Regular exercise is among the best ways to lower blood sugar, improve insulin sensitivity and reduce diabetes-related complications.

However, the reality is that many people with diabetes have never exercised, and you can't expect someone to go from being totally sedentary to athletic just by saying that he/she should.

A coach looks for ways to ease people into exercise. For example, you might take a 10-minute walk after each meal—but even that might be too much, particularly for someone who's obese or has other health issues. How about standing up during TV commercials? Even this small step can make a difference. Marching in place is even better. Don't feel like standing? Try tapping your feet while you sit. From a health coach's perspective, any activity is better than none.

•**Investigating blood sugar spikes.** Let's say you take diabetes medication and check your blood sugar every day. The readings have generally been good, but lately your glucose has been consistently testing high. What changed?

It could be many things. For example, have you had a recent illness? A bacterial infection may raise glucose levels. Maybe you've gotten careless with your diet because you're not testing often enough.

Your coach can help you figure it out. He will look at all of the factors that affect blood sugar—not in general terms, but those that affect you personally.

•**Help with carb counting.** It's among the most effective ways to manage after-meal glucose levels. Counting carbohydrates is particu-

larly important for people taking insulin—they often need a higher dose for a carbohydrate-rich meal.

But carb counting can be tricky. Carb plans are individualized, but generally patients are advised to have between nine and 13 carbohydrate choices a day, with each "choice" equaling 15 g of carbohydrate. A coach can help you fine-tune your carb plan when your glucose is running high.

Example: Many people depend on "eyeball estimates"—they look at the size of an apple or another food and make a quick mental calculation about the carbohydrates. You might be great at estimating...or not so great. If there's been an unexpected change in your readings, inaccurate carb counting could be to blame. Your coach might recommend that you take a more scientific approach, such as using a scale or measuring cups.

•**Real-life monitoring.** Many people don't realize that their glucose is high because they're not checking their blood sugar levels often enough (the full cost of test strips isn't always covered by insurance). A diabetes coach will always ask how often and when you're checking your glucose—and help you find a solution if cost is an issue.

Example: Maybe you should be checking your glucose level more than four times a day but can't afford it. A coach might advise you to check your glucose around breakfast time one day...around lunchtime another day...and at bedtime on a third day. After a few weeks, the coach will have enough information to identify, in general terms, your blood sugar trends. He can then recommend certain changes—such as eating more or less carbohydrates (see above)—to bring your readings into your target range.

•**Strategic eating.** To help keep your blood sugar levels under control, a coach may give advice not only on the foods you eat but also on the order in which they are consumed. That's because research shows that eating protein-rich foods first and saving carbs for the end of meals helps blunt blood sugar spikes. Using this strategy, a person with diabetes having a meal of, say, grilled chicken, broccoli and potatoes should consume those foods in that order to minimize the impact on his blood sugar.

HOW TO FIND A COACH

If you have diabetes, a certified diabetes educator (CDE) can give you the kind of attention you need to really get control of your disease. A CDE is a health-care professional, such as a nurse, pharmacist or dietitian, who has met the requirements of the National Certification Board for Diabetes Educators (NCBDE). This certification, which requires 1,000 hours of diabetes-management training, passing an exam and undergoing continuing education, greatly increases your chances of getting reimbursed for the cost of diabetes coaching services. Check with your insurer.

If the coaching is not covered by insurance, depending on where you live, you can expect to pay $30 (for a group) to $200 (one-on-one) for an initial consultation with a coach/diabetes educator, with an additional charge for a "service plan" that includes a certain number of visits, phone calls and/or e-mails. To find a certified diabetes educator near you, go to *NCBDE.org*.

Healthier Potatoes and Pasta for Better Blood Sugar Levels

Study of resistant starch content of potatoes by cooking method presented by researchers at the USDA Agricultural Research Service (ARS) Grand Forks Human Nutrition Research Center, North Dakota, and the University of Minnesota, Minneapolis and St. Paul, at the Federation of American Societies for Experimental Biology conference in Boston.

Study titled "Efficacy of increased resistant starch consumption in human type 2 diabetes" by researchers at University of Surrey, United Kingdom, published in *Endocrine Connections*.

To make potatoes and pasta healthier, cook in a way that increases the amount of "resistant starch," which raises blood sugar less than regular starch. *Here's how...*

Take a 100-gram serving of potatoes—about three-and-a-half ounces. Boil it, and you've got 2.6 grams of resistant starch...baked, 3.1 grams...chilled (either baked or boiled), 4.3

> ## Better Way to Eat
>
> People with diabetes who ate the protein and vegetable portions of a meal 15 minutes before starting in on their carbs reduced their one-hour postmeal glucose levels by 37%, compared with their glucose on a day when they ate carbs first. Insulin levels were also lower when they ate protein and vegetables first.
>
> *Why:* Carbs can cause glucose and insulin levels to spike, but protein appears to mitigate this effect.
>
> Louis Aronne, MD, professor of metabolic research, Weill Cornell Medical College, New York City.

---

grams—good news for potato salad lovers. Chilled and then reheated potatoes do pretty well, too—3.5 grams. The same holds true for pasta—cooking and then cooling pasta increases the resistant starch modestly.

Does it make a difference? In a British study, people with diabetes who added 40 grams of resistant starch to their daily intake didn't improve their underlying diabetes but did have a reduced blood sugar spike after meals—a healthy thing. Whether there's any blood sugar benefit to taking in, say, an additional two or three grams of resistant starch in a meal, though, just isn't known.

So go ahead and enjoy your potatoes baked rather than boiled, and even better yet, cooled. But remember these foods already start with lots of easily digested, sugar-spiking starch, so cooking them in a way that boosts their resistant starch doesn't turn them into superfoods. A baked Russet Burbank potato has a "glycemic index" (GI), a measure of how quickly it raises blood sugar, of 111—more than white bread. So cook it right, but don't make it a daily staple—and add a healthful fat, such as olive oil, to further lower the GI.

Pasta, on the other hand, already has a lower GI than spuds, because the way it's made traps starch in a matrix that takes the body a longer time to break down into sugar. The GI range—30 to 60. So enjoy your pasta cooled in pasta salads...and if you like it hot, reduce its

GI even more by cooking it al dente—slightly chewy rather than soft—and drizzling it with olive oil.

In the end, though, what matters more is how much you eat of these delicious but high-starch foods. Want to make a really healthy pasta salad? Start with whole grain pasta for extra nutrition, cook it al dente, and use just one cup of cooled pasta with three cups of chopped nonstarchy veggies with your favorite dressing. Now you're cooking.

Diabetes Food Tool

Chopsticks may lower glycemic response to carbohydrates. When people ate white rice with chopsticks, their glycemic response dropped by 16%—causing less of an insulin increase than when people ate rice with a spoon.

Possible reason: Using chopsticks means taking smaller bites and eating more slowly.

Study by researchers at Singapore Institute for Clinical Sciences, published in *Physiology & Behavior*.

Get a Barley Boost!

Anne Nilsson, PhD, associate professor, Lund University, Sweden.

Adults who ate bread made mostly with barley at each meal had lower blood sugar and insulin levels after three days—and felt full longer—than those who ate white bread, a new study reported.

Possible reason: Barley's mix of different fibers stimulates healthy gut bacteria that help to regulate metabolism and appetite, which could cut risk for diabetes and cardiovascular disease.

Other ways to enjoy barley: Add barley grains to soups and stews...or make a barley side dish instead of rice or potatoes.

Breakthrough Obesity Drug

Angela Fitch, MD, is director of medical weight management and associate professor of medicine, University of Cincinnati College of Medicine.

Liraglutide (Saxenda) is a high-dose version of the diabetes drug Victoza. Like other weight-loss drugs, liraglutide curbs appetite—but it also acts like a natural hormone to slow stomach emptying. Gastrointestinal upsets are the most common side effect. Liraglutide, which is injected daily, is used in combination with exercise and a weight-loss diet.

Whom it may help: Overweight people who have diabetes, prediabetes or another weight-related health condition.

The Best (and Worst) Diabetes Drugs—For Your Heart

Study titled "Cardiovascular Safety Profile of Currently Available Diabetic Drugs" by Debabrata Mukherjee, MD, chairman of the department of internal medicine and chief of cardiovascular medicine at Texas Tech University Health Sciences Center El Paso, and colleagues, published in *The Ochsner Journal*.

Study titled "Empagliflozin, Cardiovascular Outcomes, and Mortality in Type 2 Diabetes" by researchers at Mount Sinai Hospital, Toronto, et al., published in *The New England Journal of Medicine*.

Heart disease is the number-one killer of people with type 2 diabetes, so you would think drugs that help control diabetes would be good for the heart.

But the opposite is sometimes true—some commonly prescribed diabetes drugs actually increase your risk for heart disease.

There are many ways this can happen. Sometimes they can cause hypoglycemia—low blood sugar—which can reduce the amount of nutrients going to the heart. Sometimes they raise bad lipids and lower good cholesterol, or increase water retention, which raises blood pressure, or reduce the ability of the coronary arteries to dilate properly. And some, we don't understand why they raise the risk for heart disease.

How could these drugs be developed by the pharmaceutical industry and be approved by the Food and Drug Administration (FDA) yet make people with diabetes more likely to develop heart disease?

RESEARCHING DRUGS... WITH BLINDERS ON

Until 2008, clinical studies needed to get diabetes drugs approved by the FDA didn't have to even look at cardiovascular effects. They just had to show that the drugs lowered blood sugar (glucose). That's a crucial omission, since the risk for stroke, heart disease and death from heart disease in patients with diabetes is at least twice that of patients without diabetes. So that year, the FDA made it clear to drug manufacturers that it wanted to see new drugs for type 2 diabetes undergo clinical trials to demonstrate cardiovascular safety—in addition to blood glucose effects.

Now the results of these studies are in. One recent review found that out of the 11 classes of diabetes drugs, drugs in four of them are associated with increased risk.

FOR A HEALTHIER HEART, AVOID THESE DIABETES DRUGS

The following drugs, or drug classes, increase heart disease risk. What to do? That's simple—avoid them as frontline drugs. *The drugs...*

•*Sulfonylureas* (Glucotrol, Micronase). This class of drugs stimulates the pancreas to make more insulin, but it also causes weight gain and increases the risk for heart attacks. And it makes it harder for the body to recover after a heart attack.

•*Meglitinides* (Starlix, Prandin). This class works similarly to sulfonylureas, also causes weight gain and is associated with negative cardiovascular effects, although less severe.

•*Rosiglitazone* (Avandia). Approved in 1999, Avandia was severely restricted by the FDA in 2010 when it was shown to greatly increase the risk for strokes, heart attacks and heart failure.

•*Saxagliptin* (Onglyz). This drug has been linked with an increase in hospitalization for heart failure.

THE BEST DIABETES DRUG FOR YOUR HEART—METFORMIN

One of the oldest, safest and as it turns out, least expensive drugs is metformin. This should be the initial diabetes drug of choice for most people. "It lowers glucose, provides a little weight loss, and there's some evidence it can reduce cardiovascular events. For example, one study found that metformin, when initiated early in the disease, reduces many complications of diabetes—including heart attacks, heart failure and stroke—by 12% overall.

Metformin isn't right for everyone, however. Some patients have trouble tolerating its side effects, which include GI distress, and caution is recommended for elderly patients and for those with liver or kidney disease.

Others may do fine with metformin but need a second drug to bring blood sugar even lower. However, be cautious in trying to get your blood sugar down too low. It used to be thought that lower glucose was better. But there's a balance, and too low can lead to problems.

IF YOU NEED MORE THAN METFORMIN

If you do need another drug besides metformin, these are either neutral or positive for heart health...

•**Many DPP-4 inhibitors,** which increase insulin release after meals, are neutral and possibly positive for heart health. Examples include *alogliptin* (Nesina), *sitagliptin* (Januvia), *linagliptin* (Tradjenta) and *vildagliptin* (Galvus)—and there are combination drugs that pair a DPP-4 inhibitor with metformin.

•**GLP-1 agonists** (Byetta, Bydureon). These medications, which increase insulin release after a meal, lead to modest weight loss and a moderate decrease in the risk for cardiovascular disease.

•**Alpha-glucosidase inhibitors** (Glyset, Precose) slow the digestion of carbohydrates, moderating blood sugar rise after meals. They don't lead to weight gain and may lower blood pressure as well as cardiovascular "events," such as heart attacks.

•*Empagliflozin* (Jardiance). This new drug, an SGLT2 inhibitor, slows the rate at which glucose is reabsorbed by the kidneys, thus lowering blood sugar levels. In a recent study, it was found to reduce risk for cardiovascular disease among patients being treated for diabetes who had a high risk for heart disease. The study found a 38% reduced risk in cardiovascular mortality in those who took Jardiance compared with a placebo. In absolute figures, rates of death from cardiovascular causes were 3.7% with empagliflozin versus 5.9% with a placebo. Because of this study, almost two-thirds of physicians said they were prescribing empagliflozin for more patients with diabetes, according to an online poll conducted by *Medscape Medical News*. The drug is promising, but it is expensive and comes with other risks such as an increased risk for urinary infections. The FDA is also monitoring reports of ketoacidosis, a potentially dangerous condition that requires hospitalization.

A HEALTHIER HEART

It's best to take a balanced approach and look at the big picture. That means starting with diet and losing weight if you are overweight, which can make metformin more effective, so that you may not need to consider other options. There's so much that can be done to avoid drug therapy, such as lifestyle changes.

The good news is that the era in which drug manufacturers could just ignore heart health for diabetes has ended. But you still need to be vigilant. Talk to your doctor about the benefits and risks of any medication you are prescribed, including how it affects your weight and your cardiovascular health. After all, the goal of treating diabetes isn't to lower your blood sugar numbers but to help you live a long and healthy life—with a healthy heart.

Better Surgery Outcomes

David Mosen, PhD, MPH, health services researcher, Kaiser Permanente Center for Health Research, Portland, Oregon.

Having pharmacists manage insulin use and blood sugar in adults with diabetes who are having any type of surgery led to significantly better outcomes.

Details: Patients were 33% less likely to be readmitted to the hospital after three months and had fewer complications and better glucose control. Although proper blood sugar management is a known factor in positive surgical outcomes, doctors and surgeons are frequently too busy to focus on it.

The Best Treatments for Common Diabetic Eye Disease

Paul Sieving, MD, PhD, director, National Eye Institute, Bethesda, Maryland.
John Wells, MD, retina specialist, Palmetto Retina Center, Columbia, South Carolina.
Mark Fromer, MD, ophthalmologist, Lenox Hill Hospital, New York City.
Nazanin Barzideh, MD, chief, vitreoretinal surgery, division of ophthalmology, Winthrop-University Hospital, Mineola, New York.
U.S. National Eye Institute, news release.

People with diabetes are at risk for blurred vision or even a loss of vision from a condition called macular edema.

Three drugs for the disease—Avastin, Eylea and Lucentis—vary widely in price, but new research suggests all work equally well for patients with mild vision loss.

However, when diabetic macular edema leads to more severe vision loss, researchers found Eylea to be the better choice.

The study, funded by the U.S. National Eye Institute (NEI), "will help doctors and their patients with diabetic macular edema choose the most appropriate therapy," study lead author John Wells, MD, said in an institute news release.

"The study suggests there is little advantage of choosing Eylea or Lucentis over [much cheaper] Avastin when a patient's loss of visual acuity from macular edema is mild, meaning a visual acuity of 20/40 or better," Dr. Wells explained.

"However, patients with 20/50 or worse vision loss may benefit from Eylea, which over the course of the two-year study outperformed Lucentis and Avastin," said Dr. Wells, a retinal specialist at the Palmetto Retina Center in Columbia, South Carolina.

ABOUT MACULAR EDEMA

As the researchers explained it, diabetic macular edema can cause fluid to leak from abnormal blood vessels in the retina. This can result in blurry vision or vision loss. Drugs used to treat the condition are injected into the eye and work by blocking a substance that can trigger the leakage.

Cost is a factor, too. Although they work in similar ways, the three drugs vary dramatically in price. Based on Medicare's pricing guidelines, the per-injection cost for Eylea is $1,850, $1,200 for Lucentis and only $60 for Avastin, the news release noted.

STUDY DETAILS

The two-year clinical trial compared the effectiveness of the three drugs in 660 patients with diabetic macular edema.

According to Dr. Wells and colleagues, all three drugs performed similarly among participants with mild vision loss when the study began. On average, participants' vision improved from 20/40 vision to 20/25, the study showed.

"This rigorous trial confirms that Eylea, Avastin, and Lucentis are all effective treatments for diabetic macular edema," NEI director Paul Sieving, MD, PhD, said in the news release. "Eye care providers and patients can have confidence in all three drugs."

Patients with moderate to severe vision loss also reported significant improvements in their ability to see. Halfway through the study, however, Eylea outperformed Avastin and Lucentis. By the two-year mark, Eylea and Lucentis produced similar gains in vision, the team found.

The researchers reported that the average visual acuity was 20/32 to 20/40 among participants in each treatment group by the end of the study. Patients needed about the same number of injections over the course of the study, regardless of the type of drug taken.

The need for laser treatment varied. Of the patients taking Eylea, 41% needed laser treatment. In contrast, 64% of the patients in the Avastin group and 52% of those in the Lucentis group also needed laser treatment.

EXPERT COMMENTARY

Two experts said the study provides important guidance for patients and physicians.

"There are 7.7 million diabetic patients in the United States with approximately 750,000 of those suffering from diabetic macular edema," said Mark Fromer, MD, an ophthalmologist at Lenox Hill Hospital in New York City. "This study will help both retina specialists and patients alike understand the benefits of choosing these drugs in the treatment of diabetic macular edema."

Nazanin Barzideh, MD, is chief of vitreoretinal surgery at Winthrop-University Hospital in Mineola, New York. She said that the study findings were in line with her experience.

"I have seen my diabetic patients with macular edema having a better response to Elyea compared to other [similar] drugs available on the market, especially those patients with severe visual acuity," she said.

The study was published online in the journal *Ophthalmology*.

info The American Diabetes Association (*diabetes.org*) has more about eye complications associated with diabetes, including macular edema.

Drug Beats Laser Therapy for Retinopathy

Jeffrey G. Gross, MD, is an ophthalmologist at Carolina Retina Center, Columbia, South Carolina, and leader of a study of 305 patients, published in *JAMA*.

Retinopathy patients do better with Lucentis, reports Jeffrey G. Gross, MD. Proliferative diabetic retinopathy (PDR) can cause blindness. The standard treatment is laser therapy called panretinal photocoagulation (PRP), which preserves central vision but can damage night and side vision. In a study, the injected drug Lucentis (*ranibizumab*) did a better job of preserving vision, with fewer side effects, than PRP.

A Wearable Patch Might Help Manage Diabetes Painlessly

Hyunjae Lee, PhD, and Tae Kyu Choi, PhD, Seoul National University.

Richard Guy, PhD, professor, pharmaceutical sciences, University of Bath, United Kingdom.

Joel Zonszein, MD, director, Clinical Diabetes Center, Montefiore Medical Center, New York City.

Nature Nanotechnology, online

An experimental device might one day literally take the pain out of managing diabetes, Korean researchers say.

The new invention uses a patch to monitor blood sugar levels via sweat, and delivers the diabetes drug metformin through the skin with microneedles.

"Diabetics are reluctant to monitor their blood glucose levels because of the painful blood-gathering process," said study author Hyunjae Lee, PhD, from Seoul National University in the Republic of Korea. "We highly focused on a noninvasive monitoring and therapy system for diabetics."

Currently, people with diabetes have two options for monitoring blood sugar (glucose) levels, said Richard Guy, PhD, who wrote an accompanying editorial in the journal. He's a professor of pharmaceutical sciences at the University of Bath in the United Kingdom.

One option is a blood glucose meter that requires a finger stick to draw out a drop of blood for testing. The other option is continuous glucose monitoring, which requires that a sensor be placed underneath the skin and worn constantly. Both of these options are invasive and can be painful.

Previously, a less invasive product called GlucoWatch pulled fluid through the skin to the device to measure blood sugar levels. However, that device was never commercially successful and was taken off the market, Dr. Guy said.

ABOUT THE NEW DIABETES PATCH

The Korean research team used a substance called graphene to develop a thin, flexible patch. Graphene conducts electricity, and can be transparent, soft and very thin, the researchers explained.

The patch also contains a variety of sensors that detect humidity, sweat glucose levels, pH and temperature, the researchers said. In addition, the patch contains heat-sensitive microneedles.

The patch uses sweat to determine "sweat glucose," which can be used to figure out blood glucose levels.

Dr. Lee said the accuracy of the sweat glucose sensor is similar to that of home blood glucose meters in the United States.

Dr. Guy pointed out that someone who sweats a lot might pose a challenge for the patch.

But the researchers said they've already taken this into consideration. "We integrated a humidity sensor in the diabetes patch to check how much sweat is generated. So the person who perspires heavily wouldn't affect the sensing," said Tae Kyu Choi, another study author from Seoul National University.

Likewise, Dr. Choi said, the researchers accounted for someone who perspires very lightly.

STUDY DETAILS

The researchers tested the glucose-sensing ability of the patch in two humans and found the device was able to accurately measure blood sugar levels.

In the current version of the patch, the researchers used microneedles to deliver the dia-

blood sugar levels are as often as people with type 1 diabetes.

The researchers said their next step is to improve the long-term stability and accuracy of the blood glucose sensor. Drs. Lee and Choi estimated it would be at least five years before they could solve any remaining obstacles and commercialize the device.

Diabetes Drugs Can Cause Severe Arthritis Pain

Certain diabetes drugs may cause debilitating arthritis that results in joint pain. The four medications—*alogliptin* (Nesina), *linagliptin* (Tradjenta), *saxagliptin* (Onglyza) and *sitagliptin* (Januvia)—belong to a relatively new class of medications called dipeptidyl peptidase-4 (DPP-4) inhibitors. If you experience severe, persistent joint pain, consult your physician. Do not stop taking the drug on your own.

Osama Hamdy, MD, PhD, is director of the inpatient diabetes program at Joslin Diabetes Center, Harvard Medical School, Boston, and coauthor of *The Diabetes Breakthrough*.

Is Type 1 Diabetes Linked to Raised Risk of Certain Cancers?

Sarah Wild, PhD, professor, epidemiology, University of Edinburgh, United Kingdom.
Diabetologia

Having type 1 diabetes may raise the risk of some cancers, but lower the risk of others, a new study suggests.

A higher risk was seen for cancers of the stomach, liver, pancreas, endometrium, ovary and kidneys. But a reduced risk was seen for prostate and breast cancers, researchers reported.

"This pattern of cancer risk [seen in the study] is similar to that seen for people with type 2 diabetes and people who are overweight," said Sarah Wild, PhD, a professor of epidemiology at the University of Edinburgh in the United Kingdom. "This suggests that insulin treatment for type 1 diabetes does not itself increase risk of cancer."

And, Dr. Wild pointed out, the new findings only show an association between type 1 diabetes and an increased risk for cancer, not that type 1 diabetes is a direct cause of the increased risk.

betes drug metformin to mice. Over six hours, the drug—delivered through the skin—was able to drop blood sugar levels from 400 milligrams per deciliter to 120 milligrams per deciliter, the researchers said. For someone without diabetes, a normal blood sugar level taken randomly would generally be under 125 milligrams per deciliter, according to the U.S. National Library of Medicine.

Insulin—the hormone necessary to lower blood sugar for people with type 1 diabetes—wasn't used because it's a protein that would be difficult to deliver through microneedles because it's large, and it would be vulnerable to the heating process that allows the drug to be delivered through the skin, the study authors explained.

But, Dr. Guy said he expects that should this system go forward in development, other drugs that can lower blood sugar more effectively might be considered. "I think metformin was chosen as an example of a drug used in diabetics for the illustration of proof-of-concept," he said.

The researchers said they believe the device could be used by either type 1 or type 2 diabetics.

EXPERT REACTION

However, Joel Zonszein, MD, director of the Clinical Diabetes Center at Montefiore Medical Center in New York City, said the cost of the device might make it very impractical for people with type 2 diabetes. And, he said, people with type 2 diabetes don't have to know what their

STUDY DETAILS

For the study, Dr. Wild and her colleagues collected data from national registries on more than 9,000 cancers among people with type 1 diabetes from Australia, Denmark, Finland, Scotland and Sweden. They compared people with type 1 diabetes to people in the general population of each country.

Type 1 diabetes was linked to a 23% higher risk of stomach cancer for men and a 78% higher risk for women, the study found. For liver cancer, the risk for men with type 1 diabetes was doubled, while it was 55% higher for women, the study authors said.

However, women with type 1 diabetes were 10% less likely to develop breast cancer, Dr. Wild said.

Because many of these cancers are rare, the actual risk is slight, Dr. Wild added.

Also, the risk for cancer appeared to be highest shortly after diagnosis of type 1 diabetes, she said. During the first year after a diabetes diagnosis, the cancer risk was more than doubled for both men and women. The longer someone had type 1 diabetes, the lower the odds of cancer diagnosis, she said.

After about 20 years, the cancer risk dropped to that of the general population for men. For women, it took only five years for the cancer risk to drop to almost normal, the study found.

The reported elevated cancer risk soon after type 1 diabetes diagnosis may owe to the detection of pre-existing cancers, the researchers suggested.

Although type 1 diabetes hasn't been linked to lifestyle factors like type 2 diabetes has, Dr. Wild noted that lifestyle changes might help reduce cancer risk.

"Lifestyle changes to reduce cancer risk—such as avoiding smoking, [and improving] weight management and physical activity—are important for people with type 1 diabetes, particularly because several of the cancers are ones where these factors affect risk," Dr. Wild said.

The report findings were published in the journal *Diabetologia*.

Diabetes Heart Helper

Bryan Williams, MD, is chair of medicine at University College London (UCL) and director of UCL Hospitals National Institutes for Health Research, both in London, England.

Blood pressure drugs help diabetics even if they don't have high blood pressure. Each decrease of 10 mm Hg in systolic pressure (top number) decreases the risk for stroke and heart disease in diabetes patients by 27% and 12%, respectively. People with systolic pressure higher than 140 mm Hg had the greatest reduction—but people with lower numbers also benefited.

New Transplant Technique Might Free Type 1 Diabetics from Daily Injections

Julia Greenstein, PhD, vice president, discovery research, JDRF.
Daniel Anderson, PhD, Samuel A. Goldblith Associate Professor, chemical engineering, Massachusetts Institute of Technology, Cambridge, Massachusetts.
Nature Medicine, online.
Nature Biotechnology, online.

Using a two-pronged approach, researchers report they were able to restore normal blood sugar levels for six months in mice with induced diabetes.

But, while the research is promising, it's too soon for people with type 1 diabetes to start planning a life free of needles and injections just yet, experts said.

The first part of the treatment was using insulin-producing pancreas cells generated from human stem cells employing a technique recently developed at Harvard. But the latest breakthrough came from MIT researchers, who developed a way to encapsulate the cells—called islet cells—before they were implanted in the mice, to protect them from the immune system.

That's key for two reasons. One is that when you introduce foreign cells into the body, the immune system recognizes them as foreign and destroys them. This is why people who have organ transplants need to take immune-suppressing medications, which can cause serious side effects.

The second reason is that type 1 diabetes develops when the body's immune system mistakenly attacks healthy islet cells and destroys them—known as an autoimmune attack. When people have had islet cell transplant, the new cells eventually die off, and researchers suspect one reason why is that the autoimmune attack doesn't stop.

However, the encapsulation hides the islet cells, essentially making them invisible to the immune system, the researchers explained.

IMPLICATIONS

"They're stealth islets," said Julia Greenstein, PhD, vice president of discovery research for JDRF, a type 1 diabetes research foundation that provided funding for the study along with the Helmsley Charitable Trust and the U.S. National Institutes of Health.

"We're really excited about this. It's been a long and big effort for us to try to drive novel biomaterials," she added.

There are still a number of steps before a human trial could be done, such as scaling up the capsules for larger animals, and seeing whether or not the encapsulated islet cells can achieve blood sugar control in non-human primates, Dr. Greenstein said.

But, if all goes well, both Dr. Greenstein and the senior researcher on the project, Daniel Anderson, PhD, an associate professor of chemical engineering at the Massachusetts Institute of Technology in Cambridge, Massachusetts, predict that phase 1 clinical trials in people might just be a few years away.

CHAPTER 7

Diet, Nutrition and Fitness

Want to Lose Weight? Stop Dieting!

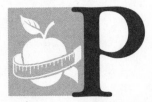

People go on a diet (or watch their weight) for a variety of reasons— to keep their hearts healthy…to avoid diabetes and other chronic diseases…or simply to look better.

But clearly something isn't working. More than two-thirds of American adults are overweight or obese. The average American dieter makes up to five weight-loss attempts a year— but within a year, two-thirds of dieters regain all of the weight that they lost…and more than 95% gain it back within five years.

Why are so many people losing the battle of the bulge?

AVOIDING THE NOT-SO-OBVIOUS TRAPS

The truth is, if we all stuck to healthful, whole foods—such as vegetables, fruits, lean meats and fish and nuts—far fewer people would ever have to go on a "diet." Have you ever seen anyone eat too much broccoli? But sticking to this principle of eating whole (not processed) foods isn't always easy. *So here are the other steps I recommend to prevent out-of-control eating…*

•**Downsize your dishes.** Have you noticed that serving dishes have gotten larger? A generation ago, the standard dinner plate was 10 inches…now it's 12 inches, and it's human nature to fill that extra real estate with bigger portions.

Even nutrition experts, who know all about these dangers, can be fooled by the so-called Delboeuf illusion, in which a food portion can seem large or small, depending on the empty space that surrounds it.

A fascinating study: Nutrition experts were given either a small bowl or a large one, along with an ice cream scoop. Those given the larger bowls took 31% more ice cream than those with

John M. Kennedy, MD, a clinical associate professor of cardiology at Harbor-UCLA Medical Center in Los Angeles, director of preventive cardiology and wellness at Marina Del Rey Hospital and founder of Encardia Wellness, a health, wellness and fitness consultancy in San Francisco. He is the author of *The Heart Health Bible: The 5-Step Plan to Prevent and Reverse Heart Disease.*

the smaller ones. The big bowl made the large serving appear "normal"—even to those who should know better.

What to do: To avoid the Delboeuf illusion, use smaller plates and bowls. Not worth the effort?

Consider this: Research shows that going from 12-inch plates to 10-inch plates reduces caloric intake by 22%.

Where to find 10-inch dinner plates: Bed Bath & Beyond…and Walmart. For fun colors in plates this size, go to *Zak.com* or *CB2.com*.

Also helpful: Some people notice that they also eat less if they start using chopsticks…or hold utensils with their nondominant hand.

•**Go with single-serves.** A study published in the journal *Appetite* found that men ate up to 37% more (women 18% more) when food came in bigger bags.

Single-serve bags typically contain one to two ounces. Admittedly, that's not very much. But if you're going to indulge now and then by having, say, potato chips, a single-serve portion has about 150 calories. Think how much more you'd get by dipping your hand repeatedly into an oversized bag!

Also helpful: If you decide to save money with bigger packages, pour the amount that you want to eat into a bowl…and don't go back for refills. To cut the compulsion to go back for another serving, take a few sips of lemon water to break the cycle of wanting to eat more.

•**Slow down.** It takes roughly 20 minutes for chemical signals of fullness to reach the brain. People who eat quickly tend to get more calories than they need—or even want.

Scientific evidence: When researchers instructed participants to either rush through a meal or take their time, the slow eaters (who took small bites, chewed their food well and put down their forks between bites) consumed 88 fewer calories. They also reported that they felt less hungry than when they ate more quickly.

What helps: When eating a meal, set a timer (or an alarm on your cell phone) for 20 minutes and pace your eating so that it takes that much time to finish.

•**Watch what you're watching!** You may know that television leads to "mindless eating"—

one study found that adults who ate pizza while watching TV consumed 36% more calories than those listening to music. The reason? They were too distracted to notice what they were doing—or when they were full. But new research shows that some types of viewing are worse than others. Action movies and sad movies are more likely to trigger distracted and/or emotional eating than more sedate viewing choices.

What helps: To avoid excessive eating when watching a movie or TV, especially an action movie or a tearjerker, sit down with some crunchy veggies instead of a bowl of buttery popcorn or other snacks.

Odd Secret to Staying Slim

Karen Larson, editor, *Bottom Line Personal*, with Marcia C. de Oliveira Otto, PhD.

I eat the same breakfast every morning—plain Greek yogurt with wild blueberries and a sprinkling of walnuts. That unvaried menu might strike you as unexciting, but it turns out my monotonous morning meals could be helping me keep off pounds.

Many people believe that it's perfectly fine to eat whatever they want as long as they don't eat too much of any treat—overindulgence is considered the enemy, not the unhealthy foods themselves. But a recent study cast serious doubt on this "everything in moderation" consumption philosophy. When researchers tracked the diets of more than 6,000 people, they found that after five years of follow-up, the waist circumferences of people who ate very varied diets increased at more than double the rate of the waistlines of people who ate the same foods frequently.

When the researchers dug deeper into the data, they discovered a potential explanation—people who eat a wide variety of foods tell themselves it's OK to have a piece of cake as long as they have only a thin slice. Those people might be right, too—except that they make the same rationalization with a single scoop of ice cream…a few pieces of candy…a snack-size bag of chips…a small soda, etc.

No Single Weight-Loss Diet Is Right for Everyone

Each person's body responds differently to identical foods. This means Atkins, Paleo, Dukan and other diets won't work for all those who try them.

Example: Bread and rice cause blood sugar increases in some people but not in others. A regimen such as the Mediterranean diet—which includes tomatoes—may be a poor choice for some people because tomatoes cause blood sugar levels to surge in certain individuals.

Study of 800 people's response to 46,898 meals by researchers at Weizmann Institute, Rehovot, Israel, published in Cell.

In theory, the solution is to eat a diverse diet and skew it toward healthy items. But according to Marcia C. de Oliveira Otto, PhD, an assistant professor at The University of Texas Health Science Center and lead author of the study, the greater the difference among foods a person consumes regularly, the more difficult it becomes for that person to eat a healthy diet even if he/she truly tries to eat healthfully.

Otto's advice: Find a few healthy foods you really like, and stick with them.

Better Breakfast

Candida Rebello, MS, RD, researcher, Louisiana State University School of Nutrition & Food Sciences, Baton Rouge.

Want to eat less at lunch? Choose oatmeal for breakfast.

Recent study: Volunteers who ate a bowl of hot instant oatmeal with skim milk reported feeling fuller longer and ate significantly less at lunch than on the days that they ate a breakfast of cold, oat-based cereal and skim milk.

Explanation: Although both the oatmeal and cold cereal consumed in the study had the same number of calories, oatmeal has more fiber, which increases satiety.

Eat This Plus That!

Tonia Reinhard, MS, RD, registered dietitian and professor at Wayne State University, Detroit. She is the program director for the Coordinated Program in Dietetics, codirector of clinical nutrition in the Wayne State University School of Medicine and past president of the Michigan Dietetic Association. She is author of Superfoods: The Healthiest Foods on the Planet *and* Superjuicing: More Than 100 Nutritious Vegetable and Fruit Recipes.

Well-chosen food pairings do more than just excite your taste buds. Consuming certain food combos or food and drink combos creates a synergy that increases the absorption of important nutrients and phytochemicals.

Here are four supercharged combinations…

FISH + WINE

The American Heart Association recommends eating fish at least twice a week. The omega-3 fatty acids in fish have been shown to reduce triglycerides, irregular heartbeats and blood pressure and slow the growth of arterial plaques. It turns out that wine can boost those omega-3 levels.

A large European study looked at the dietary habits and alcohol consumption of more than 1,600 people. The participants underwent comprehensive medical exams and gave blood samples that were used to measure omega-3 levels. Their amount of "marine food intake," defined as the total intake of fish, shellfish, cuttlefish, squid, octopus, shrimp and crab, was also measured.

The researchers found that people who drank moderate amounts of alcohol (one daily drink for women and two for men) had higher concentrations of omega-3s than nondrinkers, despite consuming similar amounts of marine food. Wine drinkers had the biggest gains, but people who drank beer or spirits (such as Scotch) also showed an increase in omega-3s.

Important caveat: The study found that heavy drinkers had lower amounts of omega-3s.

LEMON + TEA

Both black and green teas contain catechins, a group of antioxidants that are surprisingly good for cardiovascular health. A study published in *Stroke,* which looked at more than 83,000 Japanese adults, found that those who drank two to three cups of green tea daily were 14% less likely to have a stroke than those who rarely drank tea.

Tea has been found to reduce cholesterol and reduce the risk for cancer, diabetes and heart disease. But there's a catch—the catechins in tea aren't very durable. They tend to break down during digestion, leaving behind less than 20% of the active compounds.

Tasty solution: Add a squeeze of lemon to your tea. A laboratory study published in *Molecular Nutrition & Food Research* found that combining lemon juice with tea allowed 80% of the catechins to "survive" post-digestion. Orange, lime and grapefruit juices also stabilized the compounds, although not as much as the lemon.

If you prefer bottled to brewed tea, you'll get a similar effect by picking a product that includes vitamin C—listed as ascorbic acid on the label.

CITRUS + IRON-RICH FOODS

Low iron is common in people who take acid-suppressing drugs for GERD and in people who have gastrointestinal problems in which inflammation and bleeding occur (such as inflammatory bowel disease and bleeding ulcers).

Many foods contain iron. Iron-rich animal foods include beef, liver, oysters and sardines. Iron-rich plant foods include dark leafy greens such as spinach, kale and collard greens…beans…lentils…whole grains…and nuts. But iron is not the easiest mineral to absorb. The body can absorb only 2% to 20% of the non-heme iron in plant foods. The absorption of the heme iron from meats and fish/shellfish is better but still not great—typically between 15% and 35%. And certain supplements such as calcium can interfere with iron absorption.

How can you boost absorption of iron? By eating citrus fruits or other vitamin C–rich foods such as strawberries and yellow and red peppers with heme or non-heme foods.

Examples: Add orange slices to your kale salad…or yellow peppers to your beef stew. One study found that consuming as little as 63 mg of vitamin C (a little more than the amount in one orange) nearly tripled the absorption of non-heme iron.

FAT + SALAD

Salads are rich in carotenoids—antioxidants such as lutein, lycopene and beta-carotene that reduce your risk for cancer and heart disease, preserve bone density and prevent macular degeneration. A fat-based salad dressing can maximize the absorption of these carotenoids (so avoid fat-free salad dressings). Researchers at Purdue University served participants salads with dressings made from a monounsaturated fat (canola oil)…a polyunsaturated fat (soybean oil)…or a saturated fat (butter). All the fats boosted absorption of the carotenoids, but the monounsaturated fat required the least amount of fat to get the most carotenoid absorption. Another monounsaturated fat often found in salad dressings is olive oil.

You can get similar benefits by adding hard-boiled eggs to your salad. The fat from the yolks will increase your absorption of carotenoids. In a Purdue University study published in *The American Journal of Nutrition,* participants who ate a salad with one-and-a-half eggs had double the carotenoid absorption of people who had a salad with no eggs.

Awesome Avocados: New Ways to Enjoy This Tasty Superfood

Janet Bond Brill, PhD, RDN, FAND, is a registered dietitian nutritionist, a fellow of the Academy of Nutrition and Dietetics and a nationally recognized nutrition, health and fitness expert who specializes in cardiovascular disease prevention. Based in Allentown, Pennsylvania, Dr. Brill is the author of *Blood Pressure DOWN, Cholesterol DOWN* and *Prevent a Second Heart Attack.* DrJanet.com

With their silky texture, great flavor and numerous nutrients, you gotta love avocados! Technically a fruit, avocados are a potassium dynamo (one avocado contains more than twice as much blood pressure–lowering potassium as a banana). They also provide a variety of other minerals and vitamins, such as B vitamins, vitamin E and copper, and are packed with super-heart-healthy monounsaturated fat. If the only way you've ever eaten an avocado is sliced up in a salad or as guacamole, think again. These creamy gems are incredibly versatile and can be used in an array of tasty recipes. *Several different ways to use avocados plus some recipes to try…*

•**Grilled.** To grill an avocado, slice it in half, twist to pull apart and remove the pit, but leave the skin on. Brush the avocado flesh with a touch of extra-virgin olive oil and a spritz of fresh lime juice. Then place cut side down on a stovetop grill or an outdoor grill for five to seven minutes. Scoop out the flesh or serve in the skin as a tasty, warm side dish.

•**In a salsa.** Avocado salsa is a great topping.

To make: Toss one diced avocado with one diced fresh tomato and one-third cup of chopped red onion. Then drizzle with extra-virgin olive oil and fresh-squeezed lime juice, and season with salt and pepper. Spoon over your favorite grilled fish or a Mexican entrée.

•**As a substitute for mayo.** To replace artery-clogging saturated fat with a tasty healthy fat, try using ripe avocado in place of mayo on a sandwich or butter on bread. You can also make a heart-healthy green goddess salad dressing by using a ripe avocado instead of mayo and sour cream.

Ingredients: 1 cup of fresh spinach leaves…2 scallions…1 avocado…1 garlic clove…2 Tablespoons of white wine vinegar…2 Tablespoons of lemon juice…1 Tablespoon of olive oil…1 Tablespoon of fresh tarragon, chopped (or dried tarragon)…½ teaspoon of black pepper.

What to do: Put all the ingredients in a food processor or blender and mix until smooth. It's a delicious dressing for potato salad or dip for veggies.

•**In ceviche.** This delicious, easy-to-make ceviche (a cold seafood dish) features two avocados plus cilantro for zest.

Ingredients: 1 pound of cooked shrimp (peeled, deveined and chopped)…2 avocados, chopped (about 1 cup)…½ red onion,

chopped…¼ cup of fresh cilantro, minced…¼ cup of lime juice…½ teaspoon of ground black pepper…¼ teaspoon of salt.

What to do: Mix all the ingredients together in a large bowl. Chill in the refrigerator for one hour. Serve with sliced bell peppers and/or cucumbers and pita chips or whole-wheat crackers.

Yield: 16 servings (1 serving = ⅛ cup).

•**In desserts.** Bet you didn't know that you can use avocado as a substitute for butter or oil in your favorite baked goods and desserts. One-half cup of puréed ripe avocado equals about one-half cup of butter. You can also use it to make a sinfully rich, heart-healthy dark-chocolate pudding.

Ingredients: 1 avocado…1 banana…⅓ cup of honey (or agave syrup)…⅓ cup of unsweetened, dark cocoa powder…¼ cup of peanut butter (or substitute any nut or seed butter).

What to do: Put all the ingredients in a food processor or blender and mix until the pudding is smooth.

Yield: 6 servings (1 serving = ⅓ cup).

Coconut Oil May Be Healthier Than GMO Soybean Oil

Poonam Jot Deol, PhD, researcher and assistant project scientist at the department of cell biology, University of California, Riverside, in the laboratory of Frances M. Sladek, PhD. Her study was presented at the annual meeting of The Endocrine Society in San Diego.

You know that trans fats are out…so no more partially hydrogenated soybean oil. But in recent years, the food industry has genetically engineered soybean oil to be more like healthful olive oil. It's "shelf stable" (exactly what "Big Food" wants) without hydrogenation, so no trans fats. And it's appearing in more and more of the food you buy. But is soybean oil that's made to be more like olive oil good for you? Better than coconut oil? New research focuses on the possible effects on weight gain and diabetes, two emerging concerns with our cooking oils. The answers may surprise you...and motivate a quick oil change in your kitchen.

The latest approach is to genetically modify soybean oil so that it contains more oleic acid—the monounsaturated fatty acid found in large amounts in olive oil—to make a healthier, inexpensive, shelf-stable oil. What if this new GMO soybean oil weren't just good for business but also good for health?

SOYBEAN OIL COMES UNDER FIRE

Soybean oil, while relatively new to the human diet, is now the predominant oil in American food. It's everywhere, from salad dressings to baked goods to condiments and snacks—not to mention that big bottle of soybean cooking oil that you may have on your kitchen shelf. It's cheap (no wonder it's everywhere). But because regular soybean oil is so high in polyunsaturated fats, it goes rancid quickly. Hydrogenation, which keeps it from going rancid but creates trans fats, was a major health fiasco. Even without the trans problem, regular soybean oil has been losing some of its healthful glow in some circles. Some researchers have even suggested that soybean oil in general, and its primary fat linoleic acid in particular, may be contributing to obesity and diabetes.

A GENETICALLY MODIFIED...BUST

To look at these health questions, researchers fed mice one of four diets for six months. One was a very low-fat diet (5% of calories) known to minimize weight gain and reduce diabetes factors. It was compared with high-fat diets (40% of calories) rich in regular soybean oil, high-oleic-acid GMO soybean oil or coconut oil.

Result: The mice fed either kind of soybean oil gained significantly more weight, had fattier livers and had more glucose intolerance (a diabetes risk factor) than either controls or coconut oil eaters. Those fed GMO soybean oil gained less weight and had less insulin resistance (another diabetes risk factor) than those fed regular soybean oil—good news for the bioengineered stuff—but the effects on weight and the liver

were still negative. Maybe it's something in soybean oil other than linoleic acid that's a problem, the researchers speculate.

The coconut oil–fed mice did better, gaining only slightly more weight than controls on the super-low-fat diet. Researcher Poonam Jot Deol, PhD, from the department of cell biology and neuroscience at University of California at Riverside, explained that coconut oil contains medium-chain fatty acids that are metabolized more quickly than other fatty acids, so it may contribute less to weight gain, including belly fat.

WHAT SHOULD YOU DRIZZLE AND POUR?

This study has nothing to do with GMO issues, since almost all soybean oil in this country is already GMO. And the study results have nothing to do with soy foods in general. They are nutritionally very different from the highly processed oils extracted from soybeans.

Nor does this study mean that you should leap on the coconut oil bandwagon yet. Coconut oil is high in saturated fat, and while healthier than we once thought, it's not a perfect oil.

What's best for your kitchen? The researchers themselves believe that coconut oil is a healthy choice, and that extra-virgin olive oil may be even healthier. The researchers used coconut oil in this study because it's naturally low in linoleic acid, making the study design easier, but they plan to compare olive oil with GMO-modified soybean oil in their next study. Extra-virgin olive oil is not only rich in oleic acid and low in linoleic acid, but is also extracted under low-heat conditions that preserve healthful antioxidant compounds.

Dr. Deol's personal recommendations? Cook at home more, so you are in control of what you eat...use olive oil or coconut oil...and be conscious of the amount of fat or oil you use. Too much of even a "good" oil is still too much.

Good-for-You Comfort Food

Laura Cipullo, RD, CDE, a registered dietitian and certified diabetes educator in private practice in New York City. Cipullo is the author of *The Diabetes Comfort Food Diet* and is president of the New York chapter of the International Association of Eating Disorders Professionals.

As a health-conscious reader, you probably know that limiting carb intake while increasing fiber and reducing saturated fat is a healthful eating plan to follow. But you're human, and it can be oh, so hard to resist carbohydrate-laden, high-calorie comfort foods like creamy mashed potatoes and rich pasta dishes.

Good news: With a few smart tweaks and swaps, you can enjoy even the most decadent-sounding comfort foods without sabotaging your health. *Here's how...*

•**Get the right amount of carbohydrates.** You don't need to eliminate carbs entirely, you just need to eat the right amount, which is probably more than you think.

Research shows that even people with diabetes who eat small, consistent amounts of carbohydrates with every meal or snack as opposed to eating excessive carbs at each meal or eating them once a day have better control of their blood sugar levels and body weight. However, the average woman who has prediabetes or diabetes should moderate carb intake to about 45 g per meal and men should have no more than about 60 g per meal. (A health-care provider can help adjust amounts based on individual needs.) The allowance is more generous for those who don't have diabetes, but everyone can benefit from sticking to these guidelines.

Some foods with 45 g of carbs: One cup of brown rice...one and a half English muffins. Not too stingy!

•**Fiber is your secret weapon.** Fiber—especially the soluble kind—takes longer to metabolize than other carbs, so it improves blood sugar control and lowers insulin resistance in

Note: The recipes in this article were developed for people with diabetes, but those who don't have diabetes and people with other conditions can benefit as well.

both people who have diabetes and those who don't. Consistently getting the right amount of fiber can even lessen (or in some instances, eliminate) the need for diabetes medication. The American Diabetes Association recommends that women consume at least 25 g of fiber per day...men should get a minimum of 38 g daily. But aim for 44 g to 50 g a day to reap the health benefits above. Whole grains, beans, fruits and vegetables are all naturally high in fiber.

•**Don't forget healthy fats.** Replacing saturated fats and trans fats with monounsaturated fatty acids (MUFAs), such as olive oil, canola oil, peanut oil, nuts, nut butters and avocado, helps lower total and LDL "bad" cholesterol levels, improves the function of blood vessels and benefits insulin levels and blood sugar control.

The following are healthful comfort foods that meet the goals above...

CREAMY MASHED POTATOES

Instead of mashed potatoes loaded with saturated fat from butter, enjoy these mashed potatoes made with yogurt and a surprise ingredient...

What to do: In a large pot, combine 1 pound of peeled or unpeeled (I like to leave the peels on for extra fiber and nutrients) and halved russet (baking) potatoes and 1 small head of cauliflower, cut into florets. Cover with water, bring to a boil, then reduce heat to medium and simmer for 20 minutes, or until the potatoes and cauliflower are easily pierced with a fork. Drain and place in a large bowl with ⅓ cup of vegetable broth and 2 tablespoons of olive oil. Using an electric mixer on medium speed, beat until creamy. Add ½ cup of plain nonfat Greek yogurt and beat until just blended. Try adding garlic or rosemary if you desire. Makes six servings.

Traditional recipe: 250 calories per serving, 5 g saturated fat, 2 g fiber, 39 g carbs.

New recipe above: 132 calories, 1 g saturated fat, 3 g fiber, 19 g carbs.

Why it's good for you: The addition of cauliflower is a sneaky-but-healthy nutrition hack—cauliflower delivers more fiber than potatoes, while cutting the carb content of this dish in half! Plus, a 2014 study in *BMJ* offered further proof that diets high in produce are associated with lower risk for death, particularly cardiovascular mortality. Olive oil is a great source of MUFAs, and the yogurt adds creaminess and even a little protein while curbing carbs.

BROCCOLI PENNE

Instead of white, blood sugar–spiking pasta with high-fat alfredo sauce, have this healthful broccoli pasta dish with mozzarella…

What to do: Cook 6 ounces of multigrain penne pasta in boiling water. Add 2 cups of fresh broccoli florets to the pot during the last two minutes of cooking. Drain the pasta and broccoli, reserving ½ cup of the water. In a large bowl, place the pasta, broccoli, 1 cup of halved grape tomatoes, 6 ounces of fresh, part-skim mozzarella cheese cubed, ¼ cup of pesto sauce and 1 tablespoon of lemon juice. Add the reserved pasta water to the bowl, one tablespoon at a time, stirring gently until the ingredients are combined. Makes four servings.

Tip: Cook the pasta al dente (just until firm). Longer cooking times break down starches, which causes more carbohydrates to be absorbed into your blood, resulting in a faster rise in blood sugar.

Traditional recipe: 800 calories per serving, 30 g saturated fat, 4 g fiber, 69 g carbs.

New recipe above: 341 calories, 5 g saturated fat, 5 g fiber, 34 g carbs.

Why it's good for you: A 2015 study confirmed what we already knew—diets rich in whole grains protect against diabetes, while diets rich in refined carbohydrates like conventional white pasta increase risk. High-fiber broccoli and tomatoes fill you up, which enables you to halve the amount of pasta in this recipe. Flavorful olive oil–based pesto means you can pass on the alfredo sauce—full of artery-clogging saturated fat—and get a dose of MUFAs instead. (***Surprising:*** Multigrain pasta contains MUFAs, too.) Ideally, make your own pesto using fresh basil, Parmesan cheese, olive oil, crushed garlic and pine nuts. If you're using store-bought pesto, choose a local brand, which is more likely to have high-quality ingredients and fewer preservatives than a big-box brand. Grilled chicken or trout goes well with this pasta dish.

Want to Feel Less Hungry? Cut Back on Red Meat

Study titled "Adipocyte iron regulates leptin and food intake" by researchers at Wake Forest Baptist Medical Center, Salem, North Carolina, published in Journal of Clinical Investigation.

Too much dietary iron—common in diets that are heavy in red meat—stimulates the hormone leptin and boosts appetite, finds a new study from Wake Forest.

Whole Grains You Haven't Tried Yet— Some Are Gluten-Free

Julie Miller Jones, PhD, CNS, LN, certified nutrition specialist and licensed nutritionist, and distinguished scholar and professor emerita of food and nutrition, St. Catherine University, St. Paul. She regularly writes and lectures about whole grains and dietary fiber.

You know that you're supposed to eat whole grains, but many people just don't like whole-wheat pasta, whole-wheat bread or whole-wheat anything. To make sure you're eating enough whole grains, offer your taste buds more variety.

Here's what some recent studies found…

•**People who ate three or more servings of whole grains and less than one serving of refined grains** (white bread, cookies, etc.) daily averaged 10% less belly fat—linked to cardiovascular disease and diabetes—compared with people who ate the fewest whole grains and the most refined grains.

•**People who consumed the most fiber,** primarily from whole grains, were 22% less likely to die during a nine-year study than those who ate the least fiber. Fiber's protective effect was particularly pronounced in women.

•**Two recent analyses from Johns Hopkins** showed that those eating the most dietary fiber had a lower risk for death from any cause than those eating the least. For every additional 10 grams of dietary fiber, there was a 10% reduction in risk for death from any cause.

•In a Harvard study, compared with people who rarely ate whole grains, those who ate the equivalent of one bowl of oatmeal daily had a 9% reduced risk for early death...and for each additional daily ounce of whole grains, that risk was reduced by another 5%.

The problem is, fewer than 5% of Americans consume the USDA-recommended minimum of about three ounces of whole grains per day. What's the big deal? Whole grain contains the entire edible part of a grain (a.k.a., "seed")—including the germ (technically the sprout of a new plant)...endosperm (the seed's energy storehouse)...and nutrient-rich bran (the seed's outer layer). Refined grains, on the other hand, are stripped of their bran and germ layers during milling.

Enriched refined grains, however, can have a place in a healthy diet—minerals contained in the grains can be better absorbed from an enriched product than one with a lot of fiber and bran. And if a whole-grain pasta or bread that is partly enriched refined grains is more appealing, at least it gets you to eat some whole grains. But, the greater the variety of whole grains you eat, the better. Each whole grain brings different nutrients, fibers and phytonutrients to the table, so it is worth exploring and enjoying various types.

Lesser known but delicious whole grains can be found in supermarkets, health-food stores and online. *Check out these...*

•Amaranth provides protein, calcium, iron, phosphorus, potassium and many other nutrients. It's also free of gluten, a protein in wheat, rye and barley that can cause digestive upset in some people. When cooked, amaranth is pleasantly sticky and mild tasting.

To cook: Boil one cup of amaranth grains in two-and-a-half cups of water or broth for 20 minutes or until tender. If desired, season with herbs, pepper and a bit of olive oil. Or use milk as part of the cooking liquid and add sweet spices, such as cinnamon and cardamom. Also try amaranth flakes as a breakfast cereal... amaranth crackers... and amaranth flour, swapping it for one-third of a recipe's white flour.

•Buckwheat, a gluten-free grain, offers plenty of protein...the heart-healthy flavonoid rutin...plus bone-building magnesium and other minerals. It is strongly flavored, so serve it as a side dish paired with robust entrées, such as those made with red wine or balsamic vinegar. Cook the hulled, crushed kernels by simmering one cup of buckwheat in two cups of water for about 10 to 15 minutes (avoid overcooking so it doesn't become mushy)... then flavor with onions, mushrooms and whatever else you like.

•Kamut, the brand name for an ancient relative of wheat, provides protein, fiber, vitamin A, iron and zinc (it does contain gluten). With their nutty, buttery taste, kamut kernels make a great substitute for rice in recipes. Note that the cooking time is around 90 minutes...or you can soak the kernels overnight to reduce cooking time to about 30 minutes. Kamut flour can be used to bake bread, tortillas, cookies and more.

Recipes: Kamut.com.

•Quinoa is a tiny gluten-free grain rich in essential amino acids (protein building blocks that our bodies must get from dietary sources) as well as iron, magnesium, phosphorus, potassium and protein.

To cook: Simmer one cup of quinoa and two cups of water or broth for 15 minutes or until water is absorbed. Add cooked quinoa to omelets or soups...or combine with vegetables, nuts and spices for a tasty side dish.

•White whole wheat is an unrefined variety of wheat with a light-colored kernel. It has a lower gluten content than the red wheat used to make regular whole-wheat flour, so it produces foods with a softer texture and sweeter flavor. It provides nutrient and fiber content similar to

---

Bison Burgers Are Better

Order bison burgers instead of beef. Bison usually is grass-fed, not grain-fed, so it contains more healthful omega-3 fatty acids than beef does, and it has more iron.

Wayne Askew, PhD, professor emeritus, division of nutrition, University of Utah, Salt Lake City, quoted in *Self* magazine.

that of regular whole wheat, though it is lower in some antioxidants (which accounts for its lighter color).

In recipes: Substitute white whole-wheat flour for half of the refined flour or for all of the regular whole-wheat flour.

A Berry Potent Fruit!

Journal of Food Science.

The Ceylon gooseberry, grown in Brazil and used to make drinks and also eaten as a whole fruit, has even more antioxidant activity than blueberries, a well-known super fruit.

Super Superfood Match-Up: Collard-and-Kimchi Slaw

Debby Maugans, food writer based in Asheville, North Carolina, and author of *Small Batch Baking, Small Batch Baking for Chocolate Lovers* and *Farmer & Chef Asheville.*

Collard greens, meet kimchi. You're both in the cabbage family, but you're from very different worlds—collards are a mainstay of southern American cooking while spicy kimchi is an everyday feature on Korean tables.

Together, these two superfoods are extraordinarily nutritious. Collard greens contain cancer-fighting (and brain-building) sulphur compounds, plus fiber, calcium, iron, vitamin A and vitamin C. Kimchi, often made from Napa cabbage, has similar nutritional benefits—plus the added power of fermentation. The pickling process that creates kimchi gives rise to probiotics—healthy microorganisms that help our digestive system work better and support immunity.

The idea of combining these superfoods in one dish was inspired by Top Chef Edward Lee, who is of Korean origin and runs the award-winning restaurant 610 Magnolia in Louisville, Kentucky.

Lettuce: Red Beats Green

Lettuce is a rich source of antioxidants, including flavonoids, anthocyanins and vitamins A and C, which neutralize disease-causing free radicals in the body.

New finding: Red leaf lettuce contains antioxidants that work faster than those in green leaves.

Best: Eat a mix of different colors and types of lettuce for long-lasting (both slow and fast) absorption of antioxidants.

Usue Pérez-López, PhD, adjunct professor of plant biology and ecology, University of the Basque Country, Bilbao, Spain.

In his Appalachian home, tasting vinegary, salty braised collards reminded him that the two intensely flavored dishes have much in common. One of his signature dishes is braised collards and kimchi seasoned with country ham and onions.

The collard and kimchi slaw recipe below is a quick-and-easy vegetarian side dish. You can buy jarred kimchi in many supermarkets, and it's also widely available online. Collard greens have a milder taste than kale, but they have sturdier leaves. By slicing them thinly, and mixing with kimchi, they are delicious raw.

This dish is a perfect match for barbecued meats—either Southern or Korean!

COLLARD AND KIMCHI SLAW

Makes 3 cups
1 bunch fresh collard greens
1 cup drained kimchi, large pieces chopped
2 Tablespoons unseasoned rice vinegar
1 Tablespoon canola oil
1 teaspoon sesame oil
⅓ cup chopped roasted, unsalted almonds

Trim stems from collard greens. Stack leaves, roll up tightly, and cut the roll tightly into thin slices. Place in a large bowl, and toss with kimchi. Sprinkle with rice vinegar and oils. Toss well. Add almonds just before serving.

Warm Green Drinks

Sandra Woodruff, RD, LDN, a registered dietitian in Tallahassee, Florida, and coauthor of *The Complete Diabetes Prevention Plan*.

If you don't like to drink cold kale smoothies during the winter, there are tasty warm alternative drinks that use greens. You can enjory nourishing cozy drinks all winter long!

One way: Blend kale, apple, cucumber and ginger with hot green tea. You can also warm up your favorite smoothie recipe with hot herbal tea or hot water and lemon. You can make hot beverages in some high-speed blenders, just be sure to follow the manufacturer's safety instructions. Or toss some chopped spinach, kale or escarole into your favorite soup or stew during the last few minutes of cooking for a boost of nutrition, color and flavor. Vegetable soup is easy to make in your blender with veggies, low-sodium vegetable broth, diced onion and a dash of basil. Then heat it on the stove top or in the microwave.

"Beet" Altitude Sickness

Study titled "Acute dietary nitrate supplementation improves arterial endothelial function at high altitude: A double-blinded randomized controlled cross over study" by researchers at Norwegian University of Science and Technology, Trondheim, and Mid-Sweden University, Östersund, published in *Nitric Oxide*.

Flying up to the mountains? You may acclimatize more quickly if you drink a glass of beet juice before you board. It worked for high-altitude trekkers to Kathmandu. Beet juice's nitrates get converted quickly to nitric oxide, which improves the ability of blood vessels to get oxygen throughout the body.

Get a Bigger Health Boost from Dark Chocolate

Michael F. Roizen, MD, chief wellness officer of the Cleveland Clinic and chief medical consultant to *The Dr. Oz Show*. He is the author of *This Is Your Do-Over: The 7 Secrets to Losing Weight, Living Longer, and Getting a Second Chance at the Life You Want*.

As chief wellness officer at the Cleveland Clinic, there are two things I do every day to protect my health—I really get my heart pumping...and I eat three small pieces of 72% cacao dark chocolate!

By now, most of you know that dark chocolate offers many health benefits. Enjoying an ounce a day correlates with less depression, better heart health, fewer strokes and reduced rates of system-wide inflammation.

Latest research findings: Dark chocolate even curbs appetite and improves gut health. But which forms of chocolate and which products are the most healthful?

CACAO OR COCOA?

Lots of people get tripped up when chocolate products are labeled either cacao or cocoa. *What these terms mean...*

• **Cacao beans are what's used to make chocolate products.** These beans are brimming with polyphenols (including flavanols and

---

Mushrooms Boost Immunity

Volunteers who ate four ounces of cooked shiitake mushrooms daily for four weeks had better-functioning gamma delta T-cells and fewer inflammatory proteins in their blood—both signs of a stronger immune system. This could be because of beta-glucans, immune system boosters found in all mushrooms.

Susan S. Percival, PhD, is professor and chair, food science & human nutrition at Institute of Food and Agricultural Sciences, University of Florida, Gainesville, and leader of a study published online in *Journal of the American College of Nutrition*.

resveratrol), which act as antioxidants. Polyphenols enhance the production of artery-relaxing nitric oxide, blunt the effects of free radicals and turn on beneficial genes.

Once cacao beans have been fermented, dried and roasted, they're chopped up into cacao nibs (which are like chocolate chips minus the added sugar and fat). Cacao in this form is fairly bitter due to its high concentration of polyphenols, so manufacturers sometimes decrease the polyphenol content. The nibs are then mixed with sugar, milk and other ingredients—milk chocolate has more of these ingredients…dark chocolate has less.

Cacao nibs can also be ground into raw cacao powder, a fiber- and nutrient-rich superfood. Cacao powder often undergoes additional processing to give it a smoother taste, but this processing strips it of much of its nutrients and fiber (this is known as Dutch-processed cocoa).

Bottom line: The higher percentage of cacao beans in a chocolate product and the less processing involved, the higher the polyphenol content. To maximize the health benefits from chocolate, the key is to choose chocolate (nibs, powder or bars) with 70% or more cacao and little or no added sugar.

GET THE MOST FROM YOUR DAILY CHOCOLATE

Simple ways to maximize the health benefits from chocolate…

•**Get a boost by adding apples, walnuts and more.** Like dark chocolate, fruit is also high in polyphenols, so eating the two together is extra-healthful…plus, fruit helps to balance out the bitterness of dark chocolate, so less sugar is needed. I particularly like my chocolate with berries, orange slices or apples.

New finding: When paired, apples and dark chocolate are uniquely powerful, having been shown to lower blood pressure and inflammation. Be sure to eat organic apples (to avoid pesticides) and consume the peel of the apple, which contains the most beneficial nutrients.

Also: I often eat a small handful of walnuts with my chocolate to add a dose of heart-healthy omega-3s and protein. In fact, some chocolates come fortified with healthful ingredients such as probiotics, fruit and nuts.

Worth trying: Fantasy Candies Sweet Truth 72% Dark Chocolate Roasted Almond Bark with Probiotics ($7.50 for a four-ounce box). The company also makes cinnamon/chia and cranberry/chia dark chocolate bark.

•**Fun ways to incorporate cacao powder into your diet.** I like adding unsweetened dark cacao powder to spicy tomato sauce and to black beans seasoned with cinnamon and hot sauce.

Also: To make a heart-healthy chocolate mousse, I purée six dates, one-half avocado, four tablespoons of high-quality cacao powder and one to two teaspoons of water. It makes two delicious servings. The dates are a rich source of potassium and other minerals, and the avocado provides omega-3 fatty acids.

Good Cacao powder products: CocoaVia Unsweetened Dark Chocolate Powder, which can be mixed into skim milk, coffee or smoothies or used in the recipes above ($44.99 for 30 packs, each pack contains 375 mg of flavanols)…or Navitas Naturals Cacao Powder ($9.99 for eight ounces).

•**For snacking.** My favorite chocolate for eating by itself is Featherss Dark Chocolate. Each disk is 72% dark chocolate and just 22 calories ($18 for a 52-piece box).

More great chocolate choices: Theo 85% Dark Chocolate Black Rice Quinoa Crunch Bar ($4 for a three-ounce bar)…or Lindt 85% Cocoa Extra Dark Excellence Bar ($3.99 for a 3.5-ounce bar).

Better Than a Hot Toddy!

Sharon Palmer, RD, a registered dietitian based in Duarte, California, and the author of *The Plant-Powered Diet* and *Plant-Powered for Life*, from which the recipes in this article were adapted. Palmer is also the nutrition editor for *Today's Dietitian.* SharonPalmer.com

---

If cozying up with a steaming hot toddy is your idea of a perfect winter night, then here's some news for you. That quintessential winter drink is not exactly the healthiest choice you can make. While the hot toddy's shot of hard liquor may give an initial feeling of warmth, it actually lowers your core body temperature. Plus, the two tablespoons of honey used in many hot toddy recipes equals 34 g of sugar—or more than what's found in a Snickers bar!

To perk up your cold weather repertoire: Try one of these healthful—and tasty—hot drinks...

CHILE HOT CHOCOLATE

•**Cocoa,** the main ingredient in chocolate, is chock-full of flavonoids, plant compounds with antioxidant properties that help protect you from heart disease, cancer and neurodegenerative diseases.

In addition, the red chile used in this recipe adds a pleasant, warming spice and is rich in the anti-inflammatory compound capsaicin, which researchers are now investigating for its possible ability to help boost metabolism.

Ingredients (makes two eight-ounce servings)...

1 small, dried red chile pepper
(I like chile de arbol, a potent chile often found in Latin markets, as well as many supermarkets.)

1½ cups of unsweetened, plain plant-based milk, such as almond, rice or coconut milk (Substitute regular milk if desired.)

2 cinnamon sticks
(Or powdered cinnamon to taste.)

2 ounces of dark chocolate, coarsely grated or chopped
(The chocolate should be at least 70% cocoa with a low sugar content—less than 9 g per serving.)

1 Tablespoon of agave nectar
(This sweetener is a less processed alternative to highly refined sweeteners but should be used in moderation.)

What to do: To toast the chile, put it in a small pot and cook on medium for about one minute, until the chile begins to change color. Remove it, let it cool and grind the chile (including skin and seeds) in a blender, small food processor or spice grinder. Add the milk and cinnamon sticks to the same pot, and heat on low heat for five minutes, stirring occasionally, until hot and bubbly. Put the cinnamon sticks

aside. Add the chocolate, agave and ground chile (start with half—it's spicy, so you don't want to overdo it), stirring vigorously with a wire whisk until the chocolate is melted and the mixture is foamy. Serve piping hot with the cinnamon sticks.

HOT GINGER GREEN TEA

Green tea is good for your heart and brain, helps keep your blood sugar levels stable and has been linked to reduced risk for some types of cancer. What gives green tea all this disease-fighting muscle? You can thank the antioxidant compounds known as catechins. And if you've got an upset stomach, you're also in luck. Ginger can provide natural relief from nausea, indigestion, upset stomach and motion sickness.

Ingredients (makes one eight-ounce serving)...

1 green tea bag
2 lemon slices (Wash the lemon peel.)
2 slices of peeled ginger
1 cup boiling water
1 teaspoon of honey (optional)

What to do: Place the tea bag, lemon slices and ginger in a mug. Add hot water, and let steep for three to four minutes before straining. If desired, sweeten with honey.

PUMPKIN SPICE SOY LATTE

Pumpkin is a good source of vitamin A, which promotes healthy skin, teeth and vision...and vitamin K, which is needed for healthy blood clotting. Soy has been linked to heart health, and maple syrup provides antioxidant compounds.

To top it off, you'll get a classic gingerbread flavor from the cloves, which are rich in the anti-inflammatory compounds eugenol and beta-caryophyllene. And cinnamon may help with blood sugar levels in people with type 2 diabetes.

Ingredients (makes two eight-ounce servings)...

3 Tablespoons of canned pumpkin
½ teaspoon of cinnamon
¼ teaspoon of ground cloves
1 Tablespoon of maple syrup
¾ cup of unsweetened soy milk
1 cup of brewed espresso

(You can substitute strong coffee.)

What to do: Combine all ingredients in a small pot, and heat until bubbly.

Try This Chili Pepper Health Fix

Li Liming, MD, MPH, professor of public health, Peking University Health Science Center, China.

Adults who ate spicy foods almost every day had a 14% reduced risk for death from any cause compared with those who ate these foods less than once a week, according to a recent seven-year study of nearly 500,000 people. Most reported eating fresh and/or dried chili peppers, which have antioxidant and anti-inflammatory properties that help reduce risk for some cancers, high blood pressure and heart disease. Other research has found garlic and ginger to also be healthful spices.

Matcha Tea Can Be Super-Healthy—If You Heed This Warning

Health Insider research.

You know green tea is really good for you. Its antioxidant compounds show up in studies as protective against heart disease, diabetes, cancer, dementia, obesity and more. But you're probably not going to start drinking four or more cups every day—even 10 cups a day in some studies—like many Chinese and Japanese people do. How to get the bennies without all the cuppas?

The models at Fashion Week in New York City had a solution. Backstage, for energy and Zen balance, they sipped little shots of matcha green tea, a specific kind that contains unusually high levels of antioxidants. There's also matcha tea powder that has become today's "it" ingredient in everything from smoothies to latte to fruit pops to very, very green muffins. Matcha, it seems, is suddenly and literally on everyone's lips.

Does it deserve the hype? There's no question that it can be a very healthy beverage or even recipe ingredient. But now that it's a fad, and everyone's getting into the act, be careful about matcha products that are unhealthy—or even unsafe...because they are contaminated with heavy metals. So it pays to be matcha savvy. Here's what you need to know to safely benefit from this unique form of green tea.

GOOD STUFF IN A SMALL PACKAGE

For matcha, concentration is the name of the game. It's made from green tea, so it contains the powerful antioxidant epigallocatechin gallate (EGCG), responsible for many of green tea's health benefits, as well as the amino acid L-theanine, which has antianxiety properties (more about that in a moment).

It has about three times as much EGCG as standard brewed green tea, according to some estimates. It also has about as much caffeine as a cup of coffee.

How does matcha deliver this bioactive bounty? It's a combination of how it's grown and how it's prepared. Unlike with other varieties, a few weeks before harvest, the plant is covered from the sun, which causes it to produce more EGCG and L-theanine.

Another unusual step: After harvest, the leaves are ground into a fine powder. And matcha is also prepared differently. When you drink matcha, you're actually drinking a "suspension" of ground leaves infused in water, rather than a typical brew where leaves are steeped and then removed from the cup or pot. Hence, you are actually consuming the leaves and, along with them, more green tea compounds.

The L-theanine may be responsible for one of matcha's coveted benefits—a pleasant sense that users say it brings that may be described as "alert calmness." Credit caffeine for the alertness, of course. L-theanine, on the other hand, has been shown in studies to reduce anxiety.

MATCHA DOS—AND ONE BIG DON'T

Matcha has long been appreciated in the East. In Japan it forms part of the traditional tea ceremony and is the most revered form of tea. Because matcha involves consuming the entire tea leaf, however, the origin of any matcha powder you consume is extremely important for your safety. *Here's what you need to know...*

•**Tea plants** grown in soil that is contaminated with lead will absorb it into the leaves, and, because you are consuming the entire leaf, more lead may wind up in your cup. In one study from the research organization ConsumerLab, tea grown in China had high lead concentrations.

•**Your best bet—stick to matcha teas grown in Japan,** and look for brands that report consistent testing for the presence of heavy metals. In the ConsumerLab's study, for example, the one tea tested that came from Japan, Teavana, had no detectable lead.

•**The highest-quality matcha comes from the southern regions of Japan—**Kyushu, Nishio, Shizuoka and Uji.

•**Good-quality matcha is bright, vivid green and will have a find powdery consistency—**anything yellowish or coarse is not likely to taste very good.

•**Expect to pay about $26 to $32 for a standard 30-gram tin (about an ounce).** Anything cheaper is not likely to have good flavor.

•**One cup of matcha calls for about one gram of dry powder,** so a 30-gram tin should give you a cup of matcha tea every day for a month. (You can get a special measuring spoon from a matcha supplier, along with a whisk to prepare the tea in a bowl.)

•**Now that matcha has become popular in the US,** some prepared versions may have plenty of added sugar. Skip them, and make the real thing yourself.

•**Ready to try it?** Kenko Tea, an Australian brand that gets its matcha from the Nishio region of Japan and ships worldwide has a quick video tutorial on how to prepare tea at *kenotea.com. au.* Other reputable brands include DoMatcha, and MidoriSpring.

So go ahead, enjoy your own tea ceremony. Matcha has a grassy, slightly bitter flavor...some people compare it to that of kale or spinach. You can try it the traditional way or experiment with adding the powder to recipes. Just remember that tossing matcha into your 1,000-calorie ice cream milkshake doesn't suddenly turn it into a health drink!

The Vitamin D Debate

Michael F. Holick, PhD, MD, director of the Vitamin D, Skin and Bone Research Laboratory at Boston University Medical Center and author of *The Vitamin D Solution.*

Low blood levels of vitamin D have been linked to many diseases including osteoporosis, heart disease, cancer, type 2 diabetes, Alzheimer's and autoimmune diseases.

But what about recent headlines declaring that high blood levels of vitamin D can cause heart disease? They were based on a study published in *The Journal of Clinical Endocrinology & Metabolism,* which showed that people with high levels of vitamin D (25-hydroxy-vitamin D) were 30% more likely to die of a heart attack, heart failure or stroke.

As I wrote in a recent paper in the journal *Nutrients,* citing 49 studies that involved millions of people, vitamin D toxicity is rare. Yes, high levels increase calcium and phosphate, which can damage kidneys and clog arteries. But research shows that daily doses as high as 20,000 international units (IU) of vitamin D-3 (much higher than levels found in most vitamin D-3 supplements, which typically supply 400 IU to 2,000 IU) do not raise blood levels above 100 ng/mL, the level traditionally considered a sign of possible toxicity.

The reality is that many Americans have either an insufficient blood level of vitamin D (21 ng/mL to 29 ng/mL) or an outright deficiency (less than 20 ng/mL). An analysis of 73 studies on vitamin D, involving nearly 900,000 people, shows that low levels raise the risk of dying from heart disease (or any cause) by 35%.

My advice: Blood levels of vitamin D should be at least 30 ng/mL (the preferred range is 40 ng/mL to 60 ng/mL).

To achieve that level, the Endocrine Society recommends that adults take 1,500 IU to 2,000 IU of vitamin D-3 daily, even in the summer when sun exposure gives us more natural vitamin D.

Simple Ways to Correct 4 Nutrition Deficiencies...

Dennis Goodman, MD, a board-certified cardiologist and clinical associate professor of medicine in the Leon H. Charney Division of Cardiology and director of Integrative Medicine, both at NYU Langone Medical Center in New York City. He is the author of *Magnificent Magnesium*, *The Thrill of Krill* and *Vitamin K2*. Dennis GoodmanMD.com

If you eat a balanced diet, you may assume that you're getting all the nutrition you need. To play it safe, you might even take a multivitamin-mineral supplement. But is that enough? Probably not.

Four missing nutrients: Increasing evidence shows that there are four little-known nutritional deficiencies—each of which can threaten your health. The problem is, these deficiencies are not remedied by a typical multivitamin-mineral supplement and are extremely difficult to reverse through diet alone—even if you eat organic foods, which provide higher levels of some nutrients. *Here's what you're likely missing—and the nutrient fix you need...**

VITAMIN K-2

Vitamin K isn't even on most people's radar. But there are more than a dozen subtypes of this vitamin, including an important one known as menaquinone (vitamin K-2).

K-2 is crucial for your bones and heart. Without enough K-2, osteocalcin, a protein that binds calcium to bone, cannot be activated. When calcium doesn't stay in bones, it can end up clogging your arteries, causing a heart attack or stroke.

Important finding: People with the lowest blood levels of vitamin K-2 had a 57% greater risk of dying from heart disease than those with the highest levels, according to research published in *The Journal of Nutrition.* People with low K-2 levels also are at increased risk for osteoporosis and bone fractures.

K-2 is found mainly in meat, eggs and dairy. But to get a bone- and heart-protecting level of

*If you take medication, check with your doctor before trying any of these supplements to avoid potential interactions.

K-2 from animal sources, you'd have to include in your daily diet at least eight pounds of beef, a gallon of milk, eight egg yolks and a gallon of yogurt. The only good nonanimal sources of K-2—fermented soybeans, found in foods such as tamari, miso and natto—aren't eaten regularly by most Americans.

My advice: Take a K-2 supplement—at least 45 micrograms (mcg) daily. Look for MenaQ7 (MK-7), a long-acting and better-absorbed variety.

Good products: MenaQ7 from NattoPharma, *MenaQ7.com*...and MK-7 from NOW Foods, *NowFoods.com.*

Caution: If you take *warfarin* (Coumadin), ask your doctor before trying vitamin K-2—it can alter the drug's effectiveness.

COENZYME Q10

Coenzyme Q10 (CoQ10) helps the body make adenosine triphosphate (ATP), the main energy source for cellular activity. But modern life steals CoQ10. You are probably deficient in this nutrient if you take a cholesterol-lowering statin...if you're exposed to high levels of air pollutants...or if you have a chronic disease. Research links low levels of CoQ10 to heart disease, Parkinson's disease, type 2 diabetes, male infertility and fibromyalgia.

CoQ10 is found in such foods as broccoli, nuts, beef and fatty fish—but only in small amounts.

My advice: Take a 100-mg CoQ10 supplement daily. If you have side effects from taking a

---

Vitamin D Can Help with Weight Loss

Vitamin D supplements will not cause you to lose weight, but people who are vitamin D–deficient may experience muscle weakness, fatigue and joint pain, which could result in weight gain. Adults should take 1,500 IU to 2,000 IU of vitamin D a day. If you're obese, you may need more.

Michael F. Holick, PhD, MD, is professor of medicine, physiology and biophysics at Boston University School of Medicine.

statin—such as muscle pain and weakness—consider taking 200 mg of CoQ10 daily. In my cardiology practice, I recommend SmartQ10, from Enzymatic Therapy, *EnzymaticTherapy.com*.

OMEGA-3S

Chronic, low-grade inflammation underlies many chronic health problems, including heart disease, type 2 diabetes, arthritis, cancer and Alzheimer's disease.

Omega-3 essential fatty acids—found in fatty fish, such as salmon, mackerel and tuna, and in oil-rich plant foods, such as walnuts and flaxseeds—are anti-inflammatory. In contrast, omega-6 essential fatty acids—found in baked goods (such as chips, crackers and cookies), cooking oils (such as corn oil, cottonseed oil and sunflower oil) and meat (especially processed meats and non-lean red meat)—are pro-inflammatory. Because the typical American diet has far too much omega-6 and not nearly enough omega-3, the majority of us have an omega-3 deficiency.

My advice: Take 500 mg of krill oil daily. I choose krill oil for myself and my patients rather than fish oil. Krill—small, shrimplike crustaceans—are at the bottom of the oceanic food chain and mostly harvested in the pristine waters around Antarctica, so their oil is less likely to be contaminated with mercury.

Krill oil also contains phospholipids, fatty substances that optimize the absorption of omega-3s. And because of that superior absorption, you need less—500 mg of krill oil is the therapeutic equivalent of 1 g to 2 g of fish oil.

If you are allergic to shellfish: Do not take krill oil.

MAGNESIUM

Eight out of 10 Americans unknowingly suffer from a chronic deficiency of this crucial nutrient. That deficiency causes or contributes to health problems, including heart attacks and other forms of cardiovascular disease (such as arrhythmias, heart failure and stroke), some forms of cancer, type 2 diabetes, obesity, osteoporosis, fatigue, depression and anxiety, migraines, muscle cramps and insomnia.

My advice: Magnesium is the most important supplement anyone can take. I recommend that women take 400 mg to 500 mg daily...and men take 500 mg to 600 mg daily. You can take it all at once or in divided doses—just take it! (If you have insomnia, consider taking your daily dose before bedtime to help you sleep.) I recommend Jigsaw Magnesium, from Jigsaw Health, *JigsawHealth.com*. A well-absorbed form of magnesium malate, its sustained-release formula helps prevent diarrhea, a possible side effect of magnesium.

Whatever brand you use, look for magnesium malate, magnesium citrate or magnesium glycinate—the most absorbable forms. Avoid magnesium oxide—unless you want its stool-loosening effect to help ease constipation. You can also get magnesium in spray or cream forms online (check *Ancient-Minerals.com* or *Amazon.com*)—and by using Epsom salts (which is hydrated magnesium sulfate) in your bath!

Lazy Weekends Are Dangerous to Your Health

Clemens Drenowatz, PhD, MEd, MS, assistant professor, exercise science, University of South Carolina, Columbia, South Carolina.

Omar Khan, MD, medical director, community health, and service line leader, primary care and community medicine, Christiana Care Health System, Wilmington, Delaware.

Karen Anthony, MS, senior program manager, community health, Christiana Care Health System, Wilmington, Delaware.

Presentation, American Heart Association meeting, Phoenix, Arizona.

Playing couch potato on the weekends may be even worse for your weight than working at a desk all week, new research suggests.

Exercise scientists reported that even a 20-minute reduction in sedentary time on Saturdays and Sundays added up to a loss of more than 2 pounds and 1.6% of body fat after a year. But the same association was not seen with sedentary time during the weekdays.

"We know that, on average, people consume less or eat healthier diets on weekdays," explained study author Clemens Drenowatz, PhD, MEd, MS, an assistant professor of exercise science at University of South Carolina in Columbia, South Carolina

"So, they may be able to get by with less activity on weekdays because their diet makes up for it. On weekends, they're eating more, which requires more activity or less sedentary behavior to offset," Dr. Drenowatz said.

STUDY DETAILS

In a group of 332 adults aged 20 to 35, Dr. Drenowatz and his colleagues measured the time participants were sedentary by using a device that measured inactivity over a 10-day period. Participants also reported their own sedentary behaviors separately for weekdays and the weekend.

In addition, the study participants' body weight and body fat measurements were taken every three months over a one-year period.

"From what we saw, the overall sedentary time wasn't different on weekdays versus weekends," Dr. Drenowatz said. "A lot of people had sedentary occupations, like office jobs, and they didn't really make up for that on the weekends either. This suggests diet is the reason, though obviously more research needs to be done."

EXPERTS COMMENT

Two clinicians from Christiana Care Health System in Wilmington, Delaware, weighed in on the findings. They suggested that healthy workplace behaviors—such as light lunches and midday walks—may help balance out the negative effects of sitting at a desk all day.

Many people "don't really have the option of being that inactive on weekdays," said Omar Khan, MD, medical director for community health at Christiana Care. "Weekends are a whole different matter. There's a big opportunity to be healthy—or, as many of us tend to be, fairly unhealthy. With a two-day chunk of potentially being a couch potato, anything we do in that space can be fairly significant."

Karen Anthony, senior program manager for community health at Christiana Care, suggested that moving around for an extra 20 minutes on the weekends—which seemed to spur measur-

able weight loss in study participants—could lead to even more activity.

"Twenty minutes is a fraction of your weekend," she said. "It doesn't take a whole lot of extra movement to see that result."

A LITTLE MOVEMENT CAN MAKE A BIG DIFFERENCE

Dr. Drenowatz said it's important to distinguish between exercising and merely reducing sedentary time, which means less sitting.

"I'm not telling people they need to go out and exercise—that's a separate issue—but just to reduce their sedentary time. It may be just standing up and walking around a bit," Dr. Drenowatz suggested.

He and Dr. Khan also noted that a loss of 1.6% of body fat over one year simply by moving 20 minutes more on the weekends may have a positive impact on the risks for developing heart disease.

Much research in recent years has established an association between sedentary behavior—which includes time sitting watching television or using computers—with poor health outcomes, such as heart disease, diabetes, obesity and some cancers, according to the American College of Sports Medicine.

"A lot of people get caught up with body weight, but from a health perspective, body fat and where it's located actually has a bigger impact on cardiovascular disease over the long term," Dr. Drenowatz said.

The study findings were presented at an American Heart Association meeting in Phoenix. Studies presented at scientific conferences typically have not been peer-reviewed or published, and results are considered preliminary.

info The American College of Sports Medicine offers tips on reducing sedentary behaviors at *acsm.org/docs/brochures/reducing-sedentary-behaviors-sitting-less-and-moving-more.pdf*

The Two-Hour Stand-Up Challenge

John P. Buckley, PhD, professor of applied exercise science, University of Chester, UK.

New British guidelines advise office workers to be on their feet for at least two hours during the typical eight-hour workday.

How: Adjustable desks for sitting and standing…standing-based work projects…and walking breaks.

Why: Sitting for prolonged periods increases risk for heart disease, diabetes and cancer.

Caution: Too much standing may lead to low-back, knee and foot pain, so be sure to alternate sitting and standing.

The Wall Workout

Joel Harper, a personal trainer in New York City who designs workouts for Olympic athletes, celebrities, musicians and business executives. He created the workout chapters for the best-selling YOU series of books by Michael Roizen, MD, and Mehmet Oz, MD. He is the creator of the PBS best-selling DVDs *Firming After 50* and *Slim & Fit*. Harper is also the author of *Mind Your Body: 10 Core Concepts for an Optimally Balanced You*. JoelHarperFitness.com

Forget crowded gyms, clunky dumbbells and fancy exercise machines. If you have access to a wall, you can get a great strength workout using nothing more than the weight of your own body. Bodyweight exercises are a simple, no-frills way to improve strength, flexibility and posture. Because you use a wall for balance, you can hold the positions longer—important for improving endurance as well as strength.

Wall workouts are particularly helpful for those who aren't accustomed to exercise…for people with physical limitations (such as back pain or knee arthritis)…or when you're recovering from surgery or other physical problems.*

*Check first with your doctor before starting this—or any new—exercise program.

The workout below is designed to use every major muscle. To further improve your balance and foot strength, you can also do the routine barefoot. Aim to do these exercises every other day for two weeks…and if you feel the benefits, continue at the same frequency thereafter…

•**Imaginary chair.** It's a great exercise for increasing thigh and gluteal (buttock) strength, which is needed to support your spine. Unlike traditional squats, which involve lowering your body and rising back up, in this exercise you hold one position—helpful for those with knee pain or limited knee strength.

What to do: Stand with your back against a wall. While keeping your back in contact with the wall, slowly slide your back down the wall while simultaneously walking your feet forward until your legs are in right angles. Go only as far as it feels comfortable for your knees. If your knees start to ache, stop moving forward…a "higher" position is easier for beginners. Once you're "sitting," count for as long as you can comfortably hold the position. Each day, try for 10 more seconds. To help improve your posture, keep your stomach taut, your chin up and your shoulders pressed against the wall.

•**Push-ups.** They strengthen the chest, biceps, triceps and shoulders—all of which pro-

Cut Workout Time in Half!

Recent 10-week study: Adults who completed a 25-minute high-intensity workout that included cycling sprints three times a week showed similar health benefits, such as improved insulin sensitivity and cholesterol levels, as those who did a moderate-intensity cycling workout for 45 minutes five days a week.

Bonus: 80% of the high-intensity group versus 60% of the moderate-intensity group had stuck to their workouts three months later—most likely due to the shorter time commitment.

Christopher S. Shaw, PhD, senior lecturer in exercise physiology, Deakin University, Geelong, Australia.

mote good posture. Traditional, on-the-floor push-ups are often too difficult for beginners… or for those with limited upper-body strength. Wall push-ups involve the same basic movements but with less resistance—and they're good for people with back problems because they don't stress the spine.

What to do: Place your palms on a wall at about shoulder height, spaced slightly wider than the width of your shoulders. Back your feet a foot or two away from the wall—stepping farther back increases the difficulty…standing closer to the wall reduces it. Start with your elbows bent. Your face will be close to the wall.

Slowly extend your arms—while exhaling—to push away from the wall. Then inhale while returning to the starting position. Repeat as many times as you comfortably can—ideally, for 30 to 60 seconds.

•**Calf stretches.** Strong calves will improve your ability to walk and climb stairs.

What to do: Stand facing the wall, with both hands on the wall and your arms extended but slightly bent—keep this position throughout the exercise. Step back with your right foot. While holding this position, bend your left leg until you feel a stretch in your right calf. You can also slightly bend your right knee and drive it toward the same toe to increase the stretch. Relax into the stretch, and hold it for 10 seconds or more. Then switch legs and stretch the left calf.

•**Ankle strengthener.** Ankles are a commonly injured body part. People with weak ankles are more likely to have sprains. They are also more likely to have balance problems—the ankles are involved in proprioception, the body's ability to orient itself in space.

What to do: Stand facing a wall, with your feet about hip-width apart. Put both hands on the wall for support. Rise up on your toes, going as high as you can. Hold the position for a few seconds, then slowly lower your heels back down. Do this 25 times.

•**Bridge.** It strengthens the entire midsection, along with the hamstrings, glutes and lower back—all needed for good posture.

What to do: Lie on your back, with your buttocks 12 to 18 inches from the wall. Start by planting the soles of your feet flat against the wall so that your legs make a right angle. Then, while squeezing your abdominal muscles, lift your hips while keeping your shoulder blades flat on the floor. Lift all the way up so that there is a straight line from your knees to your shoulders, then drop down one inch. This is the height to rise up to each time. Hold the pose for about 10 seconds, then lower back down—but don't let your bottom rest on the floor. Keeping it slightly elevated between movements will increase the intensity of the workout. Do this 25 times.

Exercise After Surgery

Wayne Westcott, PhD, director of exercise science, Quincy College, Massachusetts.

If you're recovering from bunion surgery… or any other kind of surgery that prevents a daily walk…there are several ways you can keep in shape.

When foot issues prevent you from performing your normal weight-bearing aerobic activities, substitute exercise that does not involve supporting your body weight, such as swimming or deep water running. In the gym, choose an upright or recumbent stationary bicycle and/or a rowing machine. The seat in these machines supports body weight, and the external resistance against the feet and leg muscles can be adjusted to lower or higher levels according to your physical ability and comfort level.

You can also do resistance exercises while seated that will provide excellent upper-body conditioning while burning (somewhat fewer) calories. Use a resistance band to perform arm curls, arm extensions and chest presses.

Important: Get your doctor's OK on the right time to resume exercise after surgery. You may also benefit from a physical therapy program to improve the range of motion in your foot.

7 Ways to Plank for Strength, Flexibility And Balance

Lee Jordan, certified American Council on Exercise (ACE) health coach and personal trainer based in Jacksonville, Florida.

Jim White, registered dietitian, certified fitness instructor, and owner, Jim White Fitness & Nutrition Studios, Norfolk, Virginia. He is spokesperson for the Academy of Nutrition and Dietetics, Chicago.

The Plank. We're not talking about carpentry or what pirates make prisoners walk off, but an amazing exercise that simultaneously strengthens many of your body's most critical muscles—your core.

It tightens your belly…provides better support for your lower back…increases flexibility in your shoulders and the arches of your feet and your toes…improves your posture…and helps you keep your balance when you're out and about during your busy day.

How can one single exercise that you do for only 30 seconds to a minute do all this? We'll tell you. *And we'll show you seven ways to do it, from easy to challenging, with variations to strengthen different muscle groups…*

PLANK 101

The main focus for any plank pose is on the area between your hips and your shoulders—your core. All of the plank positions below work your core, and all but the last one work your gluteals—your butt muscles. The variations target specific muscle groups—to strengthen the muscles in your chest, shoulders, arms, legs and back.

The first one, the High Plank, is the basic form. It's the best one to get started with—and also the easiest one to customize. If you want a little more challenging core workout, try the Front Plank.

With each position, start by holding it for 10 to 15 seconds. As you get stronger, increase the time—aiming for a goal of one minute. Start with the stationary poses first. Once you can hold a stationary pose for one minute, challenge yourself with one or more of the mobile poses. It's fine to increase your planking time if you want even more challenge!

STATIONARY PLANKS

•**High Plank.** Tones your core and gluteals (butt muscles).

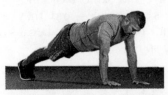

Lying on your stomach, lift your body so that you're supported on your hands (flat on the floor) and your toes, arms straight. It looks like a push-up. Pay attention to keeping your abdominals taut and maintaining your body in a straight line from your head to your ankles.

•**Front Plank.** Tones your core and gluteals and also your chest, shoulders, arms and legs.

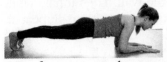

Lying on your stomach, lift your body so that you are supported by your forearms and your toes. Your elbows should align under your shoulders. Maintain your body in a straight line from your head to your ankles, making sure not to lift your head or arch or curve your lower back. Squeeze your gluteal and abdominal muscles while pressing your elbows into the floor.

•**Side Plank.** Tones your core and gluteals and also your obliques (muscles on the side of the torso that help you turn from side to side) and hips.

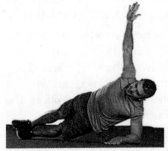

Lying on your right side, prop yourself up on your right elbow and forearm, with your elbow aligned directly under your shoulder and your feet stacked. Now tighten your abdominals and lift your hips off the floor. Your head, shoulder, hips and feet should line up straight. As you lift your hips, push your elbow into the floor for stability.

Switch sides and repeat.

MOVING PLANKS

•**High Plank with Alternating Shoulder Touch.** Tones your core and gluteals and also your upper chest, back and legs.

Start with the High Plank. In a smooth, alternating movement, balance on your left hand only and touch your right hand to your left shoulder…then bring your right hand down, and touch your left hand to your right shoulder. Repeat for one minute (or however long you can).

•**Plank Jacks.** Tones your core and gluteals and also your legs.

While holding a Front Plank position, continuously move your legs together and then apart—as if you were doing jumping jacks. Keep your upper body stable, maintaining a straight line…avoid raising your hips out of alignment.

•**Mountain Climber Plank.** Tones your core and gluteals and also your upper arms and legs.

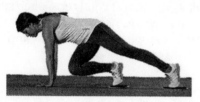

While holding a High Plank position, bring your left knee in toward your chest, pointing your toe, and then extend it back to its starting position. Bring your right knee in toward your chest and extend back to start. Continue alternating legs in a smooth movement while maintaining your upper body in a stable position.

•**Twisting Plank.** Tones your core and also your obliques, shoulders and arms.

Begin in a Front Plank position. Then turn your body so that you're supported on just your right forearm and lift your left arm straight up toward the sky. Bring your arm back down into the Front Plank…then turn and do the same on your left side, lifting your right arm toward the sky. Alternate side to side, aiming for a goal of holding for 30 seconds on each side.

Here's to happy planking—and a stronger, more supple, flexible and injury-resistant body!

Note: The images in this story that demonstrate High Plank, Side Plank, and Mountain Climber Plank are used with permission, courtesy of the American Council on Exercise. You can see more in their Exercise Library.

5 Exercises That Make Everyday Life Better… and Keep Your Body Younger

Beth and Lee Jordan, both certified American Council on Exercise (ACE) health coaches and personal trainers based in Jacksonville Beach, Florida.

Jim White, registered dietitian, certified health fitness instructor, and owner, Jim White Fitness & Nutrition Studios, Norfolk, Virginia. He is spokesperson for the Academy of Nutrition and Dietetics, Chicago.

What are your fitness goals? Amazing endurance? Extraordinary strength? Lightning speed? If so, more power to you—literally. But many of us just want to stay healthy so we can keep doing the activities we need to do…and activities we love to do…for a good long time.

Try this test: Can you put your socks on standing up? Can you stand up from a chair without using your arms, sit back down, and repeat another 11 times within 30 seconds? Can you stand on one foot for 30 seconds? These are tests of functional fitness, sometimes called neuromotor or neuromuscular fitness.

The good news is that you can improve your functional fitness level with simple exercises. The goal is to increase your ability to do the activities that you need to do every day at home, at work and during recreational fun…such as lifting work files or children or grandchildren… carrying the laundry down to the basement and back…bending down to garden…keeping your balance getting in and out of the tub and when you're out for a nice hike. It's a combination of balance and power.

"Functional fitness exercises combine upper- and lower-body movements into what are known as compound exercises, while emphasizing core stability," explain Lee and Beth Jordan, a husband-and-wife team of personal trainers with the American Council on Exercise (ACE). "They often mimic real everyday movements."

These exercises are especially important as you age, when your muscles weaken and simple activities can feel more difficult. All the things you used to barely give a thought to can become challenging if you don't give those muscles some extra attention.

Get started with these five functional exercises designed to help you keep living the active life you enjoy…for a long, long time.

BENT-OVER DUMBBELL ROW

What it helps you do: Bend over to reach things…and pick up an object such as a laundry basket, package of mulch or bag of groceries.

How to do it: Use a dumbbell with a weight that challenges you but that you can lift repeatedly. Stand next to a bench or chair and, 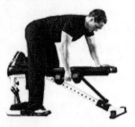 holding the dumbbell in your right hand, bend at a 90-degree angle so that your back is parallel to the floor. Brace your left hand and left knee on the bench or chair. Your weight will be on your right foot, and your right hand should hang down directly under your shoulder, holding the weight. Keeping your back straight, head in line with your spine and abdominal muscles taut, pull the dumbbell up toward your shoulder as far as you can. Your elbow should remain higher than the dumbbell. Then lower the weight by straightening your arm toward the floor. Repeat several reps and then switch sides.

SINGLE-LEG SQUAT

What it helps you do: Control and balance your own weight when walking on unstable ground, going up and down stairs, getting out of bed and getting up out of a chair.

How to do it: Start by standing with your feet hip-width apart, one foot several inches in front of the other, with feet parallel. Slowly squat down as far as you're able to, without losing balance and keeping your bent knee of the leg in front behind your 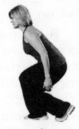 toes. Your hands can dangle below your hips or your arms can be extended straight out in front of you. Rise to your starting position. Perform several reps and then switch legs.

FORWARD LUNGE

What it helps you do: Move with ease during activities such as yard work, vacuuming and putting groceries in your cupboard.

How to do it: Start in a standing position. Keeping one leg in place, step your other foot out in front of you and bend your knees—your ultimate goal is for them to both reach 90-degree angles. (Once you get good 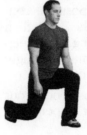 at this, your front thigh and back shin should be parallel to the floor). Push off with your front leg to return to your starting position. Maintain a straight spine and taut abdominals throughout the movement, keeping your arms at your sides or your hands on your hips. Perform several reps, alternating legs with each lunge. (Once you're comfortable with the forward lunge, try side lunges and walking lunges with twists.)

SUPERMANS

What it helps you do: Maintain a healthy posture while sitting, standing and walking.

How to do it: Lie on your stomach, facing straight down, with your head in line with your spine, legs extended straight, toes pointing, and your arms extended straight out in front of you, palms facing each other. Simultaneously, lift both your arms and your legs a few inches off the floor. Make sure your head stays aligned with your spine during the entire movement, and avoid arching your back or lifting your head. Hold the lift for a few seconds, and then gently return your arms and legs to the starting position. Perform several reps.

FARMER'S WALK

What it helps you do: Increase your grip strength and improve coordination when walking and carrying items at the same time.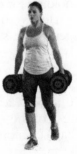

How to do it: You'll need to walk during this exercise. Don't worry if you don't have much space—this is fun if you have a lawn, driveway or walkway to use, but you can also just go in circles inside. Start in a standing position with a dumbbell beside each foot. (Choose a weight that's challenging for you but not so heavy that you can't lift it.) Keeping your back straight, squat down and grip the handles of the weights, lifting them as you stand back up, keeping your weight on your heels. Then take short, quick steps as you walk for up to 100 feet. Remember to breathe throughout the walk. Set the weights back down on the floor. Rest and repeat.

GETTING STARTED WITH A FUNCTIONAL FITNESS ROUTINE

How often should you do these exercises? The American College of Sports Medicine recommends about two or three 20-to-30-minute sessions each week. You'll still want to keep up a regular routine of aerobics, strength training and flexibility exercises, too.

As with any new exercise routine, it's always a good idea to check with your doctor before getting started…and that's especially true if you have any joint problems or other physical challenges. And as with any physical activity, if it starts to hurt, stop.

Are these five exercises the only way to improve functional fitness? Of course not. Yoga and tai chi are also great, and they "count" toward the recommendations. You can even do functional exercises with a paper towel tube.

But if you're looking for a streamlined routine, the five exercises above all work together to improve your ability to do the things that matter every day.

Note: The images in this story that demonstrate each exercise are used with permission, courtesy of the American Council on Exercise. You can see more in their Exercise Library.

CHAPTER 8

Digestive Disorders

Secrets to Staying "Regular"

With so much attention being focused these days on irritable bowel syndrome, colitis, diverticular disease and other gastrointestinal (GI) problems, many people forget about the granddaddy of them all—constipation.

It's hands down one of the most common GI challenges, and 15% of American adults regularly suffer from the condition. And if you believe TV and magazine advertisements, more fiber (often from a supplement) is the solution.

What you're not being told: While fiber is helpful, it's not always the answer. In fact, constipation isn't as straightforward as most people imagine. There are many common mistakes that prevent some people from getting relief from constipation—and cause others to worry unnecessarily.

Among the most common…

MISTAKE #1: Assuming that "normal" means daily. Constipation is usually defined as having fewer than three bowel movements a week. But there's a wide range of "normal"—some people routinely have three bowel movements a week…others go three times every day.

Doctors usually do not worry about a few missed bowel movements. There is almost always a simple explanation—travel, a new medication (see next page), changes in diet or simply a busy schedule that causes people to delay using the toilet.

When to be concerned: When constipation is persistent—especially when it occurs along with other symptoms, such as lumpy, hard stools, straining to have a bowel movement and/or feeling as though you can't completely

Anish Sheth, MD, a gastroenterologist at Princeton Medical Group and an attending physician at the University Medical Center of Princeton at Plainsboro, New Jersey. He is a member of the American Gastroenterology Association, American College of Gastroenterology and the American Association for the Study of Liver Disease, and coauthor of *What's Your Poo Telling You?*

empty the stool from your rectum. It's also cause for concern when someone's normal bowel habits suddenly change for no obvious reason. This could indicate irritable bowel syndrome, a thyroid condition or even colon cancer.

MISTAKE #2: Not taking medication into account. Many prescription and over-the-counter drugs as well as supplements can cause constipation as a side effect. People who aren't aware of this may resort to treatments, such as enemas, that they don't really need—or book unnecessary visits with their doctors.

Psychiatric medications, including tricyclic antidepressants, such as *imipramine* (Tofranil) and *amitriptyline* (Elavil), are notorious for causing constipation.

Other offenders: Blood pressure drugs, including calcium channel blockers and beta-blockers…narcotic painkillers…antihistamines such as Benadryl…and iron supplements.

My advice: If a new medication is causing constipation, ask your doctor if you can get by with a lower dose—or switch to a different drug. If that's not possible, you might need to be more aggressive with lifestyle changes—such as drinking more water and getting more exercise—both help keep stools soft and intestinal muscles active.

MISTAKE #3: Depending only on fiber. Getting more fiber from plant foods (especially pears, apples and sweet potatoes—all with skins on—and cooked greens) will usually increase the frequency and comfort of bowel movements…but not for everyone.

A form of constipation known as slow-transit constipation (STC) occurs when the intestinal muscles contract less often and with less force than normal. Some patients with STC improve when they get more fiber, but others will still need laxatives or other treatments.

My advice: If you have constipation that hasn't responded to dietary changes, ask your doctor

How to Talk About Bowel Movements

If you've been constipated or your doctor simply asks about your bowel movements, how do you describe them? You might feel awkward or at a loss for words, but help is available.

The *Bristol Stool Form Scale* is a detailed guide to the usual textures and shapes.

Check this link for descriptions of the different types of bowel movements: Bowel Control.nih.gov/bristol.aspx.

whether you might have STC. You may need a colonic transit study, which involves swallowing a capsule containing a small amount of material that can be traced with X-rays to show its movement over a period of several days. This test will help your radiologist and gastroenterologist determine how quickly stool moves through your colon.

MISTAKE #4: Rejecting laxatives. Many people have the mistaken notion that laxatives should always be avoided. Admittedly, some of the laxatives used in the past were harsh—people who took them were nervous about being more than a few steps away from a bathroom. But newer laxatives are much gentler.

I usually recommend one of the osmotic laxatives, such as polyethylene glycol 3350 (MiraLAX) or good old Milk of Magnesia. They help stool retain fluid, which softens stools and stimulates bowel movements. It's obviously preferable to have "natural" bowel movements, but these laxatives are gentle enough for long-term use (under a doctor's supervision) and can be a good choice for those with health problems (such as Parkinson's) that often cause constipation.

Note: People with heart or kidney failure should avoid these laxatives—they can cause dehydration and/or a mineral imbalance.

MISTAKE #5: Not checking the bowel. Some people would rather not see what comes out (others closely examine their stools). I advise patients to take at least a quick look before they flush. The appearance of stools can provide important information about your GI health.

Color is a big one. Stools that are extremely dark could be a sign of intestinal bleeding. Bright red can indicate a recent meal of beets, a bleeding hemorrhoid or even colon cancer. Gray can mean that something's obstructing the flow of bile to the intestine.

Texture/shape is also important. Stools that are hard and pelletlike can indicate more severe

Chronic Constipation Can Signal Disease

According to recent research, patients with chronic constipation were five or more times as likely as other people to have gastrointestinal cancers, diverticulitis or ischemic colitis.

Self-defense: Talk to your physician. He/she may do a rectal exam and prescribe a colonoscopy or other diagnostic test.

Lauren Gerson, MD, is director of clinical research, gastroenterology fellowship program, California Pacific Medical Center, San Francisco. Her study of 12,838 patients was presented at the American College of Gastroenterology meeting.

constipation, which could have many underlying causes, including chronic conditions such as thyroid problems, diabetes or Parkinson's disease. "Floaters" are usually normal (they're caused by gas in the stools) but can also be a sign of conditions that impair fat absorption, such as pancreatitis. (For more on different types of stool, see the box on the previous page.)

MISTAKE #6: Avoiding enemas. Simple fixes might not help when you haven't had a bowel movement for a week or two. Stools that stay that long in the intestine can become almost rocklike and painful to pass. Enemas are also the best treatment for fecal impaction, a hard-stool blockage that's usually caused by lengthy constipation.

An enema, available as an over-the-counter saline laxative, increases the flow of water into the intestine. It softens hard stools and usually promotes a bowel movement within a few minutes. Follow package instructions. Fecal impaction that is not relieved by an enema may require a health-care provider to manually remove stool.

MISTAKE #7: Not eating enough prunes. Your grandparents were right—prunes (and prune juice) are an effective treatment for constipation. Prunes are high in fiber, but the main benefit comes from sorbitol, a sugar that draws water into the intestine. Two servings of prunes (about 10 fruits) contain 12 g of sorbitol…and eight ounces of juice has about 15 g.

Note: Drinking warm prune juice seems to be more effective at relieving constipation in some people. If you don't like prunes, consider trying rhubarb, artichokes and/or peaches—all of which promote regular bowel movements.

Important: If you're prone to constipation, limit your intake of processed foods, cheese and meat—these foods can slow down your digestive system.

Drug-Free Constipation Cure

Ryan Abbott, MD, visiting professor of medicine, David Geffen School of Medicine, University of California, Los Angeles.

Applying self-pressure to the perineum (area between the anus and genitals) significantly reduced constipation for 72% of adults in a recent study. Patients also used traditional methods, such as increased fiber intake and stool softeners, but those who added this form of daily acupressure saw the most improvement.

How it works: Applying moderate pressure to the perineum for even a few seconds when you feel the urge to defecate can break up stools and relax the anal sphincter muscles.

What's Really Causing Your Gas and Bloating?

Douglas A. Drossman, MD, codirector emeritus at the University of North Carolina Center for Functional GI and Motility Disorders and professor emeritus of medicine and psychiatry at the University of North Carolina School of Medicine in Chapel Hill. He is also the president of the Rome Foundation, an international nonprofit group that develops guidelines for the diagnosis and treatment of functional GI disorders.

Ugh! Here comes another gas attack. Or maybe it's bloating that's got you feeling so out of sorts. If you're lucky, you can avoid gas and/or bloating by forgoing the usual triggers—carbonated drinks…some high-fiber foods such as beans…chewing gum…and artificial sweeteners and the fruit sugar fructose.

But sometimes the source of this all-too-common gastrointestinal (GI) discomfort isn't so obvious. If your symptoms don't ease within a few weeks…or they have no apparent reason and tend to come and go, you and your doctor may need to do some investigating. *The following health problems can cause gas and/or bloating but often go undetected—especially in the early stages…*

•**Aerophagia (air swallowing).** Swallowing too much air can stretch the stomach and cause bloating. This often occurs when people are experiencing anxiety or can even become an unconscious habit. It can also happen when chewing gum, using a straw or drinking carbonated beverages.

What to do: Consider stress-reducing activities like deep breathing, meditation or yoga. If symptoms are severe, see a counselor for stress-management techniques.

•**Irritable bowel syndrome (IBS).** As many as one in five adults experiences the chronic symptoms of IBS—abdominal pain, bloating, gas, diarrhea and/or constipation—to some degree. IBS can have many causes, but typically nerves in the GI tract are extremely sensitive to food and gas passing through the bowel, triggering discomfort.

What to do: An IBS diagnosis includes regular abdominal pain that is relieved by a bowel movement, along with symptoms of bloating, diarrhea and/or constipation.

If you have IBS, your doctor may prescribe antispasmodics, such as *dicyclomine* (Bentyl) and *hyoscyamine* (Levsin), that may help relieve your symptoms. Since stress can trigger IBS symptoms, try to manage it with yoga, massage, meditation and counseling, if needed.

•**Functional dyspepsia.** After eating, the stomach in a healthy adult can expand in volume up to four times its normal size. But with functional dyspepsia, the muscles don't relax properly and the stomach remains small, leaving you feeling full and bloated after just a few bites.

What to do: If symptoms are stress-related, relaxation techniques, such as deep breathing or biofeedback, may be effective. An antianxi-

ety drug, such as *buspirone* (BuSpar), can also help because it helps to relax the stomach.

•**Celiac disease.** People with celiac disease are sensitive to gluten, a protein in wheat, barley and rye that can produce inflammation in the bowel, resulting in bloating, gas, abdominal cramps and diarrhea.

What to do: If you suffer from the digestive symptoms described above—especially if you also have any nutritional deficiencies and/or experience frequent fatigue—see your doctor. Celiac disease is diagnosed with a blood test followed by an endoscopic biopsy. By avoiding foods and products that contain gluten, most sufferers can eliminate symptoms. For a list of hidden sources of gluten, go to *Celiac.org*.

More serious but less common causes of gas and/or bloating…

•**Diverticulitis.** This condition occurs when small pouches in the walls of the colon become inflamed and/or infected—often due to small tears caused by stool trapped in the pouches. It not only causes gas and bloating but also pain in the lower left side of the pelvis, where pouches get infected.

What to do: If you're having severe abdominal pain with fever and vomiting, see your doctor right away—you could have a serious infection that requires antibiotics and possibly emergency surgery. Sometimes, however, diverticulitis is mild, and symptoms may improve if you apply heat to the painful area…go on a liquid diet—including clear broth, clear fruit juice (such as apple), gelatin and plain tea—for a few days to "rest" your digestive system…and/or take antibiotics if needed to treat an infection.

•**Gallstones.** They often cause no symptoms, but if gallstones block the duct where the gallbladder empties, the gallbladder stretches, resulting in distension and pain, as well as bloating and gas.

What to do: If you suffer bloating and gas, pain in the upper-right abdomen (where the gallbladder is located), nausea and fever, see your doctor. He/she will perform an ultrasound to check for gallstones. Gallstone removal, which is routinely performed via laparoscopic surgery or, in some cases, endoscopy, is often recommended.

•**Certain cancers.** With advanced colorectal cancer, the bowel can become blocked, which leads to gas, bloating and blood in the stool. Ovarian cancer often causes subtle symptoms that may include bloating and feeling full quickly.

What to do: With colorectal cancer, regular colonoscopies after age 50 (or after age 40 if a close family member has had the disease) will catch suspicious polyps before a malignancy develops. Women who experience the symptoms described above for more than two or three weeks—especially if they are accompanied by pelvic pain and/or an urgent or frequent need to urinate—should see a gynecologist.

QUICK RELIEF

If your gas and/or bloating is only occasional, consider trying…

•**Probiotics,** which promote the growth of "good" bacteria in the bowel. One study found that Lactobacillus acidophilus and Bifidobacterium lactis helped bloating by replacing the bad (gas-causing) bacteria with good (gas-relieving) bacteria in people with bowel disorders, such as IBS or functional dyspepsia. In another study, probiotics were found to relieve intestinal gas.

What to do: Try a daily probiotic in supplement form or via probiotic-rich fermented foods and beverages such as kefir, miso or kimchi.

Before You Give Up Gluten, Try a Low-FODMAP Diet

Peter Gibson, MD, professor and director of gastroenterology, Alfred and Monash University, Melbourne Australia. He is a recipient of the Gastroenterological Society of Australia's Distinguished Research Prize. For more information on FODMAP diets, check his department's website.

These days just about everyone has a friend who has gone on a gluten-free diet and raves about it. Perhaps you've tried it yourself. Perhaps digestion improves, and so does well-being. Does that mean that you or your friend is sensitive to gluten?

Maybe not. Surprisingly, you may actually be reacting to a different ingredient in wheat…and in many other foods. Avoiding this particular class of hard-to-digest carbohydrates, called FODMAPs, may improve digestive symptoms in people who believe that they are sensitive to gluten.

That's not to say that gluten is suddenly fine for everyone. It's pure poison for the two million Americans with celiac disease, a digestive disease in which the body can't digest gluten, a protein found in wheat, rye and barley. Nor does it mean that non-celiac gluten sensitivity (NCGS) isn't real. It's just that the population with NCGS may be smaller than once believed—and certainly fewer than the 30% of Americans who currently try to avoid gluten in their diets.

The good news is that a careful plan to remove just the FODMAPs that are causing your particular reaction may lead to a less restrictive diet than a gluten-free one—and be more effective in fixing your digestion.

IS FODMAP THE NEW GLUTEN?

To understand the FODMAP/gluten story, step back to 2011. Australian researchers studied people who didn't have celiac disease but did have irritable bowel syndrome (IBS), with its symptoms of bloating, stomach pain, and diarrhea and constipation. (As many as 20% of Americans experience these symptoms in this often-undiagnosed and poorly understood condition.) In a randomized placebo-controlled study, the Australians reported that gluten made the 34 study participants' IBS symptoms worse and that a gluten-free diet reduced symptoms.

That very influential study helped establish the concept of non-celiac gluten sensitivity and boosted the popularity of gluten-free diets.

But then a couple of years later, the same researchers revisited the topic. They examined whether gluten was indeed the cause of symptoms in a group of people who had NCGS. These 37 patients "felt that gluten was the cause of their gut symptoms" says the study's lead author, Peter Gibson, MD, professor and director of gastroenterology at The Alfred and

Monash University in Melbourne, Australia. The study also looked at the effects of FODMAPs, which stands for fermentable oligosaccharides, disaccharides, monosaccharides and polyols. They're found in many foods, and some studies were starting to find that they could trigger IBS symptoms.

What the Australians found was surprising…

•**A low-FODMAP diet significantly reduced gastrointestinal symptoms.**

•**Participants who had reported improvements in GI symptoms** on a gluten-free diet before the study had even fewer symptoms on a low-FODMAP diet.

•**When the researchers "challenged" 37 of the participants by giving them food that contained either no gluten,** a small amount of gluten (2 grams), or a large amount of gluten (16 grams, about the amount in 10 slices of wheat bread), there was no difference in symptoms. In other words, gluten had no effect on symptoms.

While the study had a small number of subjects (as did the 2011 one), it was carefully designed to provide reliable clinical results. Not only was it double-blind, so that neither researcher nor subject expectations could affects the results, and placebo controlled, but it was a "cross-over re-challenge" study—each participant got each one of the different diets. "This kind of study is the gold standard way of determining whether a food is causing symptoms," says Dr. Gibson. "If gluten was the cause of the symptoms, then it would cause greater symptoms than the placebo. It did not. That is why gluten is unlikely to be the culprit in those subjects studied."

THE LOW-FODMAP DIET
TAKES OFF

Since that study was published, the benefits of a low-FODMAP diet for people with digestive symptoms has become even clearer. Researchers who've been looking for ways to help people with IBS, for example, are almost giddy with excitement—well, as giddy as scientists get in print—with editorials such as "Diet as a Therapy for Irritable Bowel Syndrome: Progress at Last." One 2014 study of the low-FODMAP diet for IBS concluded: "This high-quality evidence

supports its use as a first-line therapy." A recent study of dietitians found that in their experience, a low-FODMAP diet helps patients with GI symptoms better than the old advice to "eat a healthy diet" while restricting lactose-containing foods and cutting back on caffeine.

To be sure, the debate over whether NCGS is a distinct clinical diagnosis, unrelated to FODMAP sensitivity, at least for some people, continues. One 2015 scientific review concluded that it is not clear whether what is thought to be NCGS is caused by gluten or FODMAPs, for example. However, Alessio Fasano, MD, director of the Center for Celiac Research and Treatment at the MassGeneral Hospital for Children in Boston, pointed out in a 2015 scientific review that people with NCGS often have immunological reactions to wheat and other grains—not just stomach problems. NCGS may contribute to other conditions including chronic fatigue syndrome and autoimmune diseases, he argues. To make matters even more complicated, there are other ingredients in wheat, rye, and barley, such as amylase-trypsin inhibitors (ATIs), that may trigger immune response–related symptoms. He believes a better name for NCGS is non-celiac wheat sensitivity. Going on a low-FODMAP diet wouldn't address these concerns.

For now, though, if you have unresolved digestive symptoms, it's clearly time to give a low-FODMAP diet a close look. "Our advice is to try reducing FODMAPs first, since this is an easier diet than a gluten-free diet," says Dr. Gibson. Based on research, he estimates that about 70% of people with IBS symptoms will benefit.

HOW TO GO ON
A LOW-FODMAP DIET

"The major argument against the low-FODMAP approach is that it is too difficult, but that is the opinion of people who do not know much about how easy the low-FODMAP diet is to implement," says Dr. Gibson.

It is true that FODMAPs are very common in a typical Western diet. FODMAPs include fructans, found in wheat as well as onions and garlic…fructose, high-fructose corn syrup, and some fruits such as apples and pears…lactose, the sugar in milk and other dairy products… polyols, found in the sweetener sorbitol and in stone fruits such as plums and cherries…and galacto-oligosaccharides, found in beans, lentils and soybeans. However, many individuals are more sensitive to some FODMAPs than others. It's also the dose of FODMAPs that counts—a little bit is OK but a lot will cause symptoms. So you may need to reduce FODMAPs a small amount to feel better. (That's why it's a "low-FODMAP" diet, not a "FODMAP-free diet.")

That's good, because many of these foods are very nutritious. It's best, by far, to get help from a dietitian if you want to see whether you would feel better on a low-FODMAP diet—a dietitian will guide you through a FODMAP-elimination process in which you will get rid of most or all FODMAPS and then carefully add each type back, in turn, to see which ones cause your symptoms. A dietitian can also help make sure you eat a nutritious diet even if you need to eliminate certain classes of foods. To learn more, Stanford University has a good list of FODMAPs *stanfordhealthcare.org/medical-clinics/nutrition-services/resources/low-fodmap-diet.html* and Monash University has created a low-FODMAP diet app, *med.monash.edu.au/cecs/gastro/fodmap/iphone-app.html* with information on low- and high-FODMAP foods as well as meal plans.

If you continue to have problems and suspect gluten, on the other hand, do get it checked out. The first action is to find out if you have celiac disease, and there are well-established tests for this. Don't give up gluten until you know, because having eaten gluten is key to the diagnosis. You may also want to check for a wheat allergy, which is a different beast entirely. If the FODMAP diet doesn't help and other conditions such as Crohn's have been ruled out, you may want to consider gluten. Unfortunately, there aren't lab tests that can establish gluten sensitivity, but you can work with your doctor to go on a gluten-free diet to see if it helps your symptoms. But that should be your last step in this process—not your first!

Don't Let Them Tell You Gluten Intolerance Isn't Real

Study titled "Small Amounts of Gluten in Subjects with Suspected Nonceliac Gluten Sensitivity—a Randomized, Double-Blind, Placebo-Controlled, Cross-Over Trial," by researchers in the department of internal medicine at University of Pavia, and the department of medical and surgical sciences at University of Bologna, both in Italy, published in *Clinical Gastroenterology and Hepatology*.

You may have been told that unless you have the autoimmune disorder celiac disease, you're not gluten intolerant, and the pain and bloating you blame on sensitivity to gluten is all in your head. Meanwhile, the gluten-free food industry is booming as never before, and many people are singing the benefits of a gluten-free life. So…is gluten sensitivity real? Or is it just the latest craze?

GLUTEN SENSITIVITY IS REAL—BUT NOT ALWAYS

According to a new study, it is entirely possible to be sensitive to gluten without having a wheat allergy or celiac disease. But it's also possible that gluten exerts a "nocebo" effect on some folks. A nocebo effect is an ill effect caused by the suggestion or belief that something—in this case gluten/wheat—is harmful.

The study, conducted by researchers from the Universities of Pavia and Bologna in Italy, involved 59 participants who had self-described gluten intolerance. They reported symptoms such as bloating, gassiness, diarrhea, headache and brain fog. Before starting the study, all of the participants had blood work and biopsies of the small intestine to rule out wheat allergies and celiac disease.

To identify whether gluten was actually causing symptoms, the researchers put participants on a strict gluten-free diet for five weeks, and during part of that time had them take one of two daily pills—either wheat gluten or a placebo. Participants switched off during the study so that everyone had a chance to take gluten pills and placebos during different weeks (but without knowing which was which, of course).

Each gluten pill contained about the amount of gluten found in two slices of white bread.

Participants completed daily questionnaires that measured the severity of a wide range of symptoms on a scale of zero (not affected) to three (severely affected). In addition to intestinal symptoms, such as pain, bloating and gas, non-intestinal symptoms frequently associated with gluten intolerance, such as headache, tiredness, malaise, brain fog and anxiety, were also asked about.

The results: The participants' total average symptom severity score was 30% higher during the week they were given gluten compared with the week they received placebo pills, showing that gluten did make a difference for some. However, when the researchers plotted each participant's weekly scores on grids to view correlations between how each person felt during gluten and gluten-free weeks, they found that about half of the participants complained about symptoms to the same degree whether they were receiving gluten or not. The remaining participants either logged in more symptoms when they were receiving gluten or placebo. Of the nine patients who recorded more symptoms while on gluten than placebo, three (amounting to 5% of the study group) had scores that consistently showed symptom flares when exposed to gluten but not placebo. Symptoms of bloating, abdominal pain, brain fog, depression and canker sores—the most common intestinal and nonintestinal symptoms experienced across the board—were consistently and significantly worse during the week of gluten exposure in these patients compared with the rest of the study group. The researchers commented that these participants likely had true gluten intolerance despite lack of wheat allergy or celiac disease and that the other six participants may have had a lesser level of gluten sensitivity. They also point out that the dose of gluten given was low, and so higher amounts might have shown greater sensitivity in more of the participants.

DO YOU REALLY NEED TO BE GLUTEN-FREE?

These study findings add weight to both sides of the argument…yes, gluten intolerance does seem to occur in a small percentage of people.

On the other hand, gluten may not actually be behind symptoms that many people experience and attribute to gluten intolerance.

If you notice that you have abdominal pain or bloating, fogginess or low mood after eating foods with gluten, you can test whether you are truly sensitive to it by going gluten-free for one or two weeks, evaluating whether symptoms improve and then reintroducing bread or pasta back into your diet and again evaluating symptoms. A better strategy, though, would be to consult a dietitian or naturopathic doctor who can expertly evaluate your symptoms and guide you through a diet regimen to correct the problem without compromising nutrition—whether that means avoiding gluten or following some other strategy.

Alert: The Worst Antibiotics for Your Gut Health

Study titled "Same Exposure but Two Radically Different Responses to Antibiotics: Resilience of the Salivary Microbiome versus Long-Term Microbial Shifts in Feces" by researchers at University of Amsterdam, VU University Amsterdam, Swammerdam Institute for Life Sciences, The Netherlands, et al., published in the American Society for Microbiology's journal *MBio*.

How bad are antibiotics for your digestion and gut health, really?

Here's the answer: Worse than you may have ever imagined.

The latest study finds that the damage from certain common kinds of antibiotics may unsettle the beneficial bacteria in your gut for months, even a year—in ways that could lead to diseases such as inflammatory bowel disease, even increase risk for colon cancer.

But some other antibiotics disturb your gut for only a week or so. Here's information on which antibiotics are the most dangerous for your gastrointestinal health—and how to protect yourself from them.

HOW FOUR COMMON ANTIBIOTICS AFFECT YOUR GUT

We humans are more colonies than individuals. We rely on multitudes of beneficial bacteria in our gut and our mouths to thrive. To find out what happens to our gut microsystem during a single course of antibiotics, Swedish and British researchers gave healthy adults either a placebo or an oral antibiotic. They collected samples of saliva and feces before and after a course of antibiotics.

Four common types were studied...

●**Amoxicillin.**

Class: Penicillin-like. It's prescribed to treat bronchitis, gonorrhea and infections of the ears, nose, throat, urinary tract and skin.

●**Minocycline.**

Class: Tetracycline. It's prescribed to treat respiratory infections, acne and other skin conditions, as well as urinary and genital infections.

●**Ciprofloxacin.**

Class: Fluoroquinolone. It's prescribed to treat urinary tract infections, as well as anthrax. It's commonly called "Cipro."

●**Clindamycin.**

Class: Lincomycin. It's prescribed for infections of the lungs and skin and for vaginal infections.

Not surprisingly, all of the antibiotics knocked out many of the beneficial bacteria both in the study participants' saliva and in feces. The good news is that in the mouth, the "good" bugs repopulated pretty quickly after all four kinds of antibiotics.

But the gut didn't do so well. For the amoxicillin, the concentration of good gut bugs was disturbed for about a week. For monocyline, it was about a month. But for the heavy hitters ciprofloxacin and clindamycin, the damage was more lasting. They wiped out many of the beneficial bugs.

In particular, they destroyed several kinds of common gut bacteria that produce a short-chain fatty acid called *butyrate*—which is increasingly being recognized as one key to a healthy colon. Butyrate inhibits inflammation, acts as a powerful protective antioxidant and helps stop cancer from forming. When good-for-you bugs are killed and stop producing butyrate, other studies have shown, that can contribute to digestive disorders such as inflammatory bowel disease.

Vinegar for Gut Health

Mice with ulcerative colitis had fewer symptoms when vinegar was added to their drinking water.

Possible reasons: Vinegar may increase levels of beneficial intestinal bacteria, while suppressing pro-inflammatory proteins.

Journal of Agricultural and Food Chemistry

In this study, ciprofloxacin and clindamycin wiped out the butyrate producers for several months—and in some cases, as long as a year.

Does this study mean you should never accept a prescription for these antibiotics? That's going too far, since some infections that can be treated by these and other antibiotics can be life-threatening. But if you are prescribed antibiotics in the fluoroquinolone or lincomycin classes, discuss with your doctor if there are alternative classes of antibiotics that may work for your specific infection.

And there are many situations where antibiotics are prescribed when they're not needed at all. That contributes to the worldwide epidemic of antibiotic resistance, may increase the risk for diabetes—and, according to this study, may in some cases damage the digestive system in ways that can contribute to long-term health problems.

So take 'em if you really need 'em. But never take them lightly—and consider your alternatives.

---

5 Secrets for a Super Liver

Michelle Lai, MD, MPH, an assistant professor of medicine at Harvard Medical School and a hepatologist at Beth Israel Deaconess Medical Center, both in Boston. Dr. Lai is coauthor of *The Liver Healing Diet*. Her research frequently appears in peer-reviewed journals such as *The New England Journal of Medicine* and the *Journal of Hepatology*.

Most people assume that liver disease happens only to people who abuse alcohol. But that is not true.

Surprising facts: More than 30 million US adults suffer from chronic liver disease—and many of these people don't even know that they have it. Liver problems can be caused by a number of conditions such as fatty liver disease (see below) and hepatitis C and hepatitis B. The result can range from mild dysfunction to cirrhosis, liver failure and liver cancer.

An under-recognized problem: A condition called nonalcoholic fatty liver disease (NAFLD). Affecting as many as one in four adults in this country, it is marked by a buildup of extra fat in the liver cells. This can allow a more serious condition to develop that can result in liver scarring and cirrhosis—problems that may lead to liver failure or cancer, requiring a liver transplant.

KEEPING YOUR LIVER HEALTHY

Your liver is one of the hardest-working—and underappreciated—organs in your body. It's responsible for more than 500 critical functions, ranging from digesting and storing nutrients to processing and excreting toxic substances that sneak into your body via food, drink and air. If your liver gets sick, you get sick——it's that simple.

Fortunately, there are simple steps you can take to help protect your liver health. *My advice…*

•**Fight unwanted weight gain.** This is key to liver health. For most people, a crucial part of maintaining a healthy body weight is to cut back on their sugar intake.

Besides promoting system-wide inflammation and weight gain, excessive sugar (typically from sweets, soda, fruit drinks and other flavored beverages) can cause your liver to become fatty and inflamed—thus contributing to NAFLD.

Household Toxins

A healthy liver functions like a fortress, defending your body from toxins. A frequently overlooked source of toxins: Household cleaning agents.

Every time you spray your counter or wipe down a table, you release irritating chemicals (such as chlorine, ammonia, alcohol and others), which are inhaled. *Fortunately, safer alternatives are readily available…*

•**For an all-purpose cleaner,** (good for appliances, counters and inside the refrigerator), dissolve four tablespoons of baking soda in one quart of warm water.

•**To polish stainless steel,** olive oil works great.

Still want the convenience of a store-bought cleaner? Choose brands labeled "phosphate-free"…"VOC-free"…and/or "solvent-free." Also, look for products with the green-and-white USDA Organic Seal or ones with nontoxic, plant-derived ingredients. For more cleaners, see page 323.

Important: The just-released 2015–2020 edition of the federal Dietary Guidelines calls for us to limit our added sugar intake to less than 10% of daily calories—the equivalent of roughly 10 to 15 teaspoons of sugar per day.

Some easy ways to cut back on sugar in your diet: Switch from flavored yogurt to plain Greek yogurt topped with fruit…and substitute unsweetened applesauce for refined white sugar when baking.

•**Drink coffee.** Scientific evidence continues to shore up coffee's protective effect on the liver—perhaps due to its inflammation-fighting properties.

Important recent findings: A March 2015 World Cancer Research Fund study found that each cup of coffee you drink per day reduces your risk for liver cancer by 14%. An analysis of other studies showed that drinking two cups of coffee per day may reduce risk for cirrhosis by 44%.

Helpful: Opt for caffeinated coffee and, if possible, have it black. Sugar, of course, causes inflammation, and decaf java has not been shown in research to have the same liver-friendly benefits.

•**Try wheat germ.** With its mild, nutty taste, wheat germ is an excellent source of vitamin E. Two tablespoons of ready-to-eat wheat germ provide 5.4 mg of vitamin E—about one-third of your daily needs. Why is this vitamin so important? Animal studies suggest that wheat germ can help protect the liver against toxins. While human data is limited, a study of 132,000 Chinese adults found that as vitamin E intake rose, the likelihood of liver cancer dropped.

Wheat germ is also rich in essential fatty acids, potassium and magnesium—all of which help ease oxidative stress on the liver by protecting the body's cells from free radical damage.

Helpful: Sprinkle wheat germ over oatmeal, yogurt or popcorn…or mix it into meatloaf or smoothies. For other good sources of vitamin E, try almonds, spinach, avocado and sunflower seeds.

•**Choose seafood wisely.** Fish is an excellent source of protein, vitamins and minerals and heart-healthy omega-3 fatty acids. However, many types of fish can accumulate heavy metals, such as mercury, lead and cadmium, from the water and the aquatic life they consume. When we eat such fish, we ingest these toxins, which, over time, can cause liver damage.

Self-defense: Select seafood that is less likely to contain heavy metals. For example, you can safely enjoy 12 ounces a week of smaller fish such as anchovies…catfish…flounder…herring…perch…wild salmon…sardines…and trout.

Caution: Limit your intake of fish that may contain higher levels of heavy metals such as Chilean sea bass…grouper…mackerel…and yellowfin and white albacore tuna to less than 18 ounces per month.

Avoid large fish such as marlin…orange roughy…ahi tuna…and swordfish—these fish usually contain the highest levels of heavy metals.

Helpful: Visit the Natural Resources Defense Council at *NRDC.org* for a complete list of the safest seafood options.

•**Don't forget water!** Water makes the liver's job easier by helping flush toxins out of the body. It's also a sugar-free substitute for juice, soda, sweetened tea and other sugar-enhanced beverages.

Helpful: Keep a glass of water on your nightstand, and start your morning with it, then continue sipping all day long. To jazz up your water, try adding freshly cut slices of citrus.

Help for Bowel Incontinence

Arnold Wald, MD, professor of medicine, University of Wisconsin School of Medicine and Public Health, Madison.

Bowel incontinence device now available. The FDA recently approved an implantable device called the Fenix Continence Restoration System that helps patients who have not responded to other treatments for bowel incontinence, such as dietary changes and/or medication.

How it works: An interlinked ring of titanium beads is surgically fitted internally around the patient's anal sphincter, creating a magnetic bond that opens temporarily and automatically closes again after elimination.

Good News for IBS Sufferers

Mark Pimentel, MD, director of the GI Motility Program and Laboratory at Cedars-Sinai Medical Center in Los Angeles, where he specializes in irritable bowel syndrome and its relationship to small intestinal motility and bacterial overgrowth. He is the creator of the IBS blood tests described in this article. (Disclosure: Dr. Pimentel receives consulting fees from Commonwealth Laboratories, which produces the tests.)

If you're unlucky enough to get hit by a day or two of diarrhea, you can write it off as a short-lived bit of unpleasantness. But for those with irritable bowel syndrome (IBS), diarrhea—as well as constipation and/or other digestive problems—can be a way of life.

Imagine that you are afraid to leave the house because you might get caught without a bathroom. You suffer from gut-wrenching abdominal pain…daily bloating…and/or frequent (and unpredictable) bouts of diarrhea or constipation—or both. That is what it's like to live with IBS.

A CHALLENGE TO DIAGNOSE

IBS is the most common gastrointestinal problem in the US. Studies estimate that 10% to 15% of adults—as many as 37 million Americans—are affected to some degree. But without a definitive test, the approaches to diagnosis and treatment have been scattershot.

Problem: The same symptoms that occur with IBS can also be caused by other, more serious conditions (such as inflammatory bowel disease, ulcerative colitis and diverticulitis). As a result, IBS patients often undergo a multitude of tests (including stool analyses, blood tests and imaging tests) as well as doctor visits to rule out what's not causing their problems.

Because IBS has traditionally been so difficult to diagnose, many doctors have not fully understood the disorder and blamed their patient's IBS symptoms on stress, anxiety and/or depression…or told them that their symptoms are "all in your head" and recommended psychological counseling.

Now that's all about to change.

Latest development: Rather than spending months—or even years—going from doctor to doctor seeking help for this condition, new blood tests allow IBS patients to learn within a matter of days what's causing their symptoms so they can begin treatment much sooner.

UNCOVERING THE CAUSE OF IBS

The underlying cause of IBS was not known until pioneering research at Cedars-Sinai Medical Center in Los Angeles recently found that the majority of IBS patients were at some point infected with Salmonella, Escherichia coli or other harmful (and often food-borne) bacteria.

The bacteria secrete toxins that damage the intestinal nerves that control motility, the synchronized contractions that move digested food through the intestine. The nerve damage, which persists long after the infection is gone (and perhaps indefinitely), explains all of the typical IBS symptoms.

The blood tests that researchers have developed identify evidence of past infections that can cause IBS. This means that patients can describe their symptoms to a doctor, receive the new blood tests and get an accurate diagnosis after a single visit to a doctor.

Doctors send the patient's blood samples to a laboratory (Commonwealth Laboratories, IB Schek.com) to be analyzed. The results are generally available within 24 hours.

Typical cost: $500, which is usually covered by insurance.

HOW YOUR DIET CAN HELP

If you get a diagnosis of IBS, what you eat can affect how well you manage your symptoms. (If you simply suspect that you have IBS but have not been diagnosed with it, it's also worth trying the dietary changes below.) *What helps…*

•**Avoid "FODMAP" foods.** Scientists have identified a class of hard-to-digest carbohydrates that ferment in the small intestine and increase IBS symptoms. These so-called FODMAP (shorthand for fermentable oligosaccharides, disaccharides, monosaccharides and polyols) foods include wheat, dairy, onions, apples, high-fructose corn syrup, beans, stone fruits (such as apricots, nectarines and cherries) and artificial sweeteners (such as sorbitol and mannitol).

There's some evidence that people who feel better when they give up gluten are actually responding to the reduction in FODMAPs that occurs when they go on a gluten-free diet. No one loves restrictive diets—and a low-FODMAP diet is restrictive. But it can help if you stick with it. For a comprehensive list of FODMAP foods, go to *IBSDiets.org*.

•**Get less fiber.** In the past, doctors advised IBS patients to eat a lot of fiber to firm up stools and reduce diarrhea as well as constipation. We now know that too much fiber can increase bacterial overgrowth in the small intestine.

My advice: Limit your daily fiber intake to no more than 20 g to 35 g. For example, eat

---

Pantry Heartburn Remedy

Chew one to two teaspoons of uncooked oat flakes before swallowing. Oatmeal may help absorb the stomach acid that contributes to heartburn.

David Foley, medical herbalist, *TheNaturalWayBlog.blogspot.com*.

white bread (such as Italian) instead of whole wheat…avoid super-high-fiber cereals (more than 8 g of fiber per serving)…and limit beans, whole grains and other high-fiber foods.

MEDICATION THAT HELPS

While many IBS sufferers get relief from the dietary changes described in the main article, medication is usually also necessary. Until recently, there were only two drugs specifically approved for IBS—*alosetron* (Lotronex) for diarrhea-predominant IBS, or IBS-D…and lubiprostone (Amitiza) for constipation-predominant IBS, or IBS-C.

New options: In May, the FDA approved two new drugs, which may benefit a greater number of IBS patients…

•***Rifaximin*** **(Xifaxan).** This drug is an antibiotic, but it isn't used to treat the infections that cause IBS (those infections are usually long gone by the time patients develop symptoms). Instead, it curtails the bacterial overgrowth in the small intestine that results from months or years of impaired motility that typically accompanies IBS symptoms. Rifaximin is taken orally three times a day, for 14 days. It is expected to become the first-line therapy for IBS-D, since it has far fewer side effects than Lotronex.

•***Eluxadoline*** **(Viberzi).** This medication is an antidiarrheal. It targets opioid receptors in the intestine, while having little effect on similar receptors in the brain. This means that it's less likely to cause drowsiness or other side effects than other medications used to treat diarrhea. It improves stool consistency and reduces abdominal pain/cramping.

A Vitamin for IBS?

Simon Tazzyman, PhD, postdoctoral researcher, The University of Sheffield, UK.

There's no known cure for the diarrhea, constipation and/or urgency of irritable bowel syndrome (IBS), but a new study found that 82% of IBS sufferers were also low in vitamin D (less than 20 ng/mL). Most of those whose vitamin D levels returned to normal after tak-

ing a supplement for 12 weeks had improved IBS symptoms, but more research is needed to statistically link the two.

Psych Therapies May Have Long-Term Benefits for Irritable Bowel Patients

Vanderbilt University, news release.

Doctors have long known that psychological therapies such as relaxation and hypnosis can temporarily ease the symptoms of irritable bowel syndrome (IBS). But, new research suggests they could also offer long-term benefits.

IBS is a gastrointestinal disorder that affects up to 16% of the US population. It causes chronic abdominal pain, discomfort, bloating, diarrhea or constipation. There's currently no cure, but dietary changes, medication and psychological interventions can provide symptom relief, the study authors noted.

"Our study is the first one that has looked at long-term effects," said the study's senior author, Lynn Walker, PhD, a professor of pediatrics at Vanderbilt University Medical Center, in Nashville.

"We found that the moderate benefit that psychological therapies confer in the short term continue over the long term. This is significant because IBS is a chronic, intermittent condition for which there is no good medical treatment," she said in a hospital news release.

The researchers analyzed results of 41 clinical trials involving more than 2,200 IBS patients.

The analysis found several different psychological therapies—including relaxation, hypnosis and cognitive behavioral therapy—equally beneficial in helping people change the way they think. Regardless of the length of treatment, the researchers found the effects may last at least six to 12 months after treatment ends.

Online treatments were just as effective as those conducted in person, the study, published recently in *Clinical Gastroenterology and Hepatology*, found.

The study's first author, Kelsey Laird, a doctoral student in Vanderbilt's clinical psychology program, said, "Western medicine often conceptualizes the mind as separate from the body, but IBS is a perfect example of how the two are connected."

"Ho-Hum" Herbs for Better Digestion

Jamison Starbuck, ND, is a naturopathic physician in family practice and a guest lecturer at the University of Montana, both in Missoula. She is a past president of the American Association of Naturopathic Physicians and a contributing editor to The Alternative Advisor: The Complete Guide to Natural Therapies and Alternative Treatments.

Too often, there's an assumption that the newest and most advanced medical treatments are the best. But in my experience, seemingly ordinary remedies often produce extraordinary results. Certain herbs are a good case in point. Ones that are often considered "ho-hums" of the botanical world are, in fact, surprisingly powerful medicines you can use to safely treat a number of common complaints, especially digestive health. *My favorite ho-hum herbs…*

•**Chamomile.** While many people think of drinking a cup of chamomile tea to help them relax or sleep (which it does), this herb also has several lesser-known benefits. For example, as an antispasmodic, chamomile helps control muscle spasms, as may occur with irritable bowel syndrome or diverticulitis pain. The herb also has antiseptic (germ-fighting), carminative (digestion-supporting and gas-reducing) and analgesic (pain-fighting) properties. For example, dried chamomile flowers can be used to make a topical compress that relieves the pain, irritation and/or infection of sties, pinkeye, bug bites, acne, eczema, burns and hemorrhoids.

What to do: In a pot, pour three ounces of boiling water over one tablespoon of dried chamomile flowers. Cover and let sit for 10 minutes, then put the moist flowers and remaining liquid in gauze and place it directly over the skin condition you want to treat. Cover with a dry towel, and leave in place for 15 minutes. Repeat this hourly as needed. You can also use chamomile tea bags to make a compress.

How: Put as many tea bags as you need to cover the affected area in a pot, and moisten thoroughly with boiling water. Let cool slightly, then apply over the area and cover with a dry towel. Let sit for 15 minutes.

Caution: People who are allergic to ragweed may also be allergic to chamomile.

•**Peppermint.** If your digestion is sluggish or you've overeaten and feel bloated and too full, have a strong cup of peppermint tea. Or add 60 drops of peppermint tincture to four ounces of hot water and sip as you would tea. This remedy helps relieve motion sickness, too.

Note: Don't drink peppermint tea if you have gastroesophageal reflux disease (GERD) since it could worsen symptoms.

For headache pain: Put a drop of peppermint essential oil on each temple (mix with unscented baby oil if your skin is sensitive), and if possible, cover your forehead and temples with a moist, warm towel, and lie down for 15 minutes. Repeat as needed.

•**Licorice.** Many people steer clear of licorice because it can worsen high blood pressure. But if you've got high blood pressure, you can still use licorice—it just needs to be "deglycyrrhizinated" licorice. This type of licorice has had the constituent responsible for blood pressure concerns (glycyrrhiza) removed. While the deglycyrrhizinating process reduces some of licorice's medicinal benefits, this herb remains very useful for ulcers, colitis, diverticulitis and gastritis.

What to do: Get chewable tablets or powdered deglycyrrhizinated licorice capsules. Take two tablets or capsules three times a day, away from meals, until your digestive condition is better. If your gastrointestinal pain is severe, lasts for more than three days, or you notice any rectal bleeding, seek medical attention. You could have a serious condition such as an infection.

Diabetes Drug Improves Gut Bacteria

Oluf Borbye Pedersen, MD, professor, Center for Basic Metabolic Research, University of Copenhagen, Denmark. University of Copenhagen, news release.

The diabetes drug *metformin* appears to trigger favorable changes in intestinal bacteria, a recent study finds.

Researchers analyzed the intestinal bacteria populations in 784 people with and without type 2 diabetes who lived in China, Denmark and Sweden.

The results showed that taking metformin had positive effects on the intestinal bacteria of people with type 2 diabetes. Specifically, the drug improved the ability of the bacteria to produce certain types of short-chain fatty acids that reduce blood sugar levels in different ways.

The researchers also found that patients who take metformin have more coliform bacteria in their intestines, which may explain why the drug causes side effects such as bloating and increased flatulence.

"We weren't able to show that other types of anti-diabetic drugs had any actual impact on the gut microbiota. When studying type 2 diabetes patients not being treated with metformin, we did, however, discover that they—irrespective of whether they were from Denmark, China or Sweden—had fewer of the bacteria which produce the health-promoting short-chain fatty acids," said senior study author Oluf Borbye Pedersen, MD, a professor with the Center for Basic Metabolic Research at the University of Copenhagen in Denmark.

"Whether the lack of certain combinations of fatty acid-producing intestinal bacterial species is one of the factors contributing to type 2 diabetes is currently being investigated," he said.

The study was published recently in the journal *Nature*.

info The American Diabetes Association has more about type 2 diabetes at *diabetes. org*.

When Omeprazole Fails for GERD, Endoscopic Fundoplication Is an Option

John G. Hunter, MD, department of surgery, Oregon Health & Science University, Portland. His article was published in *Gastroenterology*.

The use of drugs for gastroesophageal reflux disease (GERD) has more than doubled in the past decade...but about 40% of GERD-drug users still experience severe heartburn or regurgitation. And long-term use of the drugs, called proton pump inhibitors or PPIs, such as Prilosec, Prevacid and Nexium, can have bad side effects. These are the reasons some GERD sufferers are resorting to an invasive treatment called laparoscopic antireflux surgery, which involves pumping the abdomen up with carbon dioxide to make it expand and then making several small incisions in it to access and operate on the valve between the stomach and esophagus.

Are you picturing that now? No wonder less than 10% of affected patients and physicians opt for it, preferring to simply put up with less-than-adequate PPI relief. But another GERD procedure that doesn't involve drugs or surgical incisions is actually available.

It is called transoral incisionless fundoplication (TIF), and it is the only tried-and-true endoscopic alternative to laparoscopic antireflux surgery introduced in the past two decades. (Other techniques have been introduced but were discontinued either because they were ineffective or unsafe.) In TIF, an endoscope is inserted into the mouth through the esophagus to the stomach. Then a tool is passed through the endoscope to place a few stitches in the esophageal sphincter (the valve between the esophagus and stomach) to tighten the sphincter and prevent acid reflux. Patients, on average, spend about a day in the hospital to recover, whereas the hospital stay can range from two to five days for laparoscopic surgery. Recovery is also quicker, with patients often returning to most of their regular activities in a few days instead of weeks.

A recent clinical trial sponsored by the makers of TIF technology (called EsophyX) compared the effectiveness of TIF with *omeprazole* (Prilosec) to confirm that the procedure could be an alternative for people who do not get adequate relief from PPIs. It included 129 participants who were taking omeprazole but still had GERD symptoms. The participants were randomly assigned to a real TIF procedure and a placebo pill or sham surgery and real omeprazole therapy. They filled out questionnaires about their symptoms before and then periodically for six months after the study began, and the researchers periodically assessed the participants during this time. If severe GERD symptoms continued in a patient after three months, the treatment received was considered a failure, and, for ethical reasons, the participant was offered the alternative treatment.

The results: Although a relatively sizeable proportion of participants who had sham surgery plus omeprazole therapy—45%—reported that their symptoms had improved, a greater proportion of those who received TIF—67%—reported symptom improvement. As for treatment failures, after three months, they included 36% of sham surgery/PPI users but only 11% of patients who received TIF.

Through their periodic health assessments of participants, the researchers found that TIF reduced the incidence of reflux by an average of 30% and improved stomach pH (a measure of acidity). Despite the fact that 45% of participants in the sham surgery/PPI group said that their symptoms had improved, their health assessments showed no actual change in incidence of reflux or stomach pH.

SIDE EFFECTS TO EXPECT

TIF, like all medical interventions, does have some potential side effects, but serious complications are uncommon. In this study, two people in the TIF group experienced temporary stomach pain lasting two to four weeks, two had trouble swallowing for up to a week after the procedure, one patient had chest pain for three days and another had musculoskeletal pain for one day after the procedure.

TIF is available at surgical centers around the country and is being used worldwide as a safer alternative to other forms of GERD surgery. If you have had no luck getting relief from GERD with natural lifestyle remedies, drugstore medications or prescription drugs, or if you are concerned about the long-term effects of PPI use, such as malabsorption of vitamins and bone loss, you may want to discuss TIF with your doctor.

Chew This Too for Heartburn

Joe Graedon, MS, a pharmacologist, and Terry Graedon, PhD, a medical anthropologist. The Graedons are coauthors of *The People's Pharmacy Quick & Handy Home Remedies* and cohosts of *The People's Pharmacy* public radio program. PeoplesPharmacy.com

In a study published in the *Journal of Dental Research*, acid reflux patients were fed lunches that included whole milk, lots of cheese, chips and salad with mayonnaise—fare that would give almost anyone heartburn. Some subjects were then given sugar-free gum to chew for 30 minutes.

Result: Two hours later, the gum chewers had significantly lower acid levels than people who hadn't chewed gum.

Explanation: Chewing gum stimulates saliva production, which helps rinse the esophagus of acid.

What to do: If you frequently suffer from heartburn, try chewing gum after meals. Be sure to choose sugar-free gum to keep cavities at bay.

Note: Mint gum or gum with sorbitol can cause digestive upset in some people.

CHAPTER 9

Emotional Well-Being

How the World Is Making You Anxious

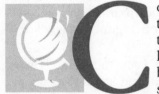

Could the worries of a troubled world be taking a toll on your life? It's one thing to be anxious about personal and family matters—Will my medical test come back positive? How will I pay my bills? Will my troubled son ever find his way? We all know that living with such anxieties can hurt our health and happiness.

Recently, however, many of us have been feeling extreme stress over far less personal problems—disturbing national and global developments that repeatedly draw our attention. And this stress, while perhaps rooted in events far from home, still can hit home in severely damaging ways—it can hurt our sleep and our health...and even shorten our lives.

Examples: Global terrorism increasingly feels like an omnipresent danger. US politics, as reflected in the recent presidential contest, has devolved in a way that triggers extreme emotions, including anger, fear and even hatred. Financial markets worldwide have become much more volatile, sparking fears of economic upheaval. Confrontations involving police have fueled racial tensions. Refugee crises around the world show us horrific suffering. The threat of nuclear proliferation and attack seem reignited as Iran and North Korea beat their chests. The Zika virus and, before it, the Ebola virus rise up as health threats. And never-ending cyber attacks threaten our privacy and security.

But are the dangers any more extreme than in the past, and must they disrupt our daily lives? Here's why global and national problems can cause anxiety disproportionate to their true risk—and how to stop these anxieties from standing in the way of living a calm and happy life...

Robert L. Leahy, PhD, director of the American Institute for Cognitive Therapy and a clinical professor of psychology at Weill Cornell Medical College, New York City. He is past president of the Association for Behavioral and Cognitive Therapies and author of *The Worry Cure: Seven Steps to Stop Worry from Stopping You.*

UNDERSTANDING GLOBAL ANXIETY

The human mind is very good at providing warnings about risks. Unfortunately, it can stumble when it comes to evaluating and prioritizing those risks. *For example, we tend to overestimate risks when…*

•**We hear about them frequently.** The more often someone hears about a threat, the more likely that person is to conclude that the threat must be substantial. This translates into out-of-proportion anxieties about global and national threats that are discussed endlessly in the media.

•**The images are hard to forget.** Troubling events often are accompanied by shocking pictures and/or video—including such recent images as shootings, beheadings and dead bodies—that can trigger deep emotional responses.

•**We don't know what we can do to stop the threat.** Worried about your family's finances? There's probably something you can do to mitigate the risks and ease your fears, such as economizing, adjusting your investment portfolio and/or earning additional income. But there is little you can do to reduce global dangers or to head off a recession or a market meltdown.

The threats are relatively new. The longer a threat is around, the more comfortable people grow with it. Heart disease and cancer have always been around, so people tend not to consider them pressing dangers—even though they kill far more Americans than terrorism does.

•**We perceive malicious intent.** People tend to overestimate risks related to forces that seem to want to cause them harm. That's another reason we might worry more about ISIS or North Korea than about a car accident—there is no "bad guy" trying to crash our car.

CONTROLLING GLOBAL ANXIETY

An important step in overcoming anxiety is to realize which problems actually are responsible for your worries. It can be especially difficult to pinpoint the source of anxiety when global problems are to blame because these problems are far removed from daily life.

What to do: Consciously monitor your emotions throughout the day. When you experience moments of anxiety, anger or sadness, jot down what you are doing, reading, discussing or thinking. Within a few days, you should see trends appearing.

Example: I often find myself feeling anxious when I think about one of the candidates who might win the presidential election.

If you discover that national or global problems cause you anxiety…

•**Carefully weigh the odds that what you fear actually will turn into reality.** If your anxieties revolve around terrorism, for example, your specific worry likely is that you or someone you love will be killed in an attack. If your anxieties revolve around an economic meltdown, your specific worry might be that you will lose your job and not be able to find a new one or that your retirement savings will disappear. As a next step, estimate the chance that this event actually will occur on a scale of 0% to 100%.

To do this, consider what evidence you really have that the risk is great—and keep in mind that people experiencing anxiety often inflate risks. If you fear not being able to find work, for example, consider that three of every four Americans in the labor force remained employed even at the deepest depths of the Great Depression. You may be surprised to find that the risk of your feared event occurring is not quite as high as you had automatically assumed.

Next, think of a person you know and respect who is not especially concerned about this particular national or global worry, and imagine how that person would estimate your risk on the same 0% to 100% scale. Now list some reasons why your worry will not come true. Ordinarily you might struggle to list reasons why something you fear will not come true—but this should become a bit easier after you take a moment to see things from the perspective of someone who sees little risk. Refer to this list when you experience anxiety on the subject in the future—it could help calm your fears.

•**Determine what productive action, if any, you can take.** You might not be able to stop a global threat, but there may be something you can do to stand in opposition to it…or to minimize the damage that it will do to you should it occur. Taking this step should ease your anxiety by helping you regain some sense of control.

Make a list of potential productive actions, and refer to this list whenever your anxieties arise.

Example: If there is a political candidate who frightens you, you could campaign for or make donations to that candidate's opponent. If terrorism frightens you, you could attend a rally for a cause that terrorists would despise—perhaps something related to religious freedom or equal rights.

•**Schedule daily time to confront this concern.** Believe it or not, if you cannot stop yourself from worrying about an issue, you still can minimize the impact that the issue has on your life by scheduling a specific time to worry—it actually works. To do this, select a 20-minute window each day during which you are "allowed" to worry about the troubling topic. If you catch yourself experiencing anxiety about it at other times, reassure yourself that you will sort through these thoughts during the designated worry time, and then turn your attention back to something else. But don't just sit around worrying during these 20 minutes. Use at least some of this time to review the other steps described here.

•**Reduce your exposure to negative news,** negative political commentary and negative social-media interactions. If something chronically discussed on the TV news, on the radio or in newspapers causes you anxiety, reduce your time spent engaging with these media outlets and do something more calming instead.

•**Consider the evidence that the US and the world actually are improving.** If you think that the US and the world are headed in the wrong direction, you're not alone—polls suggest that the majority of Americans would agree. But despite all the bad news we encounter, evidence suggests quite the opposite…

•Violent crimes are in the news every day—but what the news rarely mentions is that the violent-crime rate in the US actually is very low by historical standards. For example, the per-capita homicide rate has fallen by more than 50% in the past 25 years.

•Horrible diseases such as Zika and Ebola are frequently in the news, too—but Americans are living longer, healthier lives.

•Authoritarian regimes such as North Korea and ISIS are in the news, as is the bloody conflict in Syria—but the world is, overall, more democratic than ever…and by historical standards, global war deaths per capita have been very low for the past quarter century.

Probiotics, Happy Moods and Preventing Depression

Study titled "A randomized controlled trial to test the effect of multispecies probiotics on cognitive reactivity to sad mood" by researchers at Leiden University, Leiden Institute for Brain and Cognition, and University of Amsterdam, all in The Netherlands, published in *Brain, Behavior, and Immunity.*

Is a healthy stomach the key to happiness? It's beginning to seem that way. A healthy gut population of beneficial bacteria is increasingly being found to have not just physical but mental health benefits. In the latest study, researchers found that probiotics actually seem to chase away bad feelings.

It's all about the "brain-gut axis"—the two-way communications network between the intestines and the brain that affects the nervous system, hormones and immunity. In previous research, a few small human studies had found that either probiotic supplements or probiotic-rich foods such as yogurt reduce stress, reduce anxiety or improve mood. What's particularly interesting about the latest study is that it focused on the kind of bad moods that are linked with an increased risk for depression—even in psychologically healthy people. And anything that can help with depression and that is also totally safe, well, that's exciting.

THE MIND-ALTERING POWER OF PROBIOTICS

In the placebo-controlled, randomized study, researchers at Leiden University in The Netherlands assigned 40 healthy adults without mood disorders to take either a daily probiotic supplement or a placebo supplement for four weeks.

Each probiotic supplement contained a mixture of bacterial strains known to be important for a healthy human gut, including Bifidobacterium and Lactobacillus. The placebo was basically starch. Before and after the four-week pill period, participants answered survey questions to gauge their moods as well as vulnerability to depression and anxiety.

The result: Participants who took probiotic supplements were less prone to "rumination"—the tendency to dwell excessively on negative events or feelings—and had less aggressive feelings when they did feel sad. That's important, the study authors note, because a tendency to ruminate "is sufficient to turn mood fluctuations into depressive episodes." And aggressive thoughts are associated with depression and the risk for suicide.

PREVENTION IN A PILL?

Does this study mean we can prevent depression by eating the right foods or taking the right supplements? We can't know yet. It's more than a stone's throw to go from improved moods to actual prevention of depression or anxiety disorders. Frankly, we're just beginning to understand the connection. In a way, that's what makes it so fascinating—and promising. We have more to learn before health professionals can use specific probiotics as a way to help people protect themselves from depression—or to treat it. But that may be the future.

Nor was this study designed to answer the "how" question—but the researchers do suggest possible mechanisms based on research. One theory is that healthy gut bacteria increase blood levels of tryptophan, an amino acid that boosts brain levels of the mood-boosting chemical serotonin (which often are too low in people with depression). A second theory is that healthy gut bacteria make it less likely that toxins in the gut will "leak" out and activate inflammatory pathways that play a role in depression. The third theory is that gut bacteria may directly improve gut/brain signaling in ways that enhance positive emotions.

Whatever the mechanisms, it seems clear now that a healthy gut is good for the mind as well as the body. We already know probiotics have been shown to prevent or treat infectious diarrhea, traveler's diarrhea, antibiotic-associated diarrhea, irritable bowel syndrome, yeast infections, eczema and other conditions. Now there may be a new benefit—more happiness and less risk for depression.

So go ahead and enjoy probiotic-rich foods such as yogurt and kefir, pickled vegetables such as kimchi and sauerkraut, tempeh and miso. If you choose to supplement, look for products that contain both Bifidobacterium and Lactobacillus acidophilus, which colonize the human gut and so may provide benefits even after you stop taking them, according to naturopathic doctor Andrew L. Rubman.

Whatever you do, don't just stop taking any medication that was prescribed by your doctor and start taking a probiotic supplement instead. If you have a mood problem that lasts more than two weeks, especially if it is interfering with your life, don't put off seeing your doctor.

Should You Be Screened For Depression?

US Preventive Services Task Force, CNN, National Public Radio.

If you're an adult over age 18, the answer is emphatically yes—at least once in your life. That's true even if you feel fine and have no known risk factors.

So recommends the US Preventive Services Task Force, an independent group that has great influence over the practice of medicine—and what insurance companies will cover.

Their latest advice is to screen everyone. Why? Depression is so widespread that it is the leading cause of disability in the US. It also shortens lives through suicide and makes it harder for people with health conditions to take care of themselves.

The Task Force also advised that doctors screen all women who are pregnant or have recently given birth for postpartum depression. That's new, too.

Better Depression-Fighting Regimen

Depressed adults who completed 30 minutes of meditation followed by a half-hour of moderate-intensity exercise twice a week (on a treadmill, stationary bike or elliptical machine) lowered depressive symptoms by an average of 40% after two months—regardless of whether they were taking an antidepressant. Researchers theorize that the combination of meditation and exercise may result in brain changes that reduce negative feelings.

Brandon Alderman, PhD, assistant professor of exercise science, Rutgers, The State University of New Jersey, New Brunswick.

Diabetes Med for Depression

Natalie L. Rasgon, MD, PhD, is a professor of psychiatry and behavioral sciences at Stanford University Medical Center, Stanford, California, and leader of a study published in *Psychiatry Research*.

Diabetes medicine can improve depression. Among people who had depression for more than a year and who also were insulin-resistant, those given a 12-week course of the diabetes medicine *pioglitazone* (Actos) showed improvement in their symptoms of depression. Nondiabetic patients who have been treated with antidepressants for more than six months and still have symptoms should ask their doctors to be evaluated for insulin resistance. If found, they should discuss adding a diabetes medicine to their treatment.

Quick Depression Relief

Molecular Psychiatry

In a new animal study, an experimental drug relieves depression in hours, compared to weeks or months with standard antidepressants. It could lead to a new class of fast-acting antidepressants—and help those who don't improve with older drugs.

Roseroot Is a Safe Alternative to Treat Depression

Study titled "Rhodiola rosea versus sertraline for major depressive disorder: A randomized placebo-controlled trial," by researchers in the departments of family medicine and community health, biostatistics and epidemiology, psychiatry, and investigational drug service, Perelman School of Medicine, University of Pennsylvania, published in the journal *Phytomedicine*.

Roseroot (Rhodiola rosea), also called golden root, has a long history in traditional folk medicine of boosting energy and treating depression. Now a high-quality study of people with mild-to-moderate depression has found that roseroot has many fewer side effects than the popular antidepressant *sertraline* (Zoloft). That's key because many people quit taking antidepressants due to side effects such as nausea, headache, weight gain and loss of sex drive. And it could be great news for people with depression who would like to escape dependence on pharmaceuticals. But the question is—how well does roseroot actually work?

MILDER BENEFITS, FEWER SIDE EFFECTS

The research team recruited 57 adults with mild-to-moderate depression and randomly assigned them to take either roseroot, sertraline or placebo for 12 weeks. Before the study and at intervals during it, the participants took a diagnostic psychological test called the Hamilton Depression Rating Scale (HAM-D) and kept a log of medication side effects. The study was randomized and placebo-controlled—the subjects didn't know what they were taking, and neither did the researchers.

The results: At the end of the study, depression scores had dropped for all the participants—including those taking the placebo. They had dropped the most with the drug sertraline, while roseroot worked only slightly better than placebo.

So does that mean roseroot was a bust? It does not. One reason is the design of the study. Researchers gave subjects a very small dose of roseroot/sertraline/placebo to start, then gradually increased doses after two weeks, then again after four weeks and yet again after six weeks—assuming the participants didn't have problems with side effects. The small sample size, and the fact that it took subjects six weeks to reach the target dose, limited the study— only really dramatic improvement would have shown up.

But when the researchers went back and calculated what the emotional benefit would have been if subjects had taken higher doses throughout the 12 weeks (in which case, results of those higher doses would have been reflected in the depression measurements), both sertraline and roseroot looked better. Sertraline still had an edge—the odds that there would have been significant mood improvement were 90%. But the odds with roseroot for significant improvement were an impressive 40%.

Why would anyone choose a 40% chance of significant improvement over a 90% chance? Because sertraline's benefits came with much higher incidence of side effects. While no one had truly serious adverse effects, nearly two-thirds (63%) of those taking sertraline reported adverse side effects. For roseroot, it was 30%...and for placebo, 17%. What's more, the sertraline side effects, which included nausea, sexual dysfunction, appetite change, insomnia, palpitations and gastrointestional disturbances, were serious enough that two of the subjects stopped taking the drug. For roseroot, the only side effects were nervousness and dizziness, and no one felt the need to stop taking it.

IF YOU WANT TO CONSIDER ROSEROOT

This small study doesn't definitively answer whether roseroot is a safe and effective addition to botanical depression treatments. Like many studies, it opens up a path for the next bit of research. The next step is a larger study that can more conclusively answer the question of relative effectiveness—including whether a higher dose of roseroot might work better and still have few side effects. (Even the highest doses in this study were on the lower end of doses in other recent studies.)

If you are interested in trying roseroot to relieve depressive symptoms, consult a naturopath or other qualified health-care provider who can evaluate whether you are a good candidate for roseroot and can recommend the best dosage and brand for you based on your symptoms. A mental health specialist can help you find the right kind of therapy, including talk therapy, for your depression. And never reduce or quit an antidepressant drug on your own without consulting your physician—that can have dire consequences.

Antidepressants and NSAIDs Don't Mix

Byung-Joo Park, MD, PhD, professor of preventive medicine, Seoul National University, South Korea.

Adults taking any type of antidepressant who also used nonsteroidal anti-inflammatory drugs (NSAIDs) such as *ibuprofen* (Motrin) were 30% more likely to suffer internal brain bleeding than adults who didn't take this drug combination, a study of more than 4 million people found.

Why: Both drugs slow blood clot formation.

If you take an antidepressant: Ask your doctor to monitor your blood-clotting ability if you also take an NSAID regularly...and adjust the dose or replace either drug if needed to reduce bleeding risk.

How Safe Are Antidepressants?

Erick Turner, MD, associate professor in the department of psychiatry and the department of pharmacology at Oregon Health & Science University (OHSU) School of Medicine in Portland. He is also a senior scholar with OHSU's Center for Ethics in Health Care.

In 2001, a major study funded by the manufacturer of the antidepressant *paroxetine* (Paxil) found that the drug was safe and effective for adolescents suffering from depression. Since that time, doctors have written millions of prescriptions for depressed teens to take this drug.

Now: A re-analysis of that study conducted by an independent research group has come to a strikingly different conclusion: Paroxetine was not helpful in treating depression in teens and, in fact, increased their risk for suicide.

How could such a disparity exist in the interpretation of the evidence—and what does it mean for people of all ages who may be taking an antidepressant?

To find out, we spoke with Erick Turner, MD, a psychiatrist who has extensively studied scientific reporting methods within the psychiatric literature.

How can an independent analysis of the drug manufacturer's research come to such a different conclusion from the earlier findings?

One problem that affects the findings is a way that the data is interpreted if someone drops out of the study. It could be that 20% to 30% of patients don't make it to the end of the study, and there are various methods for handling that. One method—a misleading one—is to analyze data only from patients who make it to the end of the study. That way, you wind up with a skewed sample because people may have dropped out because the drug wasn't working for them or they were experiencing side effects. If those people are excluded from the overall analysis, then it makes the drug look more effective for depressed patients than it actually is, which makes the drug look better to doctors.

Also, regarding the issue of suicidal thinking and behavior, it's all about the coding. Suppose there's a patient who was angry one moment, crying the next and then thinking about jumping off a building. If the researchers code that as "emotional lability" (the opposite of "emotional stability"), but don't code the suicidal behavior, then it gets brushed aside and doesn't get counted the way it should. Coding differences of this sort led to different findings in the new report. This basic level of research can be subjective, so different parties can arrive at different conclusions.

Should adults who take Paxil or another antidepressant now be concerned about the safety and effectiveness of these drugs?

This is just one study among many. The totality of the evidence may tell a different story. The real message with this new study is this—if an independent party gets access to the raw data at the granular level, they can reach very different conclusions and it can depend on whether the researcher has a vested interest in the study's results.

In general, then, how effective and safe are antidepressants for depression?

You can't count on these drugs to be a magic bullet. You may have an excellent response, or you may not. You'll likely need some persistence—you might need to try a second or third type of antidepressant or consider a combination of drugs. You can also start treatment with psychotherapy and consider medication later.

And in terms of safety, the FDA has found that the risk regarding suicidal tendencies seems to decrease with age. The risk is highest with people under age 18 and somewhat less among those ages 18 to 25. For people 25 and older, the risk seems to be neutral—the drugs are even protective after age 65.

What are the possible side effects of antidepressants?

Selective serotonin reuptake inhibitors (SSRIs), which include not only paroxetine but also *fluoxetine* (Prozac), *citalopram* (Celexa), *escitalopram* (Lexapro) and *sertraline* (Zoloft), are the ones most commonly prescribed, and they're usually pretty well tolerated. But one common side effect is sexual dysfunction. For some patients, that makes these drugs a no-go…for other patients, it's a nonissue.

Other types of antidepressants have different side effects. For example, *mirtazapine* (Remeron) tends to be sedating, which can be good for people who have trouble sleeping, but the potential downside is that it can cause increased appetite and weight gain. However, weight gain can be a welcome side effect for patients who aren't eating enough.

The dosage of an antidepressant should be gradually increased. With Zoloft, for instance, the FDA-recommended dosage for depression ranges from 50 mg to 200 mg once daily. I generally start people at 25 mg daily and continue that for a week or two...then go to 50 mg daily for a week or two...then 75 mg and then 100 mg. After a few months, the patient might need to go up to 150 mg or to the 200-mg maximum daily dose. It depends on the balance between therapeutic benefits and side effects.

Tapering off antidepressants should be done gradually, as well. If you run out of pills or stop suddenly, you could have discontinuation syndrome with side effects including nausea, dizziness and feeling teary and emotionally unstable.

So you should consult your doctor—an internist or a mental-health practitioner—whenever starting or going off antidepressants.

In general, when do the benefits of antidepressants outweigh the risks?

A number of studies have shown that you get more bang for your buck in terms of effectiveness when the depression is more severe. So if a person is severely depressed—if he/she can't get out of bed or has suicidal thinking—then it's certainly worth pulling out all the stops to help that person.

You and your doctor should be sure to review your progress after six to 12 months of treatment. It's important to remember not to stop treatment once you begin to feel better. And never stop taking antidepressants without first consulting your doctor.

But if you have mild depression, you're less likely to see a substantial benefit from taking an antidepressant. You might consider other ways to treat your depression—decreasing isolation, getting more exercise and seeking psychotherapy.

A recent study found that light therapy—sitting in front of a light box daily—helped ease

---

The Happy Spice: Vanilla

Want a quick mood boost? Go vanilla. People who ate vanilla-flavored yogurt had more positive moods, according to a new study, while those who ate fruit-flavored yogurts (strawberry, pineapple) experienced no emotional lift. Interestingly, the emotional responses to the different yogurts was unrelated to whether the subjects said they liked the tastes or not—that is, even if it's not your favorite flavor, vanilla might still make you feel happier. Earlier studies have found that the mere aroma of vanilla—even when it's barely noticeable—lowers the heart rate and eases anxiety.

Study titled "Are implicit emotion measurements evoked by food unrelated to liking?" by researchers at Wageningen UR Food & Biobased Research, the Netherlands, University of Natural Resources and Life Sciences (BOKU), Austria, and VTT Technical Research of Finland, published in *Food Research International*.

---

depression symptoms. But check with your doctor first before considering light therapy, especially if you have bipolar disorder or certain other health conditions. Your doctor can guide you on the optimal amount of time to use a light box.

Light Therapy Can Fight Depression All Year Long

Study of 122 adults by researchers in the Mood and Anxiety Disorders Program at University of British Columbia, Vancouver, Canada, published in *JAMA Psychiatry*.

Daily light therapy is the standard treatment for seasonal affective disorder, which causes depression in the darker winter months. After eight weeks, about 60% of patients with nonseasonal depression who received a combination of the antidepressant Prozac and daily light therapy reported that their symptoms went into remission, versus about 40% who were treated with light therapy alone...and 20% of those who took only Prozac.

Get Happy...Erase Years from Your Face

Sanam Hafeez, PsyD, founder and clinical director of Comprehensive Consultation Psychological Services, with offices in New York City, Forest Hills and Uniondale, New York. Her research/clinical interests include neuropsychology, behavior modification and psychopathology. She has a faculty appointment at Columbia University's doctoral program in clinical psychology. ComprehendTheMind.com

Compare the faces of two people in your life. Person One is happy, relaxed and pleased with life. Person Two is overworked, stressed and harried. Guess which face appears younger and more attractive?

Stress can add years to your looks. When you're stressed, your body churns out cortisol, the hormone that primes you for action. Some cortisol is helpful (and motivating), but too much triggers inflammation, which affects every organ in your body, including the skin.

Experts have coined a term for the link between emotions and the skin—psychodermatology. This new field is based on research that shows that chronic stress and other psychological issues can trigger or exacerbate skin changes. But you can reverse those changes using emotional strategies and other lifestyle changes.

Example: Critically ill children who were given relaxing massages showed improvements in itching, redness and other skin conditions, according to researchers at the Touch Research Institute at University of Miami.

You can spend a fortune on anti-aging products and cosmetic procedures, but unless you manage stress at the same time, you'll still look older than you should.

WHAT STRESS DOES TO SKIN

Stress can cause blotches, itching, redness and acne. The cortisol-driven rise in inflammation damages tissues and capillaries that are readily apparent in the mirror. *Stress also causes...*

•**Dryness.** The constant bombardment of cortisol in women with chronic stress can mean a drop in estrogen that's been called minimenopause. Estrogen is largely responsible for the differences in appearance between young women and older ones. Women who are frequently stressed tend to develop dryness and a loss of skin elasticity.

While women need estrogen more than men and are more impacted on a monthly basis by its regulation, hormonal imbalance also happens in men with the excess secretion of the stress hormone androgen, as well as glucocorticoids. This can cause a loss of estrogen leading to dryness in both men and women and an overproduction of sebum (an oily secretion of the sebaceous glands), which can trigger acne and razor bumps.

•**Wrinkles.** There's a reason that forehead furrows, between-the-eye creases and other wrinkles are known as "frown lines," "worry lines" or even "battle lines." Repeated expressions can etch themselves permanently in your face.

•**Circles under the eyes.** They make you look tired and can age your appearance even more than wrinkles. Some people are genetically prone to under-eye circles. They also can be caused by sun exposure, a lack of sleep or allergic skin conditions, along with stress.

What happens: Stress increases blood flow, and the tiny capillaries under the eyes become engorged. Those dark circles really are blood vessels that are visible through the skin.

•**Under-eye bags.** Like circles under the eyes, these puffy areas are partly due to genetics. But they're also common in people whose stress keeps them up at night. A lack of sleep causes fluids to accumulate under the eyes and makes your face appear puffy and tired.

WHAT TO DO

•**Take "mini-vacations."** Almost everyone can benefit from frequent "mini-vacations" that provide a break from stress. These can be as simple as a lunchtime walk…admiring a piece of art…or listening to a favorite song.

•**Eat an estrogen-enhancing diet including fresh fruits and vegetables, salmon and whole grains.** These antioxidant-rich foods fight inflammation. Fruits and vegetables also are naturally rich in phytoestrogens, plant compounds that mimic the effects of estrogen in the body. Estrogen "plumps" the skin and gives women and men a healthy glow.

•**Avoid excess sugar in all forms,** including refined carbohydrates, alcohol and highly processed foods, such as cake and cookies. These cause the body to produce advanced glycation end-products, toxins that trigger inflammation in the skin. The sugars in carbohydrates attach to certain proteins and can break down skin collagen, causing a loss of elasticity and the plumpness we associate with young skin.

•**Drink more water.** People who stay hydrated tend to have plumper, younger-looking skin. Also, water can flush excess salt from the body, which reduces under-eye puffiness. If you don't care for regular water, try coconut water. It is a natural source of electrolytes that help to keep you hydrated.

•**Relax your face.** You're probably not aware of your facial expressions, but you can learn to relax your face. When you're feeling stressed, remind yourself not to squint or frown. Be mindful of your expressions. Eventually, not frowning will become a habit. If you find yourself frowning, make it a habit to smooth your hand over your forehead and think happy, tranquil thoughts until your face naturally relaxes to a resting state.

•**Get a good night's sleep.** Even if you find that you can't log a full eight hours, at least make sure that the sleep you get is quality sleep. Relax for an hour before going to bed. Turn off the TV and computers. This puts your mind into the "sleep mode" so that it starts to shut down or cool off in preparation for bedtime. Pull the blinds or curtains so that your room is dark. If you can't fall asleep in 15 or 20 minutes, get up and do something relaxing, such as gazing out the window or holding a yoga pose. You want to stay within yourself instead of engaging with electronics or the outside world until you're tired enough to try again. If you find yourself becoming anxious about all the things you have to do, make a list of what needs to be done. You'll feel like you accomplished something and are in control of your tasks. And you won't be worried about forgetting them the next day.

Sleep with your head slightly elevated—a thick pillow will do it. The increased pull of gravity will help fluids drain away from your eyes.

•**Exercise.** Exercise relieves stress. You'll almost instantly see a difference when you attend a yoga class or go for a power walk. Your face will look smoother and younger.

Better Sleep Habits

Patrick H. Finan, PhD, assistant professor of psychiatry and behavioral sciences, The Johns Hopkins University School of Medicine, Baltimore

A late bedtime is actually better than a full night of sleep with interruptions.

New study: Adults who had a delayed bedtime experienced only a 12% reduction in positive mood versus 31% in those who were awakened several times during the night.

Explanation: The interrupted sleepers had less slow-wave sleep, the type that leaves you feeling restored and rested.

Beware the Hazards of Positive Thinking

Gabriele Oettingen, PhD, professor of psychology at New York University, New York City, and University of Hamburg in Germany. She is author of *Rethinking Positive Thinking: Inside the New Science of Motivation.* WOOPMyLife.org

We're often told to think positive. Whether we want to lose weight… quit smoking…negotiate a raise or promotion…achieve great wealth…or get elected president, we're assured that the key is to ignore self-doubt, banish pessimism and believe that we can do it.

But positive thinking leads to productive action only if we know how to handle it. If we don't, pie-in-the-sky daydreams and unbridled optimism are more likely to lead to stagnancy than success. For example, a recent study found that people were less likely to make a substantial donation to a charity if they first fantasized that the problem the charity addresses had been solved. Indulging in the positive-thinking fantasy gave their minds the same positive feelings that they would have experienced if they actually had helped solve the problem, robbing them of the drive to take action.

Or consider the presidential election. Some of the candidates have been relentlessly positive about what they could achieve if elected—an attitude that whips up crowds and attracts admirers.

The problem: The more an incoming president displays positive thinking, the worse the country seems to do. A 2014 study published in *Psychological Science* examined inaugural addresses from 1933 to 2009 and found that the more idealistic a portrait a president paints, the higher the unemployment rate and the lower the gross domestic product during the ensuing four years. That may be because an overly idealistic president might be more likely to ignore the obstacles…downplay the necessary steps to achieve the economic goals…and pursue risky ventures.

So how do you employ positive thinking as a powerful force? The key is to use it as part of the following four-step strategy, which has been shown to actually increase our odds of taking productive action and achieving a goal…

•**Identify a goal.** Choose something you would like to achieve, whether you call it a "goal" or a "wish." This could be a short-term goal—something you could accomplish today—or a long-term goal that will take much longer. Your goal should be something that you believe you can realistically accomplish but that is somewhat challenging to you. Boil your goal down to a phrase of just three to six words.

Examples: "Book a trip" or "Lose five pounds."

•**Picture the best outcome.** Now imagine what it would be like if your wish came true in the very best possible way. How would you feel? How would your life change?

Let yourself mentally experience this imagined outcome. Revel in it for a few minutes. This helps link the wish to pleasurable feelings in your mind—indulging in fantasies can feel wonderful. Your blood pressure actually might drop, enveloping you in a sense of calm and contentment.

Dreamers tend not to progress beyond this stage, but two crucial steps remain to maximize your odds of making your wish come true.

•**Picture your greatest internal obstacle.** As soon as you stop fantasizing about the best possible outcome of your wish, ask yourself, What one thing in me is most holding me back from making this wish come true?

The goal here is to uncover your main internal obstacle, not an external one. If you see an external force as your main hindrance, there's a good chance that the problem will seem insurmountable. If you see something within yourself as the main problem, there's a good chance you will be able to develop a solution.

Example: If your wish is to get a promotion at work, the first obstacle that comes to mind might be, *My boss is a fool who does not appreciate me.* This is not the obstacle you need to identify—a foolish boss is an external problem. Make this obstacle internal by rephrasing it as, *I feel resentment toward my boss that makes it hard for me to earn his respect.*

Your internal obstacle might be instantly obvious, or it might take time to figure out. If it proves elusive, seek it through quiet, private contemplation. Do not ask other people for their input—your odds of understanding and overcoming the obstacle are much higher if you discover it yourself. If you're not certain whether you have identified the critical internal obstacle, you probably haven't—there's usually a "That's it!" moment of revelation when you have discovered it.

Helpful: People often initially conclude that their main obstacle is, *I don't have time to pursue the goal.* These people may want to dig deeper into why they can't seem to find the time. For example, someone might realize that he/she cannot find time to pursue his wish because he devotes lots of time to helping other people pursue their wishes…and that he does this because he fears not being needed. That fear is a major obstacle. Someone else might realize that he is not finding time for a project because he is afraid of failing.

Boil your obstacle down to three to six words, then spend some time thinking about it. Picture how this obstacle stands in your way, stopping you from reaching your goal.

This reduces the odds that your mind will be satisfied with mere fantasy and helps you do what it takes to make the wish a reality.

Once you have identified and pictured your obstacle, you might realize that you need to modify or even switch your goal because the obstacle is so formidable that you can't overcome it—or the goal is just not worth pursuing.

Example: Your wish is to get up each morning and exercise. Your obstacle is that you feel distracted by everything you have to do during the day. Perhaps it makes sense to change your initial wish to "exercise in the evenings."

•**Develop a plan to overcome your obstacle.** This plan should fit a simple if/then format—If [obstacle X occurs], then I will [take action Y].

Example: If I feel insecure when someone questions my proposal, then I will remind myself that I am just as knowledgeable on this topic as anyone.

Developing a plan in advance to overcome your internal obstacle will not just help you overcome this obstacle…it may improve your odds of overcoming any obstacle that appears. The process of obstacle identification and if/then planning described above trains the mind to look for and get past obstacles, rather than get stopped by them on a nonconscious level.

Helpful: Find a quiet moment each day to identify your goal, your best outcome, your central internal obstacle and your if/then plan. By practicing this procedure every day, you will be much more successful in understanding your wishes and attaining your goals.

Quitting or Just Cutting Back on Alcohol? What to Expect…

Jack Canfield, cocreator of the Chicken Soup for the Soul book series and CEO of Canfield Training Group, a Santa Barbara–based corporate training company, and Dave Andrews, a leading sobriety coach and founder of The 30-Day Solution, LLC. The pair are coauthors of *The 30-Day Sobriety Solution: How to Quit or Cut Back Drinking in the Privacy of Your Own Home.* The30Day Solution.com

Nearly one-third of American adults drink excessively. Many of these drinkers eventually will decide that alcohol is harming their health and happiness and try to quit or at least cut way back. *Knowing these surprising facts could improve your odds of succeeding…*

•**If you have an alcohol problem, you have a sugar problem, too.** Alcohol is basically fermented sugar. So when heavy drinkers quit drinking, their bodies don't just crave alcohol…they also crave the large quantities of sugar that they're used to consuming.

What to do: Giving up drinking is challenge enough—do not force yourself to give up sugar at the same time. For at least your first month of your sobriety, keep your blood sugar levels up by eating whenever you feel hungry—at least once every five hours…never skipping a meal, especially breakfast…and consuming plenty of fruit, which satiates cravings for sugar, without resorting to unhealthy treats such as candy.

•**Willpower alone is never enough to overcome excessive drinking.** People who have tried to quit drinking without success in the past often conclude that they lack sufficient willpower to remain sober. In truth, no one has enough willpower to permanently stop doing something they very much want to do. The secret to giving up alcohol is to find a way to decrease your desire to drink so that you are not as dependent on willpower to quit.

What to do: Whenever you feel the urge to drink, imagine what your life will be like in five or 10 years if you continue drinking heavily, versus what it could be like if you stop. *For example, consider…*

•How healthy you could be if you quit, versus how unhealthy you could be if you continue.

•How much you would accomplish if you were always sober, versus all the hours you would have wasted drinking or being drunk.

•How much money you could have saved, versus how much you would have spent on alcohol.

•How respected you could be, versus the embarrassments you might have endured with continued heavy drinking—such as behaving like a buffoon at parties.

Drinkers tend to associate drinking with pleasure and quitting with pain—that's why it takes willpower to quit. Reflecting on the long-term pain of drinking and long-term pleasure of stopping helps reverse this association, so sobriety no longer feels like an endless struggle against desire.

•**Giving up drinking can lead to chemically induced feelings of depression.** The brains of heavy drinkers often produce the "positive thinking" neurotransmitters dopamine and serotonin only when alcohol is in the bloodstream. When these people suddenly stop drinking (or cut way back on their alcohol intake), the loss of these upbeat mood-triggering neurochemicals leaves them feeling depressed. Some inevitably conclude that they need alcohol to be happy and start drinking again.

What to do: Your brain eventually will start producing dopamine and serotonin without

Trick to Overcome Cravings

Tapping your fingers on certain spots on your body can help control alcohol cravings (other cravings, too). That might sound unlikely, but decades of research confirms that this really does work for most people. One study found that it can reduce cravings by an astonishing 83%.

How is that possible? Experiencing cravings makes people feel stressed, which causes the body to release stress hormones. Gentle tapping in certain spots encourages the body to instead release dopamine and serotonin, the positive-feeling neurotransmitters discussed in the article above.

What to do: When you feel like you need a drink, use your index and middle fingers to gently tap five to seven times on each of the following eight spots…

•**The top of your head**

•**One of your eyebrows**

•**Just beyond the outer corner of one of your eyes**

•**Just under one of your eyes**

•**Just under your nose**

•**On your chin**

•**On your collarbone**

•**In one of your armpits.**

Not coincidentally, these are among the spots that acupuncturists have been targeting with their needles for thousands of years. (For more details, search "EFT Tapping Therapy" on You Tube.)

alcohol again, but it could take as long as 90 days (or in rare cases, even longer). For at least the first three months of sobriety, regularly consume foods that contain omega-3 fats, such as wild-caught salmon, sardines, herring, anchovies and mackerel—these have been shown to significantly raise dopamine levels.

Also consume foods that contain *gamma-aminobutyric acid* (GABA), such as cherry tomatoes, shrimp and bananas—these can beneficially alter the brain's serotonin balance. Taking dietary supplements containing GABA or omega-3 could help, too. But speak to your doctor before taking supplements.

•**You could end up feeling mentally foggy.** People assume that they will feel sharper when they stop drinking, and for light drinkers and weekend bingers, this usually is true. But when heavy daily drinkers first quit, they often find their thinking becoming foggier. This stems from the chemical changes occurring in the brain as it readjusts to life without alcohol, and it generally lasts several weeks.

What to do: Exercising regularly and drinking plenty of water during this foggy brain period seems to help. Some people find that listening to or playing music helps focus the mind during this period, too.

•**You don't have to hit rock bottom to quit.** There is a common misconception that drinkers cannot successfully give up drinking until they "hit bottom," which might involve going on a prolonged bender...losing a job or spouse because of drinking...or getting arrested for drunk driving. In truth, the only reason heavy drinkers tend not to quit until they "hit bottom" is that until then they generally are not willing to admit that they have a serious drinking problem.

What to do: Stop searching for reasons why your drinking is not a problem, and instead honestly consider the question, Would my life be better without alcohol? If you answer yes, then you have a problem and should quit.

•**Quitting drinking earns you free time**—but that time could be dangerous to your sobriety. Heavy drinkers who quit often are amazed by how much more time they suddenly have. Not only does quitting free up the hours they previously spent drinking, it frees up the hours they previously spent too drunk to do anything productive—and the hours they spent sleeping off hangovers.

What to do: Find constructive and/or enjoyable things to fill this newfound time. Boredom is a sobriety killer—former drinkers sometimes return to the bottle simply because they can't think of anything else to do.

If you don't have projects and hobbies in mind, try getting exercise outdoors...learning to play a musical instrument...or starting a home-improvement project.

Or you can volunteer with nonprofits...take adult-education classes...or use websites such as MeetUp.com to find nonalcohol-related gatherings.

Activities that involve spending time with people who are not drinking are best. Excessive drinking often is at some level a substitute for love and human connection. If people you love insist on getting intoxicated when you're together, it's important to not spend time with them when they're drunk. Ultimately, if they don't change, they are going to want you to drink, so spending time with them while they are intoxicated can be risky. Without coming across as judgmental or resentful, explain that you love them but that you need to make this change for your own well-being.

Drinking Is a Problem for Seniors

Tony Rao, MD, visiting researcher, Institute of Psychiatry, Psychology & Neuroscience, King's College London, UK.

Harmful drinking is rampant among older adults, we hear from Tony Rao, MD. In an analysis of the drinking habits of nearly 28,000 adults age 65 and older, one in five drank too much—more than 21 drinks a week for men and 14 for women.

Takeaway: Alcohol tolerance decreases as we age, while risk for liver damage, falls and confusion increases. Limit drinks to no more than two a day for men...one for women.

Anti-Addiction Drug May Help Curb Painkiller, Heroin Dependence

Joshua D. Lee, MD, MSc, associate professor, Department of Population Health, NYU Langone Medical Center, New York City.

Terry L. Horton, MD, chief, Division of Addiction Medicine, Christiana Care Health System, Wilmington, Delaware.

New England Journal of Medicine, online.

The newer anti-addiction drug *naltrexone* may become an important weapon in the country's escalating addiction to opioid painkillers and heroin, a new study suggests.

Researchers found that monthly injections of extended-release naltrexone—which blocks the euphoric effects of opioids—resulted in a significantly lower relapse rate among treated addicts compared to a similar group that didn't receive the drug. Additionally, during the six-month study there were no overdoses in the naltrexone group compared to five in the other group.

Opioids—including prescription painkillers such as OxyContin, Vicodin and Percocet, as well as the street drug heroin—killed more than 28,000 people in 2014, a record high, according to the U.S. Centers for Disease Control and Prevention.

"We thought this was a good approach to relapse prevention…but I was surprised by how clearly effective this medication was," said study author Joshua Lee, MD, an associate professor in the department of population health at NYU Langone Medical Center, in New York City.

"We haven't had another study like this in the United States," Dr. Lee added. "This is potentially a very important study if a [health care] provider wasn't convinced before that they should offer naltrexone. They may be less skeptical now."

The study is published in an online issue of the *New England Journal of Medicine.*

An extended-release version of naltrexone, known also by the brand name Vivitrol, is the most recently approved product by the U.S. Food and Drug Administration to treat opiate addiction, and the only drug labeled for relapse prevention. Other anti-addiction medications include methadone and buprenorphine.

STUDY DETAILS

At five sites in four major US cities, Dr. Lee and his team administered monthly injections of naltrexone to 153 opioid-addicted adults who had had some criminal justice involvement. A similar group of 155 participants did not receive the drug but were referred for "usual care" consisting of brief counseling and referrals to community treatment programs.

After six monthly injections, 43% in the treatment group had relapsed, compared to 64% of those who didn't receive naltrexone. The average time elapsing before relapse was double in the naltrexone group.

Follow-up one year after the treatment ended found both groups were using opioids at a similar rate. And two additional overdoses had occurred in the non-naltrexone group and none in the treatment group.

IMPLICATIONS

Dr. Lee and another addiction expert agreed that these results suggest naltrexone therapy should be used longer than six months.

"Addiction is a chronic brain disorder, and the brain changes under the influence of drugs," said Terry Horton, MD, chief of addiction medicine at Christiana Care Health System, in Wilmington, Delaware. Drugs "hijack" critical parts of the brain involved with motivation and reward, and "those changes take a long time to heal," he said.

"So medications facilitate moving toward recovery," he said, "but this requires a long-term effort, as with all chronic diseases."

Dr. Horton said the new research provided "hopeful" results that were similar to those done in other countries.

"My hope is this will provide another tool in the tool chest to help care for individuals who are in the criminal justice system and moving back into society so they can address their opiate dependence," Dr. Horton said. "The models of care we see in the prison population can also be generalized to the greater population. Opiate dependence is, sadly, a disease that's cutting across all socioeconomic, racial and gender boundaries. It's affecting everyone."

In an effort to curb the national epidemic of prescription painkiller abuse, the FDA and CDC announced new initiatives. The FDA moved to label certain drugs with "boxed warnings" that notify users of the dangers of misuse, while the CDC instituted tough new guidelines for doctors prescribing prescription painkillers.

Doctors Lee and Horton agreed that more research on anti-addiction treatments is necessary, particularly to compare the effectiveness of naltrexone to other anti-addiction drugs.

"But I don't know that we need a ton more research on this to say, why don't we use these?" said Dr. Lee.

info The U.S. National Institute on Drug Abuse offers more information on opioids at *drugabuse.gov.* Search "opioids."

Wearable Electric Patch May Ease PTSD

Andrew Leuchter, MD, director, neuromodulation division, Semel Institute for Neuroscience and Human Behavior, David Geffen School of Medicine, University of California, Los Angeles.
Ron Ramirez, PTSD and TNS patient, Gardena, California.
Jeffrey Deitz, MD, assistant professor, psychiatry, The Frank Netter School of Medicine of Quinnipiac University, Hamden, Connecticut, and supervising psychiatrist, Mount Sinai Beth Israel Medical Center, New York City.
Neuromodulation: Technology at the Neural Interface.

Can a small electrical patch that jolts the brain while patients sleep offer significant relief from the debilitating effects of post-traumatic stress disorder (PTSD)?

Iraq war veteran and PTSD patient Ron Ramirez thinks the answer is yes.

In May 2006, machine gunner Ramirez was seriously injured when a roadside bomb exploded during a tour of duty.

"About a year later they figured out that I had a brain injury," recalled the 38-year-old Gardena, California, resident. And like many veterans of war, that injury was further compounded by a diagnosis of PTSD, a condition typically trig-

gered by exposure to traumatic or threatening situations that provoke extreme fear.

PTSD brought on a significant shift in Ramirez' mood, thoughts and behavior, he said, resulting in a shattered quality of life.

"I had no motivation," he said. "I had constant nightmares, and I couldn't sleep. And I would get very irritated by other people, getting into altercations, sometimes even with other patients. I couldn't even take my two daughters out on my own without an escort."

Both before and after his release from the hospital in 2009, Ramirez was offered all the standard interventions available for PTSD patients, including a "trial-and-error" array of prescription drugs, behavioral therapy, PTSD counseling and anger management sessions.

But the result was little improvement. "It just wasn't really blending very well," he said. "In all honesty, I felt useless."

ABOUT TRIGEMINAL NERVE STIMULATION

Enter an experimental electrical brain treatment for PTSD called "trigeminal nerve stimulation" (TNS).

"TNS is a new approach to PTSD," said senior study author Andrew Leuchter, MD. He is director of the neuromodulation division in the Semel Institute for Neuroscience and Human Behavior at UCLA's David Geffen School of Medicine in Los Angeles.

"The challenge," he said, "is that despite offering the best treatments that we can, most PTSD patients are left, sometimes for decades, with significant residual symptoms, like anxiety, irritability, explosive outbursts and sleep difficulty, not to mention depression."

"But with TNS we approach the brain by thinking of it as a large network," Dr. Leuchter said. "And like any electrical network it's sensitive to any energy that gets put into it. So, with TNS we pulse the brain with an external source of energy through the trigeminal nerve," a nerve tasked with transmitting sensations between the face and brain.

"The hope," said Dr. Leuchter, "is that by doing this we can reset the brain network, and offer difficult-to-treat patients some relief."

The UCLA team that developed TNS set out to address the unmet needs of the roughly 3.5% of Americans who struggle with PTSD, including survivors of rape, car accidents, domestic abuse and other traumas. That figure rises to 17% of active veterans, and as many as 30% of vets who served in Iraq or Afghanistan, according to background information from the study.

The treatment relies on a 9-volt battery that powers a low-level current that zaps the brain through an external forehead patch worn during sleep, according to the researchers. The current targets the patient's autonomic nervous system and brain regions that regulate mood, behavior and thought.

STUDY DETAILS

Eight hours a night for eight weeks, 12 civilian patients with both PTSD and "major depressive disorder" underwent TNS treatment while continuing routine therapies. Participants were between the ages of 18 and 75.

"Patients reported mood improvement," Dr. Leuchter said. "And much better sleep, less anxiety and a decreased startle response," a reflexive defensive reaction to perceived threats. On average, PTSD symptoms appeared to drop by more than 30%, while depression severity fell by more than 50%, according to the researchers.

Side effects appeared limited to skin irritation at the patch site, the researchers said.

A follow-up trial, now under way, is slated to take another two to three years, and will ultimately involve 74 veterans with PTSD. But Ramirez has already completed his eight-week run.

"The first two weeks were the hardest, because it was annoying," he acknowledged. "It would shock you with a really sharp electrical impulse if you turned a certain way. But eventually I saw that I was a lot calmer. And my sleep was the best I had had in years. It took away my nightmares. I was more motivated. Usually I would lay in bed, and never leave the house. This rejuvenated me.

"And even after the eighth week, when we were done, it seemed to keep working," Ramirez added. "I do get irritated some times, but not as bad as before. Now I can go out on my own."

EXPERT REACTION

Jeffrey Deitz, MD, is an assistant professor of psychiatry at Quinnipiac University's Frank Netter School of Medicine in Hamden, Connecticut, and a supervising psychiatrist at Mount Sinai Beth Israel Medical Center in New York City. He described the new effort as "a very significant piece of work."

"This represents a whole paradigm shift in psychiatric treatment," he said. "The notion that disorders are all about biochemical imbalances in the brain, around since the '60's, is giving way to thinking about psychiatric issues in terms of brain circuitry that's overstimulated or understimulated.

"So this is very early in the process," said Dr. Deitz. "But it's also very exciting. And makes perfect sense."

info There's more on PTSD at the U.S. Department of Veteran Affairs, *PTSD.VA.gov*.

Brain Wiring Changes Might Help Guard Against Bipolar Disorder

Mount Sinai Hospital, news release

Naturally occurring brain wiring changes might help prevent bipolar disorder in people who have a high genetic risk for the mental illness, a new study suggests.

The discovery about these brain wiring changes could help efforts to develop better treatments for the disorder, according to Mount Sinai Hospital researchers in New York City.

People with bipolar disorder experience severe swings in mood, energy and activity levels, and the ability to perform daily tasks. Genetics are a major risk factor, and people with a parent or sibling with bipolar disorder are much more likely to develop it than those with no family history of the mental illness.

Researchers used functional MRI to monitor the brains of bipolar disorder patients, their siblings who did not have the illness (resilient siblings) and unrelated healthy volunteers. The bipolar disorder patients and their resilient siblings had similar abnormalities in brain wiring that handles emotional processing, but the resilient siblings had additional changes in that wiring.

"The ability of the siblings to rewire their brain networks means they have adaptive neuroplasticity that may help them avoid the disease even though they still carry the genetic scar of bipolar disorder when they process emotional information," study lead author Sophia Frangou, MD, a professor of psychiatry, said in a Mount Sinai news release.

The study was published online in the journal *Translational Psychiatry*.

"A family history remains the greatest risk factor for developing bipolar disorder and while we often focus on risk, we may forget that the majority of those who fall into this category remain well," Dr. Frangou said.

"Looking for biological mechanisms that can protect against illness opens up a completely new direction for developing new treatments. Our research should give people hope that even though mental illness runs in families, it is possible to beat the odds at the genetic lottery," she concluded.

Uncontrollable Emotional Outbursts Signal a Condition

Marc E. Agronin, MD, vice president, behavioral health and clinical research, Miami Jewish Health Systems and the author of *How We Age*. MarcAgronin.com

Uncontrollable laughter or crying can sometimes be due to a disorder known as *pseudobulbar affect* (PBA). It is typically associated with neurological conditions such as stroke, multiple sclerosis (MS), Alzheimer's disease, Parkinson's disease, traumatic brain injury, brain tumors and amyotrophic lateral sclerosis (ALS). These conditions can affect the frontal lobe of the brain that keeps emotions under control. People with PBA may have dozens of episodes of uncontrollable laughter or crying during the day, which can be extremely distressing and embarrassing.

These sudden bouts of emotion are sometimes not connected to surrounding events or the person's true feelings and can be completely inappropriate, such as laughing during a funeral. Emotions can also quickly switch, for example, from laughter to sobbing.

A medication called *dextromethorphan* and *quinidine* (Nuedexta) have been FDA-approved for the treatment of PBA. Side effects can include changes in heart rhythm, so it may not be appropriate for people with certain types of heart disease.

Uncontrollable emotional outbursts can also reflect an underlying psychiatric condition, such as bipolar disorder, especially if they are associated with symptoms of severe depression, mania or psychosis.

Anyone who has bouts of uncontrollable outbursts should be evaluated by a neurologist to determine the cause of his or her emotional episodes.

Placebos Work

JAMA Psychiatry

People with depression who respond to placebos are more likely to improve when they take real drugs. Placebos and genuine antidepressants may act on the same brain system—a finding that could lead to better treatments.

The Anxiety Advantage

Kate Sweeny, PhD, an associate professor of psychology at University of California-Riverside

Some of us are worry warts. When we have to wait for the results of a medical test—or some other important news—we agonize over the possibility that things will go wrong. But it turns out that could be a good thing. A study published recently in *Emotion* suggests that worriers are better prepared than nonworriers to cope with bad news when it comes…and we experience greater feelings of joy when the news is good.

And there is a way to reap the benefits of waiting-period anxiety without the unpleasant prolonged anxiety, says Kate Sweeny, PhD, an associate professor of psychology at University of California-Riverside and one of the study's researchers. The trick is to assume the best for most of the waiting period, then brace for the worst just before the verdict is delivered. We receive most of the psychological advantages of anxiety as long as we are anxious in those final moments. But what if there's no clear end date to your waiting period or if you can't ever set aside your worries?

Dr. Sweeny's advice is to select activities that put us in what's known as a "flow state," where the mind is so deeply engaged that we later wonder, Where did the time go? That can be solving puzzles, playing chess, painting pictures or getting work done. These activities—not passive things such as watching TV—have the best chance of distracting us from major worries.

When nothing can take our minds off our anxieties, the best option is to prepare for the feared outcome. While waiting for the results of a medical test, for example, investigate treatment options and insurance coverage. One reason we're anxious during waiting periods is that we feel a loss of control. Preparing allows us to partially regain control.

CHAPTER 10

Family Health and Safety

Get Off That Couch Together

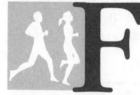

For better or worse, your significant other's health habits strongly influence your own. Got a spouse who thinks that walking to the kitchen is exercise, and you're less likely to stay fit yourself. And there's research to back this up.

Important new finding: In a study of 3,722 adults, nearly 70% of men took up physical activity if their wives did, while only one-quarter of men became active without their spouses as inspiration. Women are similarly affected by their husbands but to a lesser extent.

If you're single: Having a supportive friend who exercises may give you the incentive to get moving yourself.

MOTIVATION AND MORE

Why does it help to have an active partner? For starters, it is a great form of motivation.

Seeing your partner exercise reminds you to work out. An active partner also lends social support, acting as your cheerleader and sharing strategies for coping with setbacks such as sore muscles or trepidation when trying a new activity. Your partner can provide accountability, too—you are less likely to skip a workout if someone is planning on joining you.

An added perk: Because exercise has been repeatedly linked with better heart health and lower rates of cancer, diabetes and depression, this means that the two of you will increase your odds of having more higher-quality years together.

Working out as a team (for example, going on long walks or jogs together) allows you to talk and reconnect.

Bonus: These opportunities contribute to a satisfying and committed relationship, which

---

Mona Xu, PhD, an assistant professor of experimental psychology at Idaho State University (ISU) and director of the ISU Social, Health and Neuroscience Lab, which studies the interplay between close interpersonal relationships and behavioral health.

will help ensure that your partnership will stay strong.

Attempting shared goals, such as completing a 5K walk or run, gives you the chance to grow and celebrate as a duo. If the exercise is something novel—this could be snowshoeing, tandem bicycling or hiking a beautiful new route—you may get an extra benefit. Couples report feeling happier with their relationships and more in love with their partners after completing an exciting physical activity together… perhaps because you associate your partner with fun and adventure.

HOW TO BE THE CATALYST

If you're the more active one in your marriage—or simply the one taking the lead in making exercise a priority—your first step is to light a fire under your more sedentary partner.

Caution: Nagging him/her to join you can backfire—especially if your partner's weight is a touchy subject or if he finds exercise to be intimidating or stressful.

Helpful: Think of some activities your partner might enjoy. Then start with a low-key conversation, explaining that you're planning to try some new activities that are fun and healthy. Explain that you'd be happy for your partner to join you but that you understand if he isn't interested or wants to exercise alone. You might also offer support by, say, taking over some household chores to give your partner time to exercise.

What works well: Suggest enjoyable activities that don't seem like exercise but will improve fitness—for example, ballroom dancing, kayaking, a walk in the woods, golf or tai chi. You might also find local clubs focused on these activities.

Note: You need not exercise together in order to experience the benefits above—such as supporting one another and sharing advice on workout challenges. In fact, exercising independently is helpful when one partner prefers the meditative aspects of yoga, for example, while the other enjoys the competitiveness of basketball.

Ask your partner how you can help—maybe he would like some suggestions on finding a class or sport to try…perhaps she's anxious about shopping for the right workout gear or embarrassed about being in a gym setting.

Offer reassurance, then step back and see what happens. Resist the urge to pressure your partner…stay active yourself…and be supportive. Instead of saying, "You should work out more," try, "My hike is getting kind of stale—would you come with me and keep me company?"

MAKING IT WORK

Exercise within a marriage is not a competition. Just because your partner has been running for years, it doesn't mean that you need to attempt an hour-long run on your first day—or even that you need to run at all. If one of you is much stronger than the other and you have decided to try exercising as a team, pick activities that allow you to tailor your workout according to your own fitness level.

Good choices: Spin class, where you control the resistance on your bike…hiking (one person could wear a weighted vest)…a beginner-to-intermediate yoga class…or an indoor rock-climbing wall.

Also helpful: Use exercise as an opportunity for a date night—research shows this can strengthen a relationship. To ensure follow-through, put it on your calendar and go out for a healthy bite afterward.

The Kissing Prescription

Committed couples who increased their daily frequency of kissing reported less stress and greater relationship satisfaction after six weeks than couples who did not pucker up as often.

Bonus: The kissing couples also experienced significant drops in cholesterol levels.

Possible reason: Expressing affection as well as physical contact decreases the physical and psychological effects of stress.

Kory Floyd, PhD, professor of communication, The University of Arizona, Tucson.

TRY, TRY AGAIN...

If you and your partner are fighting as a result of your repeated efforts to motivate him to exercise, back off for a few months and re-strategize. But don't give up—suggest a new activity, offer encouragement and keep up your own exercise habit. When it comes down to it, you want your partner—and your marriage—to be healthy.

DO THIS TOGETHER...

Try this fun "full-body" move with your partner. It gives your shoulders, arms, back and legs a nice stretch, which improves flexibility before or after exercise.

What to do: Warm up with a few minutes of easy walking, then begin by sitting on the floor. Face your partner and place the bottoms of your feet against his/her feet. Each of you should grab one end of a towel or resistance band. Slowly lean backward, gently pulling the towel or band so that your partner must lean forward until he feels a stretch in his hamstrings. Hold for 10 to 30 seconds, then return to the starting position and have your partner lean back. Repeat the entire sequence three to five times.

Caution: If you've had hip or back surgery, check with your doctor before trying this stretch.

Sleep Better with a Partner

Jamison Starbuck, ND, is a naturopathic physician in family practice and a guest lecturer at the University of Montana, both in Missoula. She is a past president of the American Association of Naturopathic Physicians and a contributing editor to *The Alternative Advisor: The Complete Guide to Natural Therapies and Alternative Treatments*. DrJamisonStarbuck.com

No one will dispute the value of a good night's sleep. But when it comes to the effect that our sleep partners have on our nighttime rest, from what I've observed in the medical research and from my patients' experiences, there are a lot of myths. *Here's my take on some common ones...*

•**Sleeping with a pet.** The conventional wisdom is that sleeping with a pet is bad for your health. I can remember my grandmother forbidding our cat from sleeping with us when my sister and I were children. She was convinced that the cat would bite our throats in the night. For years, doctors have said that pets carried disease and warned that sleeping with them increased risk for asthma and allergy.

As recently as 2011, the Centers for Disease Control and Prevention reported that sleeping with pets put humans at greater risk for diseases such as parasitic infections and cat scratch fever. But now some experts are disputing that data. While it's true that sleeping with a pet can increase one's risk for asthma or an allergy, the practice does not worsen risk for most other conditions beyond what would already be present when living with a pet. That's good news because more than half of pet owners sleep with their pets some or all of the time. And a recent small study found that it may actually be a good thing. Sleeping with pets can make people feel safe, secure and relaxed—and results in a better night's sleep, according to research from the Mayo Clinic Center for Sleep Medicine in Scottsdale, Arizona.

•**Sleeping with a partner.** You may assume that if you're in love with someone, you will sleep well with him/her. Not always true! If you are in a marriage or a partnership, negotiate sleep patterns just as you would meal patterns, child care and social planning. Find common ground with one another about sleep.

•**Sleeping without a partner.** Some people who don't have a partner or spouse tell themselves that slumber time is destined to be lonely. But there are creative solutions. If you like to snuggle, a small dog may be your best bet. Cats can be great sleep partners, but they tend to be nocturnal and may not last the night with you. If you haven't got a pet or don't want to sleep with one, there's another option to consider—a full-body pillow. These long, narrow pillows are very comforting. Body pillows don't get warm the way a human sleep partner can...but they also don't perspire or roll over...or snore into your ear.

To help ensure good sleep habits, I tell my patients to write out a sleep assessment. How much room do you need in your bed to be comfortable? Do you prefer to snuggle up to something or someone? What is your body temperature when you sleep? How many blankets do you need? Use this information to help create your optimal sleep habits.

Remember: A good night's sleep is good medicine. Do it in a way that works for you!

Gratitude Solidifies a Marriage

Telephone-based study of 468 married people by researchers at University of Georgia, Athens, published in *Personal Relationships.*

Spouses who feel appreciated and who frequently thank each other have a stronger commitment to their relationship. Expressions of gratitude or thanks can pull couples out of times of conflict more quickly and effectively than other techniques. And gratitude can be an effective way to counter stressors, such as financial difficulties.

Is There an Almost-Psychopath in Your Life?

Ronald Schouten, MD, JD, director of the Law & Psychiatry Service at Massachusetts General Hospital and associate professor of psychiatry at Harvard Medical School, both in Boston. He is coauthor of *Almost a Psychopath.*

When most of us think of psychopaths, we imagine cold-blooded killers or con men who rob the elderly of their life savings without a qualm—deviant individuals we assume we have little chance of encountering. (True psychopaths make up only about 1% of the US population.) But did you ever suspect that there might be an almost-psychopath in your life?

What research is now showing: People known as almost-psychopaths are much more common—it's estimated that they make up 5% to 15% of the population.

Bad Marriage = Bad Heart

An unhappy marriage is bad for your heart. Researchers examined five years of data from married men and women, ages 57 to 85. People with spouses who were negative or critical were more likely to have heart health issues—women suffered more than men—than those with supportive partners. This effect worsened with age.

Theory: Relationship stress intensifies over time, and heart disease is harder to overcome in those who are older and more frail.

Study of nearly 1,200 married American men and women by researchers at Michigan State University, East Lansing, published in *Journal of Health and Social Behavior.*

The traits that define psychopaths and almost-psychopaths have many possible causes, including genetics and/or dysfunctional family relationships. The symptoms can also signal an underlying illness, such as depression or bipolar disorder, or certain medical conditions, such as a brain tumor or thyroid disease.

Almost-psychopaths—whose problematic behaviors don't quite meet the standard definition of a diagnosable disorder—may not wreak the havoc and harm of a true psychopath, but they can cause serious damage. And it's essential to recognize them and know how to deal with them.

TELLING BEHAVIORS

Almost-psychopaths have many of the qualities of a true psychopath but to a lesser degree. For example, they have a strong sense of self-importance, but it's not as pronounced as it is in the psychopath. Their capacity for empathy is severely stunted but not invariably defunct—they retain a glimmer of compassion for those with whom they have relationships or who can serve their needs. The stirrings of a conscience may be there, but it's weak. They also are superficially charming, lie, con and manipulate and are expert at rationalizing their misdeeds and crafting excuses for their behavior.

However, almost-psychopaths often lack the fearless sense of invulnerability that powers true psychopaths. They feel they should be above the law but generally realize that they're not and fear getting caught. This limits their capacity to hurt but also makes them harder to spot and adept at weaving a web of lies to cover their transgressions.

Unlike psychopaths, almost-psychopaths are capable of living more easily among the general population. Psychopaths may frequently be in prison for crimes, have a string of failed marriages and be estranged from their children while an almost-psychopath may, for example, be a grandiose co-worker who routinely bends the rules at work or someone who serially cheats on his/her spouse.

THE RELATIONSHIP TRAP

Their easy charm and adept lies can get you involved with—and sometimes married to—an almost-psychopath. The sense that something is seriously wrong often develops slowly and uncertainly.

What helps: Keep a private and careful record of behaviors that concern you (such as betrayals, deceptions, examples of callous actions toward you or others, or any other behaviors described in the box above) in order to determine if there's a problem. This record can also be helpful to a psychotherapist should you consult one later.

Relationships with almost-psychopaths tend to be filled with conflict. They believe that their wants are more important than anyone else's. There is typically a constant demand to accommodate the almost-psychopath's needs and desires. Additionally, there can be chronic infidelities, excessive bragging, abruptly canceled plans and extravagant expenses.

Almost-psychopaths also excel at shifting blame, turning the tables and generating self-

10 Key Signs of an Almost-Psychopath

1. He/she is superficially charming and glib.

2. There is a lack of empathy.

3. When confronted with a difficult moral choice, he more often than not arrives at a decision to act in his own self-interest.

4. He repeatedly lies, even when unnecessary and for minor reasons.

5. He is cunning and manipulative.

6. When criticized for something, it is always someone else's fault.

7. When he causes harm to others, there is a lack of true remorse.

8. There is difficulty in maintaining relationships.

9. He finds it easy to ignore responsibilities.

10. People and situations exist solely for the purpose of gratifying his needs and wants.

doubt and even guilt in those who question their honesty. *How could you even think such things?* There are numerous excuses and promises to change, given with a look of extreme innocence. Deceit and manipulation keep you perpetually off balance.

Unlike true psychopaths, almost-psychopaths can sometimes mend their ways —if they acknowledge their behaviors and want to change.

What to do if you think you're living with an almost-psychopath…

• **Acknowledge the problem and realize that there may be hope for improvement.**

• **Reach out to trusted friends or family members.** Your gut instincts are probably on target, but it helps to get another person's input and support.

• **Talk to the almost-psychopath in a calm manner (if you feel comfortable doing so) about his behaviors.** He may not be aware of them or may have grown up in a household where the behaviors were common.

• **Track progress and have additional conversations.** Once the lines of communication are open, further conversations are often easier.

• **Seek professional help if there are ongoing concerns.** Sometimes your best chance for improving the relationship is psychotherapy for your partner and/or couples therapy for both of you.

Also advisable: A visit to a primary care physician, who can rule out medical conditions that may be contributing to the situation and/or provide a referral to a psychiatrist or therapist. If your partner won't go to therapy, seek individual therapy to help you determine how to move ahead.

Warning: The threat of physical harm and/or psychological aggression is very real in a close relationship with an almost-psychopath. If a discussion leads to threats or outright violence, take steps to protect yourself—leave the situation and/or seek help from friends and, if necessary, law enforcement.

Suicide and Survivors

Study of 3,432 people by researchers at University College London, UK, published in *BMJ Open*.

Loved ones of suicide victims are 65% more likely to attempt suicide than people who were close to someone who died of natural causes.

Possible reason: People who lost a loved one to suicide tend to perceive more social stigma around the death—making grieving survivors feel more isolated and unsupported.

Save a Loved One From Suicide

Thomas Joiner, PhD, the Robert O. Lawton Distinguished Professor of Psychology at Florida State University and director of the Laboratory for the Study and Prevention of Suicide-Related Conditions and Behaviors, both in Tallahassee. Dr. Joiner is the author of *Why People Die by Suicide* and *Myths About Suicide*.

The instinct to live is hardwired in us. That's why suicidal tendencies can be so difficult—even impossible—to grasp for people who have never felt a desire to die. The more we do know, however, the better able we are to reach out to people who are at risk of dying by suicide. *To better understand suicide, it's important to know the truth behind several long-standing myths…*

MYTH: Suicide is an act of anger or revenge. Only 10% to 12% of suicides contain an element of anger or revenge. Unfortunately, these tend to draw media attention, painting all suicides with the same brush. In truth, the tendency to die by suicide can most often be attributed to two simultaneously occurring beliefs—the sense that one is a burden…and that one doesn't belong. People considering suicide often think of themselves as a liability for their families, along the lines of *They'd be better off without me.* When accompanied by a lack of belongingness—a sense of loneliness and social alienation—the result can be lethal.

MYTH: Suicide is an easy escape, one that cowards use. Suicide is very difficult to accomplish—only one death occurs for every 20 attempts. Combat soldiers and policemen, who require physical fearlessness in their work, for example, are at high suicide risk. When they experience feelings of alienation and being a burden, their bravery can turn deadly. Physicians and dentists, in particular, are also at high risk—they are so exposed to pain and injury every day that they can become inured to the natural human aversion to taking one's own life.

MYTH: People often die by suicide on a whim. When standing on top of a roof, many people experience a fleeting thought along the lines of What if I jumped? When driving a car around a sharp bend, a similar thought might occur—What if I drove off the road? It can feel like you had a sudden whim to end it all—but that's not what's happening.

That impulse is called the high-place phenomenon. It's considered to be an instinctual safety signal that causes one to pay greater attention and take precautions—for example, to back up from the rooftop. Moments later, though, your slower perceptual system kicks in and misattributes the safety signal as a kind of a death wish. It's nothing of the sort. Our studies have shown that the high-place phenomenon is, in fact, an urge to live, not die. By contrast, taking one's own life is usually preceded by detailed planning and resolve.

MYTH: Unless you're depressed, you're not at risk for suicide. While depression is a significant risk factor for suicide, it is not the only one. Mental disorders such as anorexia nervosa, schizophrenia and borderline personality disorder increase suicide risk. Additional risk factors include stressful life events (such as a death, divorce or job loss), access to firearms

Stroke Survivors at Increased Suicide Risk

Stroke survivors are twice as likely to attempt suicide as people who have not had a stroke.

At greatest risk of attempted suicide: Stroke patients who live alone, are feeling depressed and/or are younger than age 55. Men are more likely than women to attempt post-stroke suicide.

What can help: Psychosocial support, identifying and treating depression and reducing social isolation.

Marie Eriksson, PhD, is senior lecturer (associate professor) in the department of statistics, Umeå School of Business and Economics, Umeå University, Sweden, and lead author of a study of 220,336 stroke patients, published in *Neurology*.

and historical factors, including a family history of suicide, previous attempts and childhood abuse. More than one in 10 suicides are related to chronic or terminal illness.

MYTH: Most people who die by suicide leave a note. Seventy-five percent of people who kill themselves don't leave a note or other message for loved ones. Unfortunately, that helps fuel the incorrect notion that the act was impulsive.

To understand why notes are so rare, remember that people who are considering suicide are typically in a state of misery and isolation, which makes it very hard to communicate. Those who do leave notes tend to provide factual instructions about day-to-day matters rather than an emotional missive.

MYTH: Suicidal behavior peaks around the end-of-year holidays. In fact, suicides tend to occur in the spring. That's true around the world. Why? The explanation that I favor comes back to the idea that suicide requires a great deal of resolve and focus. In the spring, all living things—human, animal, even plant—become more energetic. For most people that's a good thing, but a small percentage experience symptoms such as agitation, edginess and trou-

ble sleeping. This clinical state of overarousal, combined with alienation and burdensomeness, is correlated with higher rates of suicides during the spring.

MYTH: There are more suicides in big cities than in rural areas. Not true. People who live in rural counties are 70% more likely to die by suicide than those who live in big, metropolitan areas. The reason may be that rural residents hold more physical occupations, which often go hand-in-hand with a higher level of everyday fearlessness. Another factor may be that they live far from their neighbors, resulting in social isolation. The lack of easy access to doctors and other medical professionals may also contribute.

MYTH: If people want to die by suicide, we can't stop them. A landmark study found that 94% of people who were restrained from jumping off the Golden Gate Bridge in San Francisco were still alive decades later or had died from natural causes. This was true even though they had high-risk characteristics that suggest a determined mind-set—most were men (who are at greater risk than women)…had chosen a highly lethal method (jumping from a high structure)…and were rarely referred to mental health treatment after being restrained (unfortunate but not uncommon). Yet nearly all of them chose to keep on living. This suggests that intervention can save lives.

If you or a loved one is considering suicide or shows suicidal tendencies, there is help available! The suicide hot line 800-273-TALK is a great resource—callers speak with a trained crisis worker who listens to their problems and then provides information on mental health services in the caller's area.

Another good option: Reaching out to a primary care physician who can prescribe medication and/or recommend a mental health professional.

Simple Steps Can Ease Care of Loved One With Alzheimer's

Ronald Petersen, MD, PhD, neurologist, Mayo Clinic, Rochester, Minnesota.
Mayo Clinic, news release.

As Alzheimer's disease progresses, patients find that simple tasks become difficult or impossible, but caregivers can help them maintain a sense of independence and dignity, a doctor says.

•**Create a routine that makes days more predictable and schedule the most challenging tasks**—such as bathing or medical appointments—at a time of day when your loved one is typically most calm, advised Ronald Petersen, MD, PhD, a Mayo Clinic neurologist.

•**Adapt to your loved one's needs.** If he or she insists on wearing the same clothes every day, for instance, consider buying a few identical outfits. Limiting choices will make it easier for the person to decide. Instead of a closet full of clothes, offer a choice of two outfits and do away with belts or accessories that he or she is likely to put on incorrectly.

•**Expect things to take longer than they once did.** This will help you avoid having to rush your loved one.

"Allow your loved one to do as much as possible with the least amount of assistance. For example, perhaps your loved one can dress alone if you lay out the clothes in the order they go on," Dr. Petersen said in a Mayo news release.

•**Turn off the TV and minimize distractions** during meals and conversations so your loved one is better able to focus.

•**Consider safety.** To reduce the risk of falls, remove scatter rugs, extension cords and clutter that could pose a tripping hazard. Install handrails or grab bars in appropriate locations.

"Install locks on cabinets that contain anything potentially dangerous, such as medicine, alcohol, guns, toxic cleaning substances, dangerous utensils and tools," Dr. Peterson said.

•**Lower the setting on the hot water heater** to prevent burns and keep matches and lighters out of reach. If your loved one smokes, make sure he or she is supervised while doing so.

info U.S. National Institute on Aging has more about Alzheimer's caregiving. *NIA.nih.gov/alzheimers/topics/caregiving*

Caregiver Dementia Is Real

Brenda Avadian, founder of The Caregiver's Voice, an organization that provides information and support to family caregivers, Los Angeles. She is author of the *Finding the Joy in Alzheimer's* series of books. She previously served as a caregiver for her father, who lived with Alzheimer's. TheCaregiversVoice.com

People who provide prolonged care to family members living with dementia often develop dementia symptoms themselves, including memory loss and disorientation.

This "caregiver dementia" usually is not the result of a degenerative brain condition—it stems from stress and lack of sleep. People who experience it typically recover after their caregiving duties end. But not all do—some face elevated risk for permanent dementia. A study published in *Journal of the American Geriatrics Society* found that people who care for spouses who have dementia are six times more likely to later develop permanent dementia than people whose spouses are dementia-free. The study's authors concluded that the "chronic and often severe stresses associated with dementia caregiving" might be responsible.

Four things caregivers can do…

•**Learn as much as possible about the specific disease affecting the person you care for.** Increasing your knowledge can decrease your frustration.

•**Find moments of joy with your loved one.** Give silent thanks for a quiet moment sitting together. Share a laugh when you can.

•**Take respites.** Caregivers need time off. Sometimes this can be accomplished through assistance from professional caregivers, friends and other family members. When that isn't possible, at least grant yourself five-minute respites. Step outside to take a deep breath. Walk into another room. Pet your cat or dog—research shows this is calming.

•**Replace obligation with empathy.** Reflect on how much your loved one is trying to make sense of his/her world…and how you would feel if the roles were reversed. This can help you provide care out of a sense of love rather than duty.

Defuse a Family Feud

Avidan Milevsky, PhD, associate professor of psychology, Kutztown University, Kutztown, Pennsylvania, quoted in *RealSimple*.

To *help defuse a family feud when you are stuck in the middle:* Tell each family member involved something positive you have heard about him/her from the other. This can help break through the negative feelings they have. You also can let them know how much it would mean to you if they would at least agree to meet and try to talk.

Apps That Track Family and Friends

Roundup of experts on tracking apps, reported at MarketWatch.com.

Track friends and family with free apps on an iPhone or Android phone. The apps allow users to stay in touch with elderly parents, keep track of children and find lost or stolen phones—and are used by spouses who are suspicious of their partners. These apps are becoming regular elements of divorce cases. Connect follows people you are connected to through social-media sites. Find My Friends shows contacts on a map who have chosen to share their location data. Phone Tracker and Glympse combine mapping and GPS technology to let you track your phone and one other. (The PhoneTracker upgrade allowing tracking of 10 users costs 99 cents.)

Kids and Tablets

Kids who spend lots of time using cell phones, tablets and computers may be more prone to nearsightedness (myopia). Focusing on something close to your eyes, such as a cellphone or tablet screen, contributes to myopia, especially when done in low light.

To help protect children: Encourage them to spend more time outside, where they naturally tend to focus on more distant objects

Discussion by a panel of 10 ophthalmology experts at an annual meeting of the American Academy of Ophthalmology in Las Vegas.

Fidgeting May Help Students with ADHD Learn

Michael Kofler, PhD, licensed clinical psychologist and assistant professor, psychology, Florida State University, Tallahassee.
Trevor Resnick, MD, pediatric neurologist, Nicklaus Children's Hospital, Miami
Journal of Attention Disorders

Students who have attention deficit hyperactivity disorder (ADHD) often get into trouble for fidgeting in the classroom, but that fidgeting may help them learn, recent research suggests.

"The prevailing view has been and continues to be that hyperactivity is a core deficit in ADHD," said study author Michael Kofler, PhD, an assistant professor of psychology at Florida State University in Tallahassee. "When we think of it as a deficit, we are saying it's a bad thing and it's interfering [with schoolwork]. Our work has been challenging that thought."

RESEARCH DETAILS

Dr. Kofler's team gave 25 boys and girls with ADHD, aged 8 to 12, a series of working memory tasks, observing the amount of fidgeting as the children did them. In one set, the students had to remember where a series of dots appeared on a screen and then reorder them mentally, based on color. They had to then remember a series of numbers and letters, mentally reordering them, numbers first from smallest to biggest, then the letters.

In the easier test of dots on a screen, the children knew in advance how many items they would have to remember. In the more difficult test, the amount of items they would have to remember was random so they didn't know in advance how many items they would have to remember.

The children fidgeted during all the tests, but fidgeted about 25% more when they couldn't predict how many items they would have to remember. The tests were alike in every other way, so Dr. Kofler said this shows that demands on working memory affect the level of hyperactivity in ADHD students.

The fidgeting may increase "physiological arousal," Dr. Kofler speculated, similar to what stimulant medication does for a child with the disorder. But the study didn't prove that point, he said, and the researchers don't know if the kids were fidgeting on purpose.

The study was published online in the *Journal of Attention Disorders*.

WHERE FOCUS SHOULD LIE

The findings echo some from a study published last year from the University of California, Davis. Researchers there looked at 26 children with ADHD and 18 without. They found that when the children with ADHD fidgeted more, they did better on a test. Fidgeting among kids without ADHD had no effect on test performance.

Trevor Resnick, MD, a pediatric neurologist at Nicklaus Children's Hospital in Miami, said, "We've known [intuitively] for many years that kids with ADHD often do better when they are fidgeting."

However, Dr. Resnick said, the interpretation of why they fidgeted more has not been proven. "We don't know whether they do it to help or because they are anxious, or whether it is helping," he said.

Dr. Kofler agreed, saying his team next plans research "to link the movement with the arousal and the performance, to see if we are right about that is why the movement is helpful."

Meanwhile, until more is known, students with ADHD should not have free rein to do what they want in the classroom, Dr. Kofler said.

But the new study does suggest that teachers and parents should focus less on whether a child is sitting still and more on whether the work is getting done, regardless of the movement level, he said.

info To learn more about ADHD, visit U.S. Centers for Disease Control and Prevention at *www.cdc.gov/ncbddd/adhd/facts.html*

Better Treatment for Kids' Hearing Problem

Study of 320 children, ages four to 11, led by researchers at University of Southampton, UK, published in *CMAJ* (*Canadian Medical Association Journal*).

Many young children suffer from "glue ear," in which the middle ear fills with thick fluid.

Recent finding: Asking children to blow through each nostril into a nozzle to inflate a nasal balloon is more effective than antibiotics, antihistamines, decongestants and intranasal steroids. After one month of having the treatment three times a day, 47% of participants were more likely to have normal middle-ear pressure, versus 36% of children given standard treatments. After three months, 50% of children who used the nasal balloon had normal middle-ear pressure, versus 38% of kids undergoing standard treatment.

Common Pesticides Linked to ADHD

Study of almost 700 children by researchers at Cincinnati Children's Hospital Medical Center, published in *Environmental Health*.

Pyrethroid pesticides, considered safer than other pesticides, are the most widely used for home and public-health pest control. But a recent study found an association between exposure to these pesticides and attention-deficit/hyperactivity disorder (ADHD)—although it did not find that the pesticides caused ADHD. The link was stronger in boys than girls. More research is needed, but thoroughly washing produce may help to limit pesticide exposure.

Measles Cause Long-Term Harm

Study led by researchers at Princeton University, Princeton, New Jersey, published in *Science*.

Measles weakens kids' immune systems for up to three years after recovery. Measles wipes out the immune system memory that the body uses to fight off infection day after day. That makes children who have recovered from measles more vulnerable to other serious infections, such as pneumonia and encephalitis.

Self-defense: Have your child vaccinated against measles.

Two Chickenpox Vaccines Work Best

Study by researchers at Kaiser Permanente Vaccine Study Center, Oakland, California, published in *Pediatrics*.

Chicken pox vaccine is almost 100% effective when two doses are given. A study of children from 1995 through 2009 found 1,505 cases of chicken pox among the 4,759 children who got one dose of the vaccine and no cases among 2,826 children who received two doses. A second vaccination has been recommended since 2006. Before the chicken pox vaccine became available in 1995, about 90% of the US population contracted the disease.

Bleach Can Harm Young Respiratory Systems

Bleach may increase the risk for respiratory infections. Children whose homes were cleaned with bleach at least once a week had a higher risk for respiratory and other types of infections—20% higher risk for flu at least once in the previous year...35% higher risk for recurrent tonsillitis...and 18% higher risk for any recurrent infection. Airborne components of bleach may irritate children's lungs, triggering inflammation and making it easier for infections to take hold.

Study of more than 9,000 children by researchers at Center for Environment and Health, University of Leuven, Leuven, the Netherlands, published in *Occupational and Environmental Medicine*.

Whooping-Cough Vaccine Loses Strength

Study led by researchers at the division of bacterial diseases, Centers for Disease Control and Prevention, Atlanta, published in *Pediatrics*.

Whooping-cough vaccine loses strength over time. It is 73% effective the first year after being given, but only 34% effective by the fourth year. But the Centers for Disease Control and Prevention (CDC) does not recommend changing vaccine protocols, saying that the current recommendation remains the best way to protect children against whooping cough (pertussis). The recommendation includes a five-dose vaccine series for very young children, plus a sixth dose for teens.

Reactions to Smells Help Diagnose Autism

Study by researchers at Weizmann Institute of Science, Rehovot, Israel, published in *Current Biology*.

Most people instinctively inhale pleasant smells deeply but limit breathing of un-

That Little Taste of Alcohol Is Not Harmless

Children allowed to taste alcohol are more likely to start drinking by the time they are in high school. Some parents believe introducing children to alcohol at home promotes responsible drinking later.

But: By ninth grade, 26% of kids who sipped alcohol at an earlier age had had at least one full alcoholic drink—versus fewer than 6% of those who did not try alcohol when younger.

Three-year study of 561 middle-school students by researchers at Center for Alcohol and Addiction Studies, Brown University, Providence, published in *Journal of Studies on Alcohol and Drugs*.

pleasant ones. Children with autism don't make this adjustment as quickly. In a small study, researchers were able to determine which children had been diagnosed with autism 81% of the time based on how quickly the children responded to certain odors.

U.S. Pediatricians Add Poverty to Well-Visit Checklist

American Academy of Pediatrics, news release

Pediatricians in the United States already ask parents about their child's sleep, diet and developmental milestones. Soon, they'll add poverty to the well-visit checklist.

Poverty can significantly harm a child's health, according to a new American Academy of Pediatrics policy statement.

The group says pediatricians can identify children at risk by asking parents a single question: "Do you have difficulty making ends meet at the end of the month?" Those who answer "yes" can then be directed to appropriate community resources.

"Because poverty so strongly influences children's health and development, pediatricians are asking about poverty-related stress so we can connect families to resources in their communities," Dr. James Duffee, one of the authors of the policy statement, said in an academy news release.

Studies show that severe and persistent poverty can lead to major lifelong health problems such as infant death, poor language development, and increased risk of asthma, obesity and injuries, according to the policy statement.

There is also growing evidence that childhood poverty is associated with high levels of stress that can change gene expression and brain function, and contribute to behavioral problems and chronic heart and mental health disorders, the statement added.

Census data from 2014 shows that 1 in 5 U.S. children younger than 18 lives in poverty. When families classified as poor, near poor or low-income are included, the child poverty rate rises to 43%, or more than 31.5 million, according to the academy.

Water, Please!

Analysis of data from 4,134 children ages six to 19 led by researchers at Harvard T.H. Chan School of Public Health, Boston, published in *American Journal of Public Health*.

Most kids in the US are not drinking enough water. Half of children between the ages of six and 19 are not adequately hydrated. Chronic dehydration can result in kidney problems, heatstroke, headaches, irritability, poor circulation, reduced physical performance and poor mental functioning. Children are more susceptible to dehydration than adults because they adapt to heat more slowly.

Best: Encourage kids to drink plain water, not juice or sports drinks. Infuse it with fresh fruit such as oranges…vegetables such as cucumbers…or herbs such as mint to enhance the taste without adding sugar. Serve it ice-cold when possible (or use frozen water bottles in lunch bags)—cold water tastes better to children than room-temperature water.

Football's Concussion-Prevention Efforts May Be Spurring More Leg Injuries

Robert W. Westermann, MD, chief resident, University of Iowa, Iowa City, Iowa.

Katherine Coyner, MD, assistant professor, dept of orthopaedic urgery, UT southwestern Medical Center, Dallas.

Presentation, American Orthopaedic Society for Sports Medicine.

C oncussion-prevention rules for college football players may have led to an unintended consequence—an increase in knee, thigh and ankle injuries among players, new research suggests.

"Of course concussions sustained in football can be devastating," said study author Robert Westermann, MD, chief resident at the University of Iowa in Iowa City. "But so can lower extremity injuries, which are the leading cause of disability among NFL [National Football League] retirees. So, it's important to protect the whole athlete.

"But our work," he added, "suggests that a change in the pattern of play following the new push to reduce head-to-head contact among players may be causing an increase in injuries lower down the body."

Dr. Westermann emphasized that the study was only designed to find an association between the change in football rules and an increase in leg, joint and foot injuries. It did not prove cause-and-effect.

At the time it adopted its latest concussion-related guidelines, National College Athletic Association (NCAA) data showed that college players had experienced more than 41,000 injuries overall between 2004 and 2009. Concussions—also known as mild traumatic brain injuries—accounted for more than 7% of that total, according to the NCAA.

With that in mind, the NCAA adopted several new contact rules for football in 2008. They included banning the so-called "horse-collar tackle," in which a player is pulled down by his collar or shoulder pad, and protecting players from the two-on-one "chop block" maneuver.

The revised rules also called for a focus on getting rid of all blows to the head, and all hits on defenseless players, according to the NCAA.

RESEARCH DETAILS

The new study included information collected by athletic trainers and physicians between 2009 and 2014 as part of the NCAA Injury Surveillance System.

Lower extremity injuries included those affecting the leg, knee, ankle and foot, the study authors said. Concussion risk information was also gathered.

Roughly 2,400 leg, joint or foot injuries serious enough to cause a time-out in play occurred during the study time frame. About a third involved injuries to the knee, while slightly less than that involved ankle trouble. Nearly 60% were the result of player-to-player contact, the researchers reported.

Concussion risk remained relatively "stable" over the study period, the research revealed. But, leg, joint and foot injuries rose from about 9 per 1,000 "athletic exposures" during the 2009-10 seasons (before the new rules were implemented) to nearly 13 per 1,000 by the 2013-14 season, the study showed.

Why? The investigators suggest that the rise may have been prompted by the effort to avoid head-to-head contact, causing players to target other players lower on the body.

info There's more on concussion rules at the U.S. National Collegiate Athletic Association at *ncaa.org/health-and-safety/sport-sci ence-institute/concussion-timeline*

Concussions Can Cause More Than Head Injury

Study of 102 athletes by researchers at University of North Carolina, Chapel Hill, published in *Medicine & Science in Sports & Exercise*.

A thletes are more injury-prone after suffering a concussion. They were nearly twice as likely to suffer a knee, ankle or lower-limb injury up to one year after a concussion, compared with the previous 12-month period.

Theory: A concussion may impair the brain's ability to coordinate physical movement.

Lawn Mowers Still Cause Severe Injuries to Kids

Douglas G. Armstrong, MD, professor, orthopedic surgery, and division head, pediatric orthopedics, Penn State Hershey Medical Center, Hershey, Pennsylvania.

Kevin Shea, MD, orthopaedic surgeon at Intermountain Orthopaedics, Boise, Idaho.

American Academy of Orthopaedic Surgeons meeting, Orlando, Florida.

Despite long-standing safety guidelines, US children continue to suffer severe injuries from both regular power lawn mowers and ride-on mowers, a new Pennsylvania-based study finds.

In more than half of such cases, children required an amputation, the research showed.

"People don't realize how dangerous lawn mowers are," warned senior study author Douglas Armstrong, MD. He's a professor of orthopedic surgery and division head of pediatric orthopedics at Penn State Hershey Medical Center in Hershey, Pennsylvania.

"All lawn mowers have a tremendous amount of kinetic energy given off at the tip of the lawn mower blade. It's higher than a bullet leaving the muzzle of a 357 Magnum, which means that the injuries we see are not just lacerations, they're the result of something more like an explosion or blast injury," he explained.

The researchers looked at information from all children with lawn mower-related injuries treated at Pennsylvania trauma centers between 2002 and 2013. The investigators found an average of about 16 accidents a year.

In all, the study found that nearly 200 children under the age of 18 were injured because of a lawn mower. The majority of those injured (81%) were boys, and the average age was 8 years. Nine in 10 accidents occurred during warm weather months (April through September), according to the study.

More than half of the cases (55%) involved "ride-on" lawn mowers, the investigators found.

The researchers said nearly two-thirds of the injuries involved the lower extremities. Slightly more than half of the kids had to have an amputation because of the injury. One child (age 1) died due to an incident involving a ride-on lawn mower, the study authors reported.

"The vast majority of the injuries could have been prevented if safety guidelines had been followed," Dr. Armstrong said.

Those guidelines, outlined in 2001 by the American Academy of Pediatrics (AAP), recommend that no child under the age of 16 should operate a ride-on mower, while no child under 12 should operate a powered or non-powered push mower.

The advisory further cautions parents—whether on farmland or in the suburbs—to keep all children under the age of 6 indoors when any mower is in operation. Kids shouldn't ride along as passengers on mowers operated by adults, the pediatric group said.

Following that advice would have prevented almost 70% of the Pennsylvania accidents, Dr. Armstrong said.

Sleep Loss May Be Tied to Raised Diabetes Risk in Teen Boys

Jordan Gaines, doctoral candidate, neurosciences, Penn State University, College Park, Pennsylvania.

Penn State University, news release.

Teen boys who get too little of a particular type of sleep may be at risk of developing type 2 diabetes, a recent study suggests.

The research focused on "slow-wave sleep"—an important stage of sleep that helps people store memories and recover after sleep deprivation. This type of sleep is also associated with lower levels of the stress hormone cortisol and reduced inflammation, the study authors explained.

For the study, 700 children were assessed between the ages of 5 and 12. Just over half of the participants were boys. The investigators followed up with about 420 of the kids eight years later.

Boys who lost a greater amount of slow-wave sleep between childhood and the teen years had a higher risk of developing insulin resistance than those whose slow-wave sleep totals remained fairly stable over the years.

Insulin resistance increases the risk of developing type 2 diabetes, and is also linked to more belly fat and attention problems, the study authors noted. The investigators found no link between amounts of slow-wave sleep and these problems in girls.

"On a night following sleep deprivation, we'll have significantly more slow-wave sleep to compensate for the loss," study author Jordan Gaines, a doctoral candidate in neuroscience at Penn State University in College Park, Pennsylvania, said in a university news release.

"We also know that we lose slow-wave sleep most rapidly during early adolescence. Given the restorative role of slow-wave sleep, we weren't surprised to find that metabolic and cognitive [mental] processes were affected during this developmental period," Gaines added.

The association seen in the study does not prove a cause-and-effect relationship. More research is needed to confirm the findings and determine whether there is a link between reduced amounts of slow-wave sleep and increased risk of insulin resistance in other age groups, the researchers said.

"In the meantime, we can use these findings as a springboard for future work on the sleep-health connection. The best thing we can do for ourselves today is keep a consistent sleep schedule, so as not to deprive ourselves of any more slow-wave sleep than we're already naturally losing with age," Gaines said.

info The U.S. National Institute of Diabetes and Digestive and Kidney Diseases has more on insulin resistance and prediabetes at *niddk.nih.gov*

Head Lice No Cause for Panic, Expert Says

Karen Sheehan, MD, pediatric emergency medicine specialist, Ann & Robert H. Lurie Children's Hospital, Chicago.
Ann & Robert H. Lurie Children's Hospital of Chicago, news release.

Most parents have at one time or another received the dreaded school notice: a case of head lice has been detected in your child's class.

But there's no need to panic.

Head lice don't carry diseases or indicate poor parenting or housekeeping, said Karen Sheehan, MD, a pediatric emergency medicine specialist at the Ann & Robert H. Lurie Children's Hospital of Chicago.

Children should not be sent home from school early if they're found to have lice, Dr. Sheehan added. The insects move by crawling and cannot hop or fly. So, as long as teachers keep children's heads apart, there should be no further spread of lice, she explained.

HOW TO SPOT...AND STOP... LICE INFESTATION

Would you recognize the signs of lice? Most are accurately diagnosed when a live louse is seen moving, Dr. Sheehan said in a hospital news release.

Seeing nits, or lice eggs, within one-quarter-inch of the scalp suggests a person has lice, but does not confirm an infestation, she explained. If the nits are more than one-quarter-inch from the scalp, it is likely an old infestation or not lice at all, but rather dandruff or dirt.

If head lice are discovered on one family member, all household members should be checked, according to the American Academy of Pediatrics. The use of home pesticides is not recommended, but washing pillow cases and treating natural bristle hair brushes are reasonable measures, the group said.

Also, teaching children not to share personal items such as combs, brushes and hats can help reduce the risk of head lice. Regular checks by parents can help with quick detection and treatment of head lice infestations.

PRESCRIPTION REMEDIES BEST

A recent study reported that lice in at least half of the United States have developed resistance to pyrethroids, an over-the-counter treatment product.

So, if you believe your child may have lice, ask your pediatrician for a prescription to treat them. There are several effective prescription remedies available, Dr. Sheehan said.

Lice can also be removed using a fine-tooth comb or a commercial hair treatment service.

info The U.S. Centers for Disease Control and Prevention has more on head lice at *cdc. gov/parasites/lice/head/index. html*

Dog and Cat Dangers at the Groomer

Debra Eldredge, DVM, a veterinarian based in Vernon, New York, and coauthor of *Dog Owner's Home Veterinary Handbook.*

Most trips to pet groomers go smoothly, but on rare occasions an animal is injured or killed. *Five dangers…*

Danger: Pets sometimes leap from grooming tables while wearing a hanging collar. The result can be a snapped neck or strangulation.

What to do: Ask the groomer his/her policy about monitoring pets while they are on grooming tables. The answer should be unequivocal—someone will always be with your pet the entire time it is on the table. Visit the groomer to confirm that there's always a person with any pet that's on a table.

Danger: Pets occasionally die of heat stroke in heated dryer cages. These devices generally are safe, but tragic mistakes sometimes occur.

What to do: Specify that you want your pet dried with cool air and/or towels only, not hot air. This is particularly important with brachycephalic (flat-faced) dog breeds, which can struggle to breathe in dryer cages…and with older or overweight dogs, which are especially vulnerable to heat stroke.

Danger: Some groomers sedate nervous pets. The result could be an accidental overdose or a potentially fatal allergic reaction.

What to do: Never use a groomer who sedates animals. If your pet is so anxious during grooming that a sedative truly is needed, ask your vet if he can arrange grooming right in the office so that there's a medical professional on hand.

Danger: Pets that have a strong dislike for grooming can be injured when they struggle with groomers.

What to do: Brush your pet and handle its paws in the weeks leading up to a trip to the groomer. This could increase your pet's comfort level with grooming.

Danger: Pet groomers are not licensed or regulated in most states.

What to do: Favor groomers who are certified by the National Dog Groomers Association of America (*NationalDogGroomers.com*)…International Professional Groomers (*ipgicmg. com*)…or the National Cat Groomers Institute of America (*NationalCatGroomers.com*). Or ask your vet to recommend one.

Your Dog Might Need This Vaccination

The New York Times

Dogs that have frequent contact with other dogs should have a canine flu vaccination.

Reason: A new form of the equine virus H3N2 has been reported in dogs in 25 states, with significant recent outbreaks around Atlanta and Cincinnati. The virus sickens 80% of dogs exposed to it within one week. The US Department of Agriculture has given emergency approval to a newly developed vaccine against the virus. Dogs that can benefit from the vaccine are ones that go to day care or dog parks, are boarded in kennels, are shown competitively, are groomed regularly or otherwise come into frequent contact with other dogs, as well as dogs living in areas where H3N2 has been reported. For a list of states with H3N2, go to *DogInfluenza.com*.

Your Cat Might Need This Vitamin

University of Edinburgh

How sick is your cat? Low vitamin D is linked to numerous health problems in humans—and now in cats, too.

New finding: Hospitalized cats with high levels of vitamin D have better survival rates.

Comfort Your Dog During a Thunder Storm

Nicholas Dodman, BVMS, director of the animal behavior department of the Cummings School of Veterinary Medicine at Tufts University in North Grafton, Massachusetts, writing at Rover.com.

It is not just the sound of thunder that scares dogs during thunderstorms. Studies have shown that it is the static electricity in the air that causes dogs to feel uncomfortable and get a tingling in their fur. Dogs experience numerous shocks from static electricity.

To make your dog more comfortable during a storm: Rub an unscented dryer sheet on its fur to reduce the effect of static electricity. If you have a porcelain bathtub, place the dog in the empty tub before, during and for a little while after a thunderstorm—porcelain blocks static electricity.

Protect Pets from Coyotes

Carol Cartaino, Ohio-based environmentalist and author of *Myths & Truths About Coyotes: What You Need to Know About America's Most Misunderstood Predator.*

Coyotes, once shy of humans, are becoming bolder. Though most active at night, they can be spotted at any time of day in many residential areas and parks across the US. *To stay safe…*

•**If you see a coyote, do not approach it.** Keep facing it as you move slowly toward a safe place. Do not run or crouch down. If the coyote approaches you, stand tall, wave your jacket or otherwise make yourself as big as possible. Throw something at it. Make loud noises. Brandish a stick.

•**If coyotes have been seen in the neighborhood, keep a very close eye on small children.** Never leave them unattended.

People who walk pets in places that coyotes frequent should avoid the hours between dusk and dawn.

At other times: Go with other people. Carry a stick, umbrella or other long object to keep coyotes at a distance. Avoid areas with heavy vegetation. Carry a can of pepper spray such as "Back Off"—if a coyote gets close, spray it into its face. Pick up small pets if you spot a coyote. Keep cats and small dogs inside, especially at night, even if you have a fenced yard.

•**To keep coyotes off your property,** eliminate sources of food and shelter…

•Keep garbage and compost in secure containers.

•Pick up fallen fruit instead of letting it stay on the ground.

•If pets are fed outside, remove dishes as soon as the pet is finished. Don't store pet food outdoors.

•Clean up scattered birdseed. It attracts squirrels and other rodents—which in turn attract coyotes.

•Clear out brush piles, especially around children's play areas.

•Never, never feed coyotes.

info *Useful online resources:* nhptv.org/ NatureWorks/coyote.htm and Web.Exten sion.Illinois.edu/wildlife/directory_show.cfm

CHAPTER 11

Get the Best Medical Care

Is Your Doctor Choosing the Right Care for You?

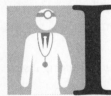If you've got symptoms that might indicate a serious medical problem, your doctor will first choose the tests that he/she believes will lead to an accurate diagnosis. Then he will choose the treatments that he thinks are most likely to work for your condition.

But how does your doctor make these important decisions? Often, there is no clear evidence and it comes down to an educated guess—but guesses aren't what you want when you're facing a life-changing decision...

BETTER MEDICAL RESEARCH

Traditional medical research has inherent limitations. Industry-sponsored studies, for example, often compare new drugs to placebos. To make real-life decisions, however, doctors and patients need to look to comparative effectiveness research (CER). This type of study makes head-to-head comparisons among existing treatments...and attempts to tailor them to individuals rather than the "average patient."

The Patient-Centered Outcomes Research Institute (PCORI), authorized by Congress in 2010, funds this type of comparative research (more than 280 studies so far) on medical conditions ranging from depression to stroke and cancer. Among recent CER findings from studies funded by PCORI or the federal government–sponsored Agency for Healthcare Research and Quality...*

KIDNEY STONES

Every year, about half a million Americans go to ERs with the fearsome pain of kidney stones. Doctors usually order an abdominal computed tomography (CT) scan to make the diagnosis.

*For recent studies funded by PCORI, go to PCORI.org and click on "Research & Results."

Harold Sox, MD, an internist, clinical epidemiologist and the director of research portfolio development at the Patient-Centered Outcomes Research Institute (PCORI) in Washington, DC. He has published numerous articles and books, including the textbook *Medical Decision Making*.

CT scans are the most sensitive test, but they're expensive…often reveal incidental (and usually harmless) abnormalities that lead to unnecessary tests…and expose patients to high doses of radiation that may increase cancer risks. Ultrasound, which is also used to diagnose kidney stones, is cheaper and safer. But until recently, experts didn't know if it was equally effective.

The study: 2,759 patients suspected of having kidney stones were randomly assigned to have CT scans or ultrasounds.

Results: Ultrasounds and CT scans were found to be equally accurate. Patients given these tests had similar rates of adverse reactions (such as subsequent complications from kidney disease). But the ultrasound patients were exposed to far less radiation than those given CT scans.

Conclusion: Ultrasound should usually be the first choice when diagnosing kidney stones.

DIABETES

More than a decade ago, the landmark Diabetes Prevention Program study found that lifestyle changes (exercise, healthful eating, etc.) reduced the risk for diabetes by 58%. The study also found that the diabetes drug metformin reduced diabetes risk by 31%.

However, few at-risk patients take advantage of either of these approaches, most likely because lifestyle improvement programs can be expensive and time-consuming. PCORI researchers wondered if it might be possible to identify those patients who would strongly benefit from these approaches.

The study: In a re-analysis of data from the original study, complex statistical models were used to correlate diabetes risk factors—age, body mass index, waist circumference, physical activity, etc.—with treatment outcomes.

Conclusion: Metformin was clearly effective, but only in the 25% of patients with the highest risk of developing diabetes (based on highest glucose levels, waist circumference and other factors). Those in lower-risk groups showed little benefit from metformin. Lifestyle changes were found to offer good protection to virtually all patients.

SPINAL STENOSIS

Spinal stenosis, an often-painful narrowing of the spinal canal that may require surgery, is typically treated with injections that combine a glucocorticoid (a type of steroid) with an anesthetic such as lidocaine. It's estimated that more than 2.2 million of these epidural injections are given every year. But the benefits have never been proved in rigorous, randomized, controlled clinical trials. Nor has it been shown that this drug combination is more effective than a single-drug injection.

The study: 400 patients with spinal stenosis were given one or two injections of either the two-drug shot or the lidocaine alone. They were then evaluated by doctors three and six weeks later.

Results: Patients given glucocorticoids plus lidocaine reported less leg pain and better physical function than those given lidocaine alone—but only at the three-week examination. At six weeks, patients in both groups had the same improvement in pain scores.

Conclusion: The steroid adds very little benefit. This is an important finding because even the short-term use of glucocorticoids can suppress calcium absorption and cause a reduction in bone density, which increases the risk for bone fracture. PCORI has funded a longer-term follow-up to this study.

STROKE

Previous studies have shown that the blood-thinning drug *warfarin* (Coumadin) can lower stroke risk for stroke survivors with atrial fibrillation (AFib), a dangerous heartbeat irregularity. But these past studies have tended to exclude the elderly and patients with more than one health problem and not taken into account the impact of warfarin on the quality of life after stroke.

The study: Researchers looked at 12,552 patients in all age groups who had AFib after a stroke to determine if warfarin decreased the number of days spent in the hospital after treatment and discharge.

Results: Patients who were treated with warfarin at discharge from the hospital had 47 more days at home during the two-year follow-up. They also had improvements in standard cardiac outcomes, such as the number of heart attacks, etc.

Conclusion: Warfarin provided these benefits to all patients studied, but the benefit was slightly stronger in women, patients older than age 80 and those who had more severe strokes (groups less likely to be treated with warfarin in the past).

Note: Warfarin can raise risk for bleeding, so risks and benefits should be carefully considered.

Don't Let Your Doctor Get It Wrong

Helen Haskell, MA, president of Mothers Against Medical Error, a nonprofit patient-safety organization. MAMEmomsonline.org

Fifteen years ago, my teenage son Lewis went to the hospital for an elective surgical procedure. After the operation, his doctors failed to notice that he was suffering from an undetected infection and blood loss from an ulcer caused by pain medication. They believed his symptoms were an indication of constipation from other pain medications he was taking. This mistake cost my son his life—he died four days after entering the hospital.

Now: I teach patients skills that can help them avoid a similar tragedy.

A "BLIND SPOT" IN MEDICINE

A groundbreaking new report from the prestigious Institute of Medicine (IOM) concluded that most Americans will experience at least one diagnostic error—that is, an inaccurate, missed or delayed diagnosis, as determined by later definitive testing—at some point in their lives.

The IOM report called diagnostic errors a "blind spot" in the delivery of quality health care. Each year, about one in 20 patients who seek outpatient care will suffer from a wrong or delayed diagnosis. According to autopsy studies, diagnostic mistakes contribute to about 10% of patient deaths. Unfortunately, diagnostic errors haven't gotten as much attention as treatment

and surgical errors—for example, operating on the wrong body part—partially because the latter are easier and quicker to identify. Now patient-safety experts are taking steps to better understand why diagnostic errors occur. *Key reasons…*

•**Tests help—and hurt.** Patients may be given a staggering number of tests—X-rays, blood tests, biopsies and more. The process of ordering, conducting and conveying the results of a test, however, can be complex and poorly organized.

•**Poor communication.** Can you count on the internist to talk to the nurse? Will the radiologist convey all of the pertinent information to the surgeon? Don't count on it. Patients also play a role. They should tell their doctors about all the symptoms they're having and whether they're getting better or worse after starting a new treatment.

•**Snap judgments.** Doctors often develop a working diagnosis within the first few minutes of hearing the patient's reported symptoms. The danger is that doctors can develop a so-called anchoring bias that leads them to cling to their initial diagnosis and prevents them from fully considering new information or looking for other possibilities.

HOW TO MAKE SURE YOUR DOCTOR GETS IT RIGHT

Major medical groups, including the Society to Improve Diagnosis in Medicine, have identified a number of institutional factors—such as stronger teamwork—to reduce errors. But no one has more at stake in these situations than the patients themselves. *Four steps you can take to avoid a misdiagnosis…*

STEP 1: Organize your thoughts. Most of the time, doctors have only 15 minutes with each patient, so you need to make the most of your time together.

Plan ahead: Your medical history—including a description of symptoms and when the problem started—is the most important part of an exam. Describe the nature and context of your symptoms in as much detail as you can. When do you feel them? What makes them worse or better? Why are you worried? Keep it concise and on topic, but include your own thoughts so the doctor can address the issues that concern you.

My advice: If possible, before you see the doctor, use the Internet to investigate your symptoms and the likely causes. Your findings should not be used to challenge your doctor, but rather as a way to have a more informed conversation. If you don't have confidence in your own abilities to do research, take advantage of a service like Expert HealthSearch (*ImproveDiagnosis. org/?page=ExpertHealthSearch*), a free service that puts you in touch with a medical librarian who can search the literature for you.

STEP 2: Don't be afraid to question test results. They are more prone to error than most people imagine. In one study, experts who reviewed biopsies of more than 6,000 cancer patients concluded that 86 had been given a wrong diagnosis. Samples can be too small or even contaminated…technicians can make mistakes…and there can be false-negatives or false-positives. Results can be misinterpreted, or even more often, they can go unreported to the patient.

My advice: If a test result seems to fly in the face of the symptoms you are experiencing, consider asking to repeat the test or have a second doctor review it. And never assume that no news is good news. Follow up to be sure that your test results have been received and reviewed and that you know what they are.

STEP 3: Ask about alternatives. Many common symptoms—such as fatigue, muscle aches and abdominal pain—are known as nonspecific symptoms. They can be caused by dozens of conditions.

My advice: To help understand your doctor's thinking, ask him/her this question: *Could you please explain your differential diagnoses?* This is a list of possible diagnoses ranked in order of likelihood. It's a thought process that helps a diagnostician avoid overlooking any likely possibilities. The most serious conditions on the list should be ruled out before settling on a less serious diagnosis, and the doctor should be looking for causes and not just treating symptoms.

What to ask: If there is any question about a diagnosis, patients can help assess the "fit"

by asking three important questions: Does this diagnosis match all my symptoms? What else could it be? Could there be more than one thing going on?

STEP 4: Don't skip the second opinion. I cannot stress this enough. In the study of cancer patients cited earlier, Johns Hopkins University researchers found that one to two of every 100 who got a second opinion with definitive testing after a tumor biopsy had gotten a wrong diagnosis the first time.

My advice: It's not always possible to get a second opinion—sometimes in medicine you have to move fast. But if you can, a second (or even a third) opinion is smart when symptoms seem severe…if your doctor is recommending surgery…or if you are told that you have a rare or fatal condition. Check first, but usually insurance will pay for a second opinion. Outside of emergencies, most of the time a brief delay in treatment while you get a second opinion will not affect your outcome.

Is Genetic Testing Right for You?

Robert Nussbaum, MD, chief medical officer at Invitae, a genetic information company based in San Francisco. He is the former director of the Cancer Risk Program at the Helen Diller Family Cancer Center, the Program in Cardiovascular Genetics and the Genomic Medicine Initiative, all at the University of California, San Francisco.

Genetic testing can save lives by alerting individuals to risk factors for diseases that may be hiding in their genes. But most patients are missing out on these benefits because the tests aren't well understood. Traditionally, genetic testing has been used to screen newborn babies for treatable conditions and by prospective parents concerned about passing on genetic diseases to their children.

What few people realize: There are now many tests that are useful for adults who may wonder about conditions, such as certain types of heart disease, cancer, Alzheimer's disease or Parkinson's disease, that tend to develop later in life. In fact, there are more than 1,000 genetic tests to detect the "variants" in genes (DNA) that can cause or complicate such health problems—before symptoms develop.

PREDICTIVE TESTING

This type of genetic testing (typically based on an analysis of blood or saliva) predicts your risk for a specific disease long before symptoms appear. A marked family history of the disease (in a first-degree relative such as a parent or sibling, for example) usually prompts a doctor to recommend the test. *Predictive testing can be helpful for…*

•**Colon cancer.** If you have a first-degree relative who had colon cancer before age 50, you may have the APC mutation, which causes familial adenomatous polyposis, a precursor to colon cancer. Or you may test positive for Lynch syndrome, a hereditary predisposition to colon cancer that carries a lifetime risk for the disease of 10% to 74%, depending on the specific gene and mutation. Lifetime colon cancer risk for the general population is about 5%.

Depending on the results of your test, you and your doctor may decide that you should…

•Have a colonoscopy every year, not every 10 years, if you test positive for the APC mutation or Lynch syndrome…or have a total colectomy (removal of the colon) as a preventive measure.

•Get more frequent screening for ovarian and uterine cancer—risk for both cancers is also significantly increased in women with Lynch syndrome. You may also consider prophylactic surgery to remove the ovaries and/or uterus.

•Receive a customized chemotherapeutic regimen proven to have greater efficacy in people with Lynch syndrome if you do develop colon cancer.

•**Heart disease.** People whose first-degree relatives have had (at any age) certain cardiac conditions (see below) may be predisposed to sudden cardiac death or heart disease. *Genetic testing is recommended for disorders including…*

•Hypertrophic cardiomyopathy, an inherited disease that causes thickening of the left ventricle, one of the four chambers of the heart… ventricular tachycardia, a faster-than-normal heartbeat that starts in the heart's lower cham-

bers…or atrial fibrillation, an irregular heartbeat caused by a misfiring of the heart's electrical system. If testing reveals one of these conditions, your doctor will be able to treat you sooner.

•**Breast and ovarian cancer.** If there is a history of breast or ovarian cancer in your family, with two or more relatives affected at a relatively young age (before age 50), ask your doctor if you should have a test for BRCA1 and BRCA2 genetic mutations.

An unexpected risk: These genetic mutations are also found in about 5% of patients with prostate and pancreatic cancer. Therefore, both men and women may want to consider the BRCA1 and BRCA2 test if these cancers have occurred in two or more of their family members before the age of 60.

GETTING TESTED

Among the issues for you and your doctor to deal with in the process of deciding to get a genetic test…

•**Usefulness of the results.** Deciding before the genetic test how you will use the results is an important part of the test process. For example, if Alzheimer's disease runs in your family, you may decide to be tested for a genetic variant in the APOE gene that indicates an increased risk for the illness.

The dilemma: If the test results reveal you have the APOE variant, there is no medicine or surgery that can address your genetic risk. However, you may be more motivated to make lifestyle changes, such as eating a Mediterranean diet or walking regularly, since studies show these can lower the risk for Alzheimer's. You might also change your long-term planning—such as moving closer to your family.

•**Health insurance.** In the APOE example above, it is likely that your insurer would not pay for this genetic test because the result would not affect your medical treatment.

Similarly, if you are concerned about breast cancer and want a test for BRCA1 and BRCA2, the insurance company may deny the request because the insurer may believe that your family history doesn't warrant the testing.

Helpful: If the test is not covered, you may try to get authorization for it by asking your doctor to write a letter indicating that the testing is a medical necessity and providing the relevant supporting data.

Good news: The Genetic Information Non-discrimination Act (GINA) of 2008 prohibits most group health insurers from denying insurance coverage or adjusting group premiums based on the genetic information of members of the group.

•**Psychological repercussions.** Before receiving a genetic test from your doctor, talk to a genetic counselor. The counselor can help determine if you need the test, provide psychological support when you receive results and also help determine whether or not family members should be informed about the results of your test, which could be meaningful for their own health. A genetic counselor can also help you through the maze of health insurance.

To find a genetic counselor: Ask your doctor for a referral or consult the National Society of Genetic Counselors (*NSGC.org*).

When to Think Twice About Medical Advice

H. Gilbert Welch, MD, MPH, an internist at White River Junction VA Medical Center, Vermont, and a professor of medicine at The Dartmouth Institute for Health Policy & Clinical Practice, where he specializes in the effects of medical testing. He is author of *Less Medicine, More Health: 7 Assumptions That Drive Too Much Medical Care.*

It's natural to assume that more health care is better than less—that checkups, tests and treatments make people healthier. But that isn't always the case.

Obviously, people who are sick need to see doctors and get the necessary tests. Those who are healthy may benefit from preventive medicine. But many of the assumed benefits of medicine don't always pan out.

Here are four common but false assumptions about medical care…

FALSE: It never hurts to get more information.

It would seem that getting as much medical information as possible would be a good thing. Not necessarily.

Example: A colleague's father was 85 years old and in good health when his doctor noticed an abdominal bulge during a checkup. He ordered an ultrasound, which showed that the bulge wasn't a problem—but the test did reveal a possible problem with the pancreas. To check it out, the doctor ordered a CT scan. The pancreas was normal, but the test showed a possible nodule on the liver. A biopsy showed that the liver was healthy, but the biopsy caused serious bleeding and other complications, necessitating a week in the hospital.

More data can produce more problems, which require more tests, which can create problems of their own. And all this can cost you real money—yet not improve your health.

More data also can distract your doctor. Minor laboratory abnormalities identified during a routine visit—such as slightly elevated cholesterol or slightly depressed thyroid function—often draw physicians away from the problems you want to talk about.

My advice: Expect more and more opportunities to get tested for a variety of conditions. Know that while all these tests may serve the financial interests of their manufacturers, they may not serve your interests. Before agreeing to any test, ask your doctor what he/she is looking for. Is there a specific problem you are likely to have? Or is it a fishing expedition? Avoid the latter—it's too easy to catch trash fish (meaningless abnormalities). Also, ask your doctor whether more information will change what you should do. If not, don't seek more information.

FALSE: It's always better to fix the problem.

All medical treatments are a bit of a gamble. You might improve when a problem is "fixed." Or things could go wrong and you could get worse. It's often better to manage a problem than to bring out the big guns.

Consider coronary artery disease. It's potentially life-threatening, so it needs to be treated. Many doctors recommend balloon angioplasty, a procedure to expand the arterial opening and restore normal blood flow. It can eliminate symptoms almost immediately, but it also carries significant risks to the patient.

With medical management, on the other hand, your doctor will treat the problem with medications and advice for a healthier lifestyle. You'll still have the underlying problem, but you'll learn to live with it.

How do the approaches compare? One large study found that patients with stable angina who had balloon angioplasty were no less likely to die or have a heart attack than those who depended on lower-risk medical management.

My advice: When you're faced with a medical decision—scheduling a test, having surgery, starting medications—tell your doctor that you want to take a stepwise approach. Start with the easiest, safest treatments first. You can always add more aggressive treatments later.

Think about upper-respiratory infections. Sure, you could get pneumonia, and you might eventually need antibiotics. But most people can just wait it out. Don't get tests or treatments unless your doctor convinces you, with good evidence, that you need them.

FALSE: It's always better to find it sooner.

The argument for cancer screening seems obvious. If you had cancer, wouldn't you want to know as soon as possible? Screening (looking for disease in large populations) does turn up a lot of cancers. Does this save lives? Less often than you might think.

Take mammography. It's been used for widespread screening for 30 years, yet the number of women who are diagnosed with metastatic breast cancer is about the same now as it was before. For every 1,000 women who get the screenings, at most three (likely closer to less than one) will avoid dying from breast cancer as a result. The numbers are roughly the same for men who are screened for prostate cancer.

The benefits are huge if you happen to be in one of these small groups, but what about the rest? They're faced with the cost and inconvenience of the initial test. Many will be advised to get biopsies or other follow-up tests. Some will have surgery or radiation for cancers that probably would have done nothing.

I'm not saying that screening tests are all bad—just that they aren't all good.

My advice: Ask your doctor if he/she is confident that you, as an individual, will benefit from screening tests.

FALSE: Newer treatments are always better.

There's a saying in medicine, "When you have a new hammer, everything looks like a nail." When doctors discover a new treatment, such as a drug or a particular surgery, they tend to want to use it again and again.

Some new drugs really are superior to old ones—but not that often. Vioxx is a good example. It's an aspirin-like arthritis drug that got a lot of attention because it was somewhat less likely than similar drugs to cause stomach bleeding. But a few years after it was approved by the FDA, it was removed from the market because it was found to increase the risk for heart attack and stroke.

New drugs are tested in relatively small numbers of people. It can take many years before their benefits and risks become fully apparent.

My advice: Unless you have to take a new, breakthrough drug, tell your doctor that you would prefer something tried and true—preferably a drug that's been on the market for seven years or more.

Smart Ways to Go Online for a Second Opinion

Trisha Torrey, a patient advocate consultant, who is founder and director of the Alliance of Professional Health Advocates in Baldwinsville, New York. She is also the author of *You Bet Your Life! The 10 Mistakes Every Patient Makes.* AdvoConnection.com

For many of us, second opinions have become an accepted, almost routine part of medical care. But what may be new to you are the many options for getting high-quality second opinions online.

WHY GO ONLINE?

For a second opinion to be truly nonbiased, it should be obtained from a doctor in a medical group and hospital system different from the doctor who made the first diagnosis. The first and second doctor shouldn't work together professionally or know each other socially. However, in a small town or even a small city, this is often impossible.

Additionally, sometimes the condition in question is so rare or the circumstances so ambiguous that sufficient medical expertise for a second opinion isn't available locally. A trip to an out-of-town medical center could be made, but sometimes mobility issues, distance, transportation difficulties and expense make this option impractical. In these situations, online second opinions can be a beneficial solution.

WHAT TO DO FIRST

Before you seek a second opinion, online or otherwise, it's important to decide what you want to know exactly. Is the accuracy of the diagnosis itself your primary concern? Do you need more information about your treatment options and their risks and benefits? Is there a specific drug or treatment you'd like to know more about? Write out all your questions.

CHOOSING A PROVIDER

Online second opinion services range from those backed by world-class health-care systems (such as Cleveland Clinic, *MyClevelandClinic.org/online-services/myconsult* and Massachusetts General Hospital, *EConsults.partners.org*)...to for-profit services (such as *Medigo.com* and *SecondOpinions.com*)...to less-than-reputable services. However, there's no objective quality rating system.

The backing of a name-brand institution doesn't always guarantee a careful, thorough approach. And a commercial service that recruits experts from a range of good hospitals can sometimes be a better choice. Online second opinions are available for most conditions, including cardiology, cancer, orthopedics and neurology.

Questions to ask...

•**How does your service handle the second opinion process?** Online second opinion services should use medical records, CT scans, MRI images and lab results to reevaluate your medical condition. They can't conduct their own physical examinations and may need to order additional tests.

•**Who will my doctors be?** No matter which service you choose, you should be able to learn the names and confirm the credentials of the doctors who will be reviewing your case.

•**How does communication occur?** You should look for a service that allows you, whenever possible, to converse directly, by phone or Skype (or something similar), with the physician who reviews your case and have the opportunity to ask questions. You have a right to understand exactly what's being recommended and why. And never use a provider that simply issues a written report without the opportunity for follow-up questions and further explanations.

•**How much will it cost?** Health insurers generally do not pay for online second opinions, and they are not covered by Medicare. A reputable online service will often post typical fees on its website, but you should ask for an estimate of the cost for your case. Prices usually start at about $550, with extra fees for radiology and pathology and/or phone or Skype consultations.

YOUR MEDICAL RECORDS

Once you decide on a service, you—not your doctor—should be the one to gather your medical records and test results and forward them to the second opinion service. (By law, you are entitled to these, but a small charge may be assessed for copying, etc.)

Although the details of your medical examinations and your doctor's clinical impressions may well be key parts of your medical record, if possible leave out the diagnosis. Even when taking a fresh look, doctors may frame information within the diagnostic label attached to it, picking out the details that confirm this preconceived notion.

THE PITFALLS

•**Conflict of interest.** Some online second opinion services work directly with employers or health insurance carriers. Your out-of-pocket costs may be minimal, but you can hardly expect a medical team that works for your insurer to be truly independent.

•**Lack of human contact.** While Skyping can provide face-to-face communication, it may not feel the same to you as in-person communication.

•**Treatment complications.** If you decide to follow the approach that the second opinion service recommends, your first doctor may not be happy about the new plan and you'll have to find a third who is agreeable. If your condition requires prompt attention, this will waste valuable time—online second opinions can take up to two weeks.

Also: If a second opinion contradicts the first diagnosis or treatment plan in a meaningful way, be sure to seek a third opinion.

IS IT WORTH IT?

A recent analysis found that second opinions can result in a significant change in diagnosis, prognosis or treatment—ranging from a new diagnosis for 10% of patients with chronic conditions to a new diagnosis and/or treatment advice for 62% of neurology patients.

Even if you get the same diagnosis and end up with the same treatment, a second opinion can give you more trust in your doctors and more confidence that you're doing the right thing.

Blood Work Follow-Up

Trisha Torrey, director of the Alliance of Professional Health Advocates, Baldwinsville, New York. AdvoConnection.com

Doctors telling patients to make a second appointment to go over routine blood test results seems to be happening to more patients and may be necessary in some cases. If your test reveals a problem or something that will require new treatment, then your doctor needs to tell you in person. But test results that are normal for you should not require a follow-up office visit.

In any case, do not ever assume the doctor will call you with your results. Let the office know how you would prefer to receive your results—phone, e-mail or postal mail—and ask when they will be ready. If your doctor still insists on an office visit, contact your insurer to see if it's covered. You can also arrange for blood work to be done before your appointment, so your doctor can go over it when you meet.

In Defense of the Annual Checkup

David Himmelstein, MD, professor, City University of New York School of Public Health at Hunter College, New York City.
Allan Prochazka, MD, professor, internal medicine, University of Colorado School of Medicine.
Annals of Internal Medicine, online

Arguments urging doctors to abandon routine physical exams are based on insufficient evidence, recent research maintains.

The case against the regular checkup has been largely based on a review of 14 trials that concluded that annual visits do not reduce either illness or risk of death, according to the paper released online in the *Annals of Internal Medicine*.

But the trials included in that review did not focus specifically on the value of the annual physical exam, and their results are being distorted, said paper lead author David Himmelstein, MD, a professor at the City University of New York School of Public Health at Hunter College in New York City.

"There's been a lot of folks saying in public that there's no need for people to see their doctor regularly," Dr. Himmelstein said. "What we're saying is no, the studies don't say that. This is a misrepresentation."

DIFFERENT SIDES OF THE CHECKUP DEBATE

The debate over the value of routine physicals has reached the point that the *New England Journal of Medicine* featured head-to-head editorials arguing for and against the time-honored practice.

Researchers questioning the worth of the regular checkup said that studies have failed to show any benefit from these periodic visits, which cost more than $10 billion a year in US health care expenses.

Doctors would do better to use electronic health records to send alerts to people who need preventive measures such as an annual flu shot, detractors say. Patients could receive regular blood tests and other screening measures from nurses or physician assistants, saving doctors time to care for people with actual medical problems, the thinking goes.

"What does one mean by an annual physical?" said Allan Prochazka, MD, co-writer of the *NEJM* piece questioning the checkup's usefulness. "From a patient perspective, it often means getting a variety of diagnostic tests."

However, the 14-trial evidence review cited as showing no benefit for patients mainly relies on clinical trials that took place in Europe, and involved people who received socialized medicine and who saw their doctor regularly, Dr. Himmelstein said.

And, he explained, the clinical trials mainly were concerned with the value of adding more tests to a regular checkup, rather than whether the checkup itself was a good thing.

"They weren't actually studies looking at routine visits to the doctor," Dr. Himmelstein said. "They added on some additional tests for people who were already seeing their doctors on a regular basis. The trials are pretty much irrelevant to what's being said about the value of routine visits."

Dr. Himmelstein's new research paper points to another systematic evidence review that focused solely on 33 more recent studies of periodic health evaluations that consisted "only of the history, risk assessment, and a tailored physical examination."

WHAT A GOOD DOCTOR VISIT DOES

This competing review showed that the periodic health exam improved delivery of some recommended preventive services, and may lessen patient worry. Some patients, especially those in vulnerable or high-risk groups, could benefit from routine visits, the review found.

Personal experience also has shown that regular checkups can help patients, Dr. Himmelstein added. He has caught skin cancers that people didn't know they had, and by building a relationship with patients has been able to

You Can Try New Drugs Without Government Approval

"Right to Try" laws give patients with terminal illnesses access to not-yet-approved medicines. About half the states have these laws. The drugs must have passed Phase I clinical trials showing that they are safe and must be in Phase II or Phase III trials evaluating their effectiveness and appropriate dosage level. For information, search online for "right to try legislation."

Charles B. Inlander is a consumer advocate and health-care consultant, Fogelsville, Pennsylvania.

detect problems such as alcoholism or depression, for which someone probably wouldn't see a doctor.

"It's penny wise and pound foolish to say we should stop people from building a relationship with their doctor before they're sick," Dr. Himmelstein said.

Dr. Prochazka said doctors may want to drag patients in regularly to get to know them, but it's unclear what patients want.

"I think most physicians believe that the routine visit does build rapport with patients, but there are few data on what patients' views are on this," said Dr. Prochazka, a professor of internal medicine at the University of Colorado School of Medicine. "Do most patients want to make an annual visit to their physician just to build rapport without getting testing?"

Dr. Prochazka and Dr. Himmelstein do agree on one point—there's not enough evidence to make a conclusive case either for or against annual physical exams, at this time.

"I agree that this issue needs more study because the physical health examination is a very common reason for medical visits," Dr. Prochazka said. "However, I don't feel that there are sufficient data to recommend the annual physical health examination for all patients."

info The U.S. National Institute on Aging has tips on choosing a doctor at *nia.nih.gov/health/publication/choosing-doctor*

Beware Online Symptom Checkers

Ateev Mehrotra, MD, MPH, associate professor of health care policy and medicine, Harvard Medical School, Boston.

Use caution with online symptom-checkers, we hear from Ateev Mehrotra, MD, MPH. The first wide-scale study of the accuracy of online tools (such as *FamilyDoctor.org*, *FreeMD. com* and *Symptify.com*) that offer a diagnosis based on a user's symptoms found that one-third of the sites listed the correct diagnosis as the first option, but only half had the right diagnosis in the top three results.

Surprising: The programs were about as accurate as telephone triage lines at primary care practices but better than a general Internet search in deciding when to seek medical care.

My Doctor Dumped Me

Trisha Torrey, founder and director, Alliance of Professional Health Advocates, Baldwinsville, New York. AdvoConnection.com

It may be difficult not to take it personally, but a doctor's decision to cull you from his/her patient list may have nothing to do with you as a patient. He may no longer accept your insurance or could be cutting back on his practice for personal reasons.

Under federal law, doctors cannot discriminate based on race, religion or sexual orientation or refuse to see patients in the midst of ongoing treatments, such as chemotherapy. But they may certainly dismiss patients who fail to follow treatment recommendations, don't show up for appointments, are rude or refuse to pay their portions of medical bills. In most states, doctors are not obligated to give patients a reason for ending their relationship.

If you really want to go back to that doctor, you can politely ask him to reconsider. But it may be better to request copies of your medical records and find another doctor.

Is It Time for a New Hospital?

Charles B. Inlander, consumer advocate and health-care consultant based in Fogelsville, Pennsylvania. He was the founding president of the nonprofit People's Medical Society, a consumer advocacy organization credited with key improvements in the quality of US health care, and is the author or coauthor of more than 20 consumer-health books.

Until recently, if you were hospitalized, odds are you would end up in a room with other patients. When you left, you might—or might not—get a discharge plan for the care you needed at home. And the only follow-up you got was a bill!

Now all that is changing. These days, one-third of doctors are employed by hospitals, which are aggressively marketing their physicians and upgraded medical facilities directly to patients. Hospitals are also focusing more on getting people well while they are hospitalized—and keeping them well after discharge—due to financial incentives and penalties associated with insurance reimbursement. *To take advantage of these changes…*

•**Ask for a private room.** Most hospitals are now either building new facilities with only single-bed rooms or converting many of their existing rooms to single beds. In a private room, you'll have a lower risk for infection and you'll get peace and quiet. However, private rooms may cost you extra—at least $100 more per night. Private rooms are covered by all insurance plans, including Medicare and Medicaid, if there are no multi-bed rooms available or your doctor deems a single-bed room "medically necessary" (which means your recovery or care is at risk in a multi-bed room).

Action step: Check the hospital(s) where your doctor has privileges to see if it charges extra for private rooms. If that hospital does charge extra, then ask your doctor whether he/

she considers a private room medically necessary for you.

•**Get thorough discharge plans.** Health insurers are now reducing hospital payments if you are readmitted within 30 days after your discharge. As a result, most hospitals are trying to provide patients with more and better information about what they need to do to stay well when they get home.

Action steps: Check with your assigned discharge planner (usually a nurse or social worker) to make sure you get a list of the medications you need to take once you're home, and ask the hospital to call your pharmacy to order those drugs before you leave. Also, ask for a list of phone numbers where you can reach hospital personnel 24 hours a day if you have a problem once you're home. If you need at-home care, make sure the hospital orders it—and any equipment you may need such as oxygen or a walker—before you are discharged. And insist that you be given instruction on any special care you may need to administer yourself, such as injections, bandages or insulin pumps.

•**Use follow-up services.** Besides buying up private doctors' practices, hospitals are also buying up many formerly independent medical services, such as agencies that provide home care and physical therapy and occupational therapy. Some hospitals even have contractual arrangements with in-store drugstore-owned clinics such as those found at CVS, Walgreens or Rite Aid stores for routine posthospital monitoring of incision sites, blood pressure, etc. While you should choose the service providers you prefer, it's often wise to consider using ones that are affiliated with your hospital to help ensure the continuity of your care (they typically have access to all your records and easy communication with the hospital).

Action step: If possible, find out before your hospital stay what follow-up services you will need and what providers are affiliated with the hospital so you can check them out in advance and request a particular provider(s) you may like and/or find convenient.

This Dangerous Moment Leads to Painkiller Addiction

Survey titled "Changes in Substance Abuse Treatment Use Among Individuals With Opioid Use Disorders in the United States, 2004-2013" published in *Journal of the American Medical Association.*

Study titled "Opioid Prescribing at Hospital Discharge Contributes to Chronic Opioid Use" published in *Journal of General Internal Medicine.*

Other sources include the Centers for Disease Control & Prevention, the Centers for Medicare & Medicaid Services and *The New York Times.*

There's a painkiller addiction epidemic—and almost anyone is vulnerable. You are vulnerable.

Don't believe it? Prescription painkillers—which don't work very well in the first place when used long-term—kill 46 Americans daily.

And you can get addicted from a hospital stay.

The primary drivers of this plague? Doctors, according to a *New York Times* piece by Richard A. Friedman, MD, director of the psychopharmacology clinic at Weill Cornell Medical College in New York. Twenty years ago, opioids were primarily used to treat acute pain such as cancer pain or post-surgery recovery, but now they are widely prescribed for chronic conditions such as low-back pain and sciatica. Opioid addiction is driving the new heroin plague, too. Many people who find it hard to get, or afford, prescription narcotics are turning to heroin, which is illegal but often cheaper.

For many Americans, the issue hits close to home—39% of us know someone personally who has been addicted to painkillers, according to the latest Kaiser Family Foundation poll.

Here's what you need to know to protect yourself—and those you love...

THE RISKIEST ADDICTION MOMENT— HOSPITAL DISCHARGE

Here's the scenario: You're not currently taking opioid medications at all. You need to have a procedure at a hospital. When you get discharged, you are given a prescription for an opioid painkiller for the pain. It might be *hydro-*

codone (Vicodin, Zohydro), *oxycodone* (Oxycontin, Percocet) or *hydromorphine* (Dilaudid).

Here's why it's risky: Compared with someone given a different kind of painkiller prescription or no prescription at all, you are five times more likely to be a chronic opioid user over the following year. So report researchers at the University of Colorado Anschutz Medical Campus in the *Journal of General Internal Medicine.* One reason, the researchers speculate—the drugs work for pain but also provide euphoria, and it's easy to get addicted even after original post-surgical pain is gone.

BETTER SOLUTIONS FOR CHRONIC PAIN

Chronic pain affects about 100 million Americans, but relying on opioid prescriptions, especially for long-term relief (more than 90 days), greatly increases the risk for adverse side effects—constipation, drowsiness, concentration problems, driving accidents, vision impairment, reduced immunity and, for men, reduced testosterone levels.

Taking opioid medications for chronic pain is a dangerous, and sometimes deadly, slippery slope. To take a different path, work with a knowledgeable practitioner to start by exploring drug-free ways to handle pain.

DO DOCTORS IN YOUR STATE OVER-PRESCRIBE OPIOIDS?

Where you live can be a risk factor, too. The states with the highest prescription opioid addiction rates, according to the Centers for Disease Control and Prevention, are Alabama, Arkansas, Indiana, Kentucky, Louisiana, Michigan, Mississippi, North Carolina, Ohio, Oklahoma, South Carolina, Tennessee and West Virginia. Similar geographical differences also show up in Medicare claims. A map from the Centers for Medicare & Medicaid Services, lets you see how your state stacks up against the national average in prescription opioid Medicare claims. Go to *www.cms.gov* and search "Opoid Drug Mapping Tool."

There are many reasons why some states have more opioid prescriptions (and addiction) than others, but one factor may be the prescription patterns of area doctors. So if you live in a high-use state, you may need to be extra-vigilant to avoid falling into a prescription addiction for chronic pain. Ask your doctor if there are better solutions for you.

Going to the Hospital for Surgery? Vitamin D May Protect Your Mind

Study titled "Association between pre-hospital vitamin D status and hospital-acquired new-onset delirium" by researchers in the department of medicine, Harvard Medical School, and Brigham and Women's Hospital, both in Boston, published in *British Journal of Nutrition.*

It's terrible what hospitals can do to you. We all know someone who checked into the hospital with his/her mind completely intact, but then quickly (especially if there was surgery) became confused and disoriented in a most disturbing way.

It's called hospital-acquired delirium. And, yeah, it's scary.

Delirium in the hospital is more common—and more dangerous—than you may think. It's a severe condition that mostly affects older patients (although not only older patients) and is often missed by hospital staff, especially in emergency rooms. If it's not treated promptly, it can lead to longer hospital stays and poor health outcomes, including permanent cognitive problems and even a higher risk for mortality. It's more common if there's already some cognitive impairment, but research shows that between 3% and 29% of "low risk" patients without any existing cognitive problems succumb to delirium after a hospital stay. A combination of surgery, infection, social isolation, dehydration, poor nutrition and mind-affecting pharmaceuticals such as painkillers, sedatives and sleeping pills can bring it on…quickly.

You can't control all of these factors, especially in the heat of the moment during emergency treatment. But researchers have discovered a nutritional factor that may protect against hospital-induced delirium…vitamin D.

D IS FOR...NO DELIRIUM

Researchers examined records of about 4,500 men and women (average age 59) who were admitted to one of two large teaching hospitals in Boston from 1993 to 2006. They included patients who had been tested before their hospitalization for blood levels of vitamin D and excluded those who had a history of delirium or dementia. Of all the patients, 198 (4%) were ultimately diagnosed with hospital-acquired new-onset delirium.

Their vitamin D levels told a story. Even after adjusting for age, sex, race, other illnesses and reason for hospitalization (medical or surgical), low preadmission vitamin D status was strongly associated with risk for hospital-acquired delirium.

Among all the patients studied, the average blood level of vitamin D was 22 nanograms per milliliter (ng/mL), which is on the low end of normal (20 ng/mL to 40 ng/mL). (A blood level of 35 ng/mL to 40 ng/mL is probably ideal, experts believe.) But those with the lowest vitamin D levels were most prone to delirium. Compared with patients who had blood levels 30 ng/mL and over, patients with levels from 10 ng/mL to 20 ng/mL were 50% more likely to develop delirium—and those with levels under 10 ng/mL faced double the risk. And that wasn't just a handful—about one in six (16%) of all the patients studied had levels under 10 ng/mL. Adjusting for other possible factors, including history of depression, calcium level and season of vitamin D testing, didn't change the results.

A NO-BRAINER APPROACH TO PROTECTING THE BRAIN

It's an observational study, which means it can't prove (or disprove) that a lack of vitamin D caused delirium, so it's possible that whatever caused delirium in these patients also made

Distractions Are Deadly

Don't talk to the nurse when he/she is preparing your medications while you are in the hospital. Each interruption raises the risk for a medication error by 12%.

Sally Rafie, PharmD, hospital pharmacist, UC San Diego Health System, quoted in *Reader's Digest*.

their vitamin D levels plummet. Nor does this study show that bringing vitamin D levels up to speed proactively prevents delirium. More studies will be needed to explore that hypothesis.

But it's a reasonable hypothesis, and there is good reason to believe that vitamin D may play a specific role in protecting the brain and the mind. The brain has vitamin D receptors throughout, and there is evidence that the active form of vitamin D may remove plaque, a hallmark of Alzheimer's, from brain cells, scientists have recently discovered. Research has shown that low blood levels of vitamin D are linked with dementia, Alzheimer's disease and depression.

In a way, though, the exact question is beside the point. Medicine is about balancing benefit and harm, and in this case, if you're vitamin D–deficient, there's no harm, and potentially much benefit, in bringing your body's vitamin D level up to normal! According to the National Institutes of Health, 77% of Americans are deficient in vitamin D, with blood levels under 30 ng/mL, and 6% have levels under 10 ng/mL. Even if you don't know your level, taking a daily supplement that contains up to 2,000 IU or 3,000 IU is considered safe.

An even better idea: Get a blood test. It's simple, quick, and inexpensive. If your level is low, your health-care provider may prescribe a higher dosage for a while or even recommend vitamin D injections to get your level up to normal quickly.

If you are going into the hospital or know someone who is, the idea of getting tested for vitamin D beforehand...and reaching a normal level with a supplement if need be...is a no brainer. It may prevent a scary form of delirium that can take hold in the hospital and lead to a downward health spiral. Even if it doesn't, it's a healthy thing to do.

MORE WAYS TO PREVENT HOSPITAL DELIRIUM

Ensuring you get enough vitamin D is something you can do before hospitalization. Once there, there are additional steps you can take to avoid delirium...or arrest it before it gets too bad. Whether it's you or a loved one, make sure that items such as eyeglasses or hearing aids

Catheter Warnings

Catheters may increase risk for blood clots. Until recently, peripherally inserted central catheters (PICC lines) were thought to be a safe way to administer long-term medication, such as chemotherapy, extended antibiotics and liquid nutrition. But patients with PICC lines have 2.5 times greater chance of developing deep vein thrombosis than patients using other types of central venous catheters.

Best: Ask about alternate intravenous (IV) options including a midline, an ultrasound-guided IV and a tunneled catheter.

Vineet Chopra, MD, MSc, is associate professor of medicine at University of Michigan Health System, Ann Arbor.

Catheters can cause infections. In a new study of more than 3,000 hospital patients in intensive care, risk for infection and blood clots was two to three times lower for those whose catheters were placed under the collarbone, compared with those who had catheters in the groin area or jugular vein (the traditional locations).

Explanation: Catheters can cause infections by allowing bacteria from the skin to enter the bloodstream—and skin in the collarbone area has fewer bacteria than either the neck or groin.

Note: A catheter under the collarbone slightly raises risk for a collapsed lung.

Jean-Jacques Parienti, MD, PhD, professor of medicine, Caen University Hospital, France.

are readily available, books and other familiar objects are nearby, and that the patient walks around if possible, stays hydrated, and gets as much sleep as possible in the sleep-depriving hospital environment. Regular visits from friends and family are key, since being (and feeling) isolated can lead to loneliness and fear that in turn can be a factor in delirium. Monitor medications carefully, especially pain and sleep drugs, which can contribute to confusion and push a patient toward delirium. If you're caring for a loved one who does become agitated, confused or disoriented while in the hospital—even if it comes and goes, a common feature of hospital-induced delirium—alert the staff and ask specifically for a delirium evaluation from a mental health care provider. Basic treatment, including making sure the patient is well hydrated and nourished…stops taking dangerous medications if possible…gets daily exercise…is surrounded by familiar objects…and stays connected to family and friends, can often turn incipient delirium around before it gets too bad.

Wrist Drop Recovery

Anne Louise Oaklander, MD, PhD, associate professor of neurology, Harvard Medical School, Boston.

Wrist drop, weakness lifting the wrist, is caused by an injury to the radial nerve that runs between the armpit and the back of the hand. The radial nerve can be damaged by an injury, such as a broken bone, or from pressure from using a crutch. Conditions such as diabetes that damage nerves can also sometimes cause wrist drop.

Patients can have difficulty raising or extending their wrist, to play tennis, for instance, or experience a loss of sensation on the back of the hand between the thumb and forefinger. A neurologist can determine the location and severity of the injury. Mild cases often recover without treatment within a few weeks, but more severe cases can take much longer or never completely heal.

Surgery to repair nerve ends can help the most severe injuries if it's done early enough. A wrist splint may be prescribed to hold up the wrist if weakness is severe. It's important to avoid anything that can slow nerve recovery, such as smoking, heavy drinking and certain medications, including some antibiotics (*nitrofurantoin* and *metronidazole*), gout drugs and megadoses (100 mg or more daily) of vitamin B-6.

CHAPTER 12

Heart and Stroke

Stop a Heart Attack Before It Happens

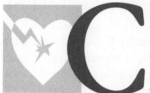

Chest pain…shortness of breath…feeling faint …and/or discomfort in the arm—or even the neck, jaw or back. If you are overcome by such symptoms and perhaps even have an intense and sudden "sense of doom," you're likely to suspect a heart attack and rush to a hospital.

But wouldn't it be better to get a heads-up beforehand that a heart attack is on the way?

What most people don't realize: For about 60% of heart attack victims, warning symptoms do occur days or even weeks before the actual heart attack. But all too often, these signs are missed or shrugged off as something trivial.

What's behind this early-warning system? The blockage that creates a heart attack often develops over time and its symptoms, though they may be mild and elusive, should not be ignored.

Knowing the early red flags—including those you might not immediately connect to a heart problem—can allow you to see a doctor before a life-threatening heart attack occurs. Women, especially, can have symptoms that do not immediately bring heart disease to mind.

Important: If these symptoms are extreme and last for more than a few minutes—especially if they are accompanied by any of the more typical symptoms such as those described above—call 911. You could be having an actual heart attack. Even if these symptoms are mild to moderate but seem unexplained, call your doctor. If he/she cannot be reached but you're still concerned, go to the emergency room.

The following are examples of the subtle symptoms that can precede a heart attack— sometimes by days or weeks…

John A. Elefteriades, MD, the William W.L. Glenn Professor of Surgery and director of the Aortic Institute at Yale University and Yale–New Haven Hospital. He serves on the editorial boards of *The American Journal of Cardiology,* the *Journal of Cardiac Surgery, Cardiology* and *The Journal of Thoracic and Cardiovascular Surgery* and is the author of several books, including *Your Heart: An Owner's Guide.* HeartAuthorMD.com

Women, Pay Attention!

After a woman goes through menopause—when the body's production of heart-protective estrogen declines—her risk for a heart attack dramatically increases.

Important facts for women: More women die of heart disease each year than men. Nearly two-thirds of women who died from heart attacks had no history of chest pain. The higher death rate for women is likely due to the fact that women don't seek medical attention as promptly as men because they are afraid of being embarrassed if the symptoms turn out to be nothing serious. Don't let this fear stop you from seeking immediate care. If the symptoms turn out to be nothing serious, the emergency medical team will be happy!

What to watch for: While most (but not all) men experience crushing or squeezing chest pain (usually under the breastbone), women are more likely to have no chest pain (or simply a feeling of "fullness" in the chest). Also, women are more likely than men to suffer dizziness, shortness of breath and/or nausea as the main symptoms of heart attack. Most women (71%) experience sudden onset of extreme weakness that feels like the flu.

•**Fatigue.** If you feel more tired than usual, it's easy to tell yourself you're just growing older or getting out of shape. But pay attention! It could be the early-warning sign of heart trouble.

If your usual daily activities, whether it's walking the dog or cleaning the house, leave you feeling more tired than normal, talk to your doctor.

•**Flulike symptoms.** If you get hit with extreme fatigue, as well as weakness and/or feelings of light-headedness, you may think you're coming down with the flu. But people report having these same symptoms prior to a heart attack.

Call your doctor if you experience flulike symptoms but no fever (a telltale flu symptom).

Another clue: The flu generally comes on quickly, while flulike symptoms associated with heart disease may develop gradually.

•**Nausea and/or indigestion.** These are among the most overlooked symptoms of a heart attack—perhaps because they are typically due to gastrointestinal problems.

But if you are feeling sick to your stomach and throwing up, it could be a heart attack rather than food poisoning or some other stomach problem—especially if you're also sweating and your skin has turned an ashen color. If indigestion comes and goes, does not occur after a meal or doesn't improve within a day or so—especially if you're using antacids or antinausea medication—this could also mean heart problems. See a doctor.

•**Excessive perspiration.** If you are sweating more than usual—especially during times when you're not exerting yourself—it could mean that there are blockages. This can cause your heart to work harder, which may lead to excessive sweating. See your doctor. Clammy skin and night sweats also can be warning signs. This is likely to be a cold sweat, instead of the heat experienced in menopausal hot flashes. If sweating occurs with any of the classic heart attack symptoms described above, don't think twice—call 911.

•**Shortness of breath.** If you notice that you are beginning to feel more winded than usual, see your doctor. Shortness of breath can be a precursor to heart attack. If shortness of breath becomes stronger or lasts longer than usual, call 911. Shortness of breath may be your only symptom of a heart attack and may occur while you are resting or doing only minor physical activity.

•**Sexual dysfunction.** Men with heart problems that can lead to heart attack often have trouble achieving and/or keeping an erection. Because poor blood flow to the penis can be a sign of possible blockages elsewhere in the body, including the heart, erectile dysfunction can be an early-warning sign to get checked for cardiovascular disease. Men should absolutely discuss this symptom with their doctors.

4 Must-Have Heart Tests

Joel K. Kahn, MD, a clinical professor of medicine at Wayne State University School of Medicine and director of Cardiac Wellness at Michigan Healthcare Professionals, both in Detroit. He is also a founding member of the International Society of Integrative, Metabolic and Functional Cardiovascular Medicine and the author of *The Whole Heart Solution*.

Heart disease is tricky. Like other "silent" conditions, such as high blood pressure and kidney disease, you may not know that you have it until you're doubled over from a heart attack.

That's because traditional methods of assessing patients for heart disease, such as cholesterol tests and blood pressure measurements, along with questions about smoking and other lifestyle factors, don't always tell a patient's whole story.

Shocking finding: In a recent study, doctors followed nearly 6,000 men and women (ages 55 to 88) who had been deemed healthy by standard heart tests for three years and then gave them basic imaging tests (see below).

Result: 60% were found to have atherosclerosis. These study participants were eight times more likely to suffer a heart attack or stroke, compared with subjects without this fatty build-up (plaque) in the arteries.

THE MUST-HAVE TESTS

Below are four simple tests that can catch arterial damage at the earliest possible stage—when it can still be reversed and before it has a chance to cause a heart attack or stroke.

My advice: Even though doctors don't routinely order these tests, everyone over age 50 should have them at least once—and sometimes more often, depending on the findings. Smokers and people with diabetes, very high cholesterol levels (more than 300 mg/dL) and/or a family history of heart disease should have these tests before age 50. *Having these tests can literally save your life...*

•**Coronary calcium computed tomography (CT) scan.** This imaging test checks for calcium deposits in the arteries—a telltale sign of atherosclerosis. People who have little or no calcium in the arteries (a score of zero) have less than a 5% risk of having a heart attack over the next three to five years. The risk is twice as high in people with a score of one to 10...and more than nine times higher in those with scores above 400.

While the American College of Cardiology recommends this test for people who haven't been diagnosed with heart disease but have known risk factors, such as high blood pressure and/or a family history of heart disease, I advise everyone to have this test at about age 50.* The test takes only 10 to 15 minutes and doesn't require the injection of a contrast agent.

Cost: $99 and up, which may be covered by insurance.

I use the calcium score as a one-time test. Unless they abandon their healthy habits, people who have a score of zero are unlikely to develop arterial calcification later in life. Those who do have deposits will know what they have to do—exercise, eat a more healthful diet, manage cholesterol and blood pressure, etc.

One drawback, however, is radiation exposure. Even though the dose is low (much less than you'd get during cardiac catheterization, for example), you should always limit your exposure.

My advice: Choose an imaging center with the fastest CT machine. A faster machine (a 256-slice CT, for example) gives less radiation exposure than, say, a 64-slice machine.

•**Carotid intima-media thickness (CIMT).** The intima and media are the innermost linings of blood vessels. Their combined thickness in the carotid arteries in the neck is affected by how much plaque is present. Thickening of these arteries can indicate increased risk for stroke and heart attack.

The beauty of this test is that it's performed with ultrasound. There's no radiation, it's fast (10 minutes) and it's painless. I often recommend it as a follow-up to the coronary calcium test or as an alternative for people who want to avoid the radiation of the coronary calcium CT.

The good news is that you can reduce CIMT—with a more healthful diet, more exercise and

*People already diagnosed with heart disease and/or who have had a stent or bypass surgery do not need the coronary calcium CT.

the use of statin medications. Pomegranate—the whole fruit, juice or a supplement—can reduce carotid plaque, too. In addition, research has found Kyolic "aged" garlic (the product brand studied) and vitamin K-2 to also be effective.

Cost: $250 to $350. It may not be covered by insurance.

•**Advanced lipid test.** Traditional cholesterol tests are less helpful than experts once thought—particularly because more than 50% of heart attacks occur in patients with normal LDL "bad" cholesterol levels.

Experts have now identified a number of cholesterol subtypes that aren't measured by standard tests. The advanced lipid test (also known as an expanded test) still measures total cholesterol and LDL but also looks at the amounts and sizes of different types of cholesterol.

Suppose that you have a normal LDL reading of 100 mg/dL. You still might have an elevated risk for a heart attack if you happen to have a high number of small, dense LDL particles (found in an advanced LDL particle test), since they can more easily enter the arterial wall.

My advice: Get the advanced lipid test at least once after age 50. It usually costs $39 and up and may be covered by insurance.

If your readings look good, you can switch to a standard cholesterol test every few years. If the numbers are less than ideal, talk to your doctor about treatment options, which might include statins or niacin, along with lifestyle changes. Helpful supplements include omega-3 fatty acids, vitamin E and plant sterols.

•**High-sensitivity C-reactive protein (hs-CRP).** This simple blood test has been available for years, but it's not used as often as it should be. Elevated C-reactive protein indicates inflammation in the body, including in the blood vessels. Data from the Physicians' Health Study found that people with elevated CRP were about three times more likely to have a heart attack than those with normal levels.

If you test low (less than 1 mg/L) or average (1 mg/L to 3 mg/L), you can repeat the test every few years. If your CRP is high (above 3 mg/L), I recommend repeating the test at least once a year. It's a good way to measure any progress you may be making from taking medications (such as statins, which reduce inflammation), improving your diet and getting more exercise.

Cost: About $50. It's usually covered by insurance.

You Don't Need CT Angiography to Diagnose Heart Disease Risk

Pamela S. Douglas, MD, professor of medicine, department of medicine, Duke University School of Medicine, Durham, North Carolina. Her study was published in *The New England Journal of Medicine.*

If you or a loved one are experiencing frightening symptoms that could be heart disease, such as chest pain, difficulty breathing, fatigue, shoulder, neck or jaw pain, palpitations or dizziness, you might be relieved when a doctor sends you for a test called a CT angiogram instead of a stress test. Unlike a stress test, a CT angiogram allows a doctor to actually see the heart's arteries and identify blockages. You might think that such a test is more accurate than a stress test. But it turns out that the long-term results using this test are no different from conventional stress tests and, in fact, a CT angiogram is potentially riskier and significantly more expensive.

CT ANGIOGRAPHY VS. STRESS TESTING

The researchers recruited 10,000 patients with symptoms typically associated with coronary artery disease, most commonly chest pain or trouble breathing with exertion. Half of the participants were randomly assigned to get traditional stress tests, and the other half to get CT angiography. After these procedures, patients were given whatever medical or surgical therapies were recommended based on their test findings and followed up at 60 days and then every six months until the end of the study for a minimum of one year. The researchers' aim was to see whether CT angiography led to better prevention of cardiovascular events than stress testing. "Cardiovascular events" included fatal

New Links to Heart Attacks

Joint Replacement

Adults age 50 and older who underwent total knee replacement were eight times more likely to have a heart attack within a month than those who did not have knee surgery…and risk was four times higher in those who had hip replacement. This risk dissipated over time. The risk for blood clots in the lungs or veins increased in the first month after surgery and continued for about one year.

Self-defense: Make sure your doctor monitors this risk after surgery and prescribes blood thinners if needed.

Yuqing Zhang, DSc, professor of medicine and epidemiology, Boston University School of Medicine.

GERD

According to a recent study, patients with gastroesophageal reflux disease (GERD), those who took proton-pump inhibitors (PPIs), such as *omeprazole* (Prilosec) or *lansoprazole* (Prevacid), were up to 21% more likely to have a heart attack than those who didn't take these drugs.

Theory: PPIs can damage the endothelium (lining of the heart and blood vessels), which can trigger atherosclerosis.

Alternative: Ask your doctor about an H2 blocker, such as *cimetidine* (Tagamet) or *ranitidine* (Zantac), which doesn't appear to have the same effect on the heart.

John P. Cooke, MD, PhD, chair of cardiovascular sciences, Houston Methodist Research Institute.

Divorce

Divorce increases heart attack risk, especially for women. Compared with people who remained married, women who had been divorced once were 24% more likely to have a heart attack, while those who had multiple divorces faced a 77% higher risk. There is no evidence that a second marriage reduced heart attack risk. Women who remarried were 35% more likely to suffer a heart attack than those who stayed married to their first husbands. Men who had been divorced two or more times were 30% more likely to have a heart attack than men who remained married or remarried once.

Study of nearly 16,000 US adults over two decades by researchers at Duke University, Durham, North Carolina, published in *Circulation: Cardiovascular Quality and Outcomes.*

or nonfatal heart attack, urgent hospitalization for chest pain or any major complication related to cardiovascular disease or diagnostic testing (such as stroke or kidney failure).

The results: Most of the patients—94%—were followed for at least a year, but some were followed for more than four years. At one year, the rates of cardiovascular events for both groups were identical—3%. And even looking at the rate of cardiovascular events at a median follow-up of two years (taking into account the patients who were followed longer), there was still no difference.

A PLACE FOR CT ANGIOGRAMS

CT angiograms do have a place in the diagnosis of coronary artery disease. When stress tests show a potential problem, patients are more likely to undergo invasive cardiac catheterization, which often does not show significant blockages. In those cases, a CT angiogram,

which would have shown the lack of blockages, has a safety advantage. And CT angiograms expose patients to less radiation than nuclear stress testing, another kind of stress test that takes a picture of the heart.

But having a CT angiogram did expose some patients to more radiation than those for whom the alternative was a treadmill stress test, which includes exercise (usually walking briskly on a treadmill) or receiving a medication to affect the heart's functioning while being hooked up to an electrocardiogram (or echocardiogram) and a blood pressure monitor. This kind of stress test does not expose patients to the potential dangers of ionizing radiation at all.

The new research underscores that CT angiograms aren't right for everyone and, when all is said and done, they don't necessarily lead to better outcomes when it comes to the real goal—preventing cardiovascular events such as heart attacks.

Don't Eat in the Evening

Joel K. Kahn, MD, clinical professor of medicine at Wayne State University School of Medicine, Detroit, and founder of The Kahn Center for Cardiac Longevity. He is author of *The Whole Heart Solution: Halt Heart Disease Now with the Best Alternative and Traditional Medicine*. DrJoelKahn.com

Research suggests that the heart (and digestive system) benefits greatly from taking an 11-to-12-hour break from food every night. One study found that men who indulge in midnight snacks are 55% more likely to suffer from heart disease than men who don't. So if you plan to eat breakfast at 7 am, consider your kitchen closed after 7 or 8 pm.

Warning: You cannot produce the same health benefits by snacking at night and then skipping breakfast. This might create an 11-to-12-hour break from eating, but skipping breakfast actually increases the risk for heart attack and/or death—by 27%, according to one study. Our bodies and minds often are under considerable stress in the morning—that's when heart attack risk is greatest. Skipping the morning meal only adds to this stress.

A Delicious Daily Snack for Your Heart

Study by researchers at Technicon-Israel Institute of Technology, led by Professor Michael Aviram of the Rappaport Faculty of Medicine and Rambam Medical Center, Haifa, Israel, published in *Food & Function*, a journal of The Royal Society of Chemistry.

Here's a really heart-healthy snack—pomegranate juice and dates. It sounds like an odd random snack, but Israeli researchers report that in animal studies the combo reduced oxidative stress in the arterial walls by 33% while decreasing cholesterol by 28%.

In the study, they included antioxidant-rich date pits, which they ground into a paste. But even without the pits, the combination of juice and pitted dates is still super-healthy, according to the researchers. Their suggestion for people who want to protect their hearts—a daily snack of four ounces (one-half cup) of pure unsweetened pomegranate juice and three dates (also with no added sugar).

18 Ways to Enjoy Heart-Healthy Walnuts

Debby Maugans, food writer based in Asheville, North Carolina, and author of *Small Batch Baking, Small Batch Baking for Chocolate Lovers* and *Farmer & Chef Asheville*.

Eating walnuts must be the tastiest way to protect your heart and your mind.

Just a handful lowers "bad" LDL cholesterol and improves the way your blood vessels function. They're rich in alpha-linolenic acid, a plant form of omega-3 fat linked with better brain function and positive moods. And even though they are high in fat and calories, research finds that people who eat them regularly don't gain weight.

Our guess: It's because they are so satisfying. At 185 calories, a daily one-ounce serving (about seven halves, or one-quarter cup) provides heart-healthy benefits without derailing your diet. We asked cookbook author Debby Maugans for new ways to include walnuts in our meals.

She gave us three recipes: Walnut Butter, Walnut Baba Ghanoush and Candied Walnuts (yes, healthful "candy!"). Be sure to read her tips at the end of this article to learn 15 more ways to enjoy walnuts.

EVEN BETTER THAN PEANUT BUTTER

Walnut Butter

This one is so delicious that it can entice even the most resolute peanut butter devotee. We tested several versions using raw walnuts, toasted walnuts, nuts with a little olive oil to make it creamier, salt and no salt. The winner was a mixture of raw and toasted walnuts, a little salt and a teaspoon of honey to smooth out any residual bitter taste from tannins in traces of walnut peel that may cling to the nut after shelling. Toasting the walnuts adds texture and aroma, too.

Makes about one cup

2 cups chopped raw walnuts

1 teaspoon honey

¼ teaspoon salt

Preheat oven to 350° F.

Spread one cup of the walnuts on a baking sheet and bake until fragrant, 8 to 10 minutes. Let cool completely.

Place remaining raw nuts and the toasted/ cooled walnuts in a food processor. Process until the mixture is a coarse paste, about 30 seconds. Add honey and salt, and process until smooth, 20 to 30 additional seconds. Scrape bowl as needed.

Store in a covered jar in the refrigerator.

A NUTTY TWIST TO EGGPLANT SPREAD

Walnut Baba Ghanoush

For these flavors to blend and develop a richer overall flavor, refrigerate the dip for 4 to 6 hours. Remove from the refrigerator 30 minutes before serving.

Makes 1⅓ cups

1 (1- to 1¼-pound) eggplant, unpeeled

3 large shallots

Vegetable cooking spray

3 Tablespoons Walnut Butter
   (see recipe above)

1 Tablespoon fresh lemon juice

½ teaspoon salt

¼ cup crushed raw walnuts

Preheat oven to 400° F.

Remove stem end from eggplant, and cut in half lengthwise. Peel shallots and cut lengthwise into quarters. Place eggplant halves on baking sheet, cut sides up, and coat with cooking spray. Place shallots on baking sheet, and coat with cooking spray. Bake, turning shallots occasionally, until eggplant is very tender when pierced with fork and shallots are golden—about 45 to 50 minutes. Let cool on baking sheet.

Remove peel from eggplant and chop coarsely. Add to food processor with shallots, walnut butter, lemon juice and salt, then process until smooth, scraping bowl as necessary. Add walnuts and pulse until well blended, 2 or 3 times.

Transfer to a bowl, cover and refrigerate 4 to 6 hours. Remove from refrigerator 30 minutes before serving with crackers, pita bread or vegetables.

A LESS SWEET TREAT

Maple Candied Walnuts

Store-bought candied nuts often are coated with loads of sugar. A little pure maple syrup gives our candied walnuts just the right amount of sweet flavor with a crunchy crystal coating.

Makes 1 cup

1 cup raw walnut halves

2 Tablespoons maple syrup

⅛ teaspoon salt

Place a dry medium-size skillet on medium heat. When it is hot, and working quickly, add walnuts, maple syrup and salt. Stir until nuts are coated and let it cook, stirring frequently, until walnuts are toasted and syrup is almost evaporated but not burned.

Scrape out onto a sheet of wax paper, and let cool. As they cool, separate walnuts with a fork. Store in an airtight container. Eat as a snack…or use as a topping, such as over yogurt, oatmeal or salad.

15 MORE WAYS TO ENJOY WALNUTS

The best way to have the freshest walnuts is to purchase them in their shells and open them as needed. The next best way is to purchase shelled walnut halves—they'll stay fresh longer than pieces. Store in a cool dry place in an airtight container.

If the appearance in a recipe is important, you can dice them. When a recipe calls for crushed walnuts, place walnut halves in a freezer ziplock bag and roll with a rolling pin to crush them. You'll end up with pieces that appear almost ground and some that are finely broken.

Here are more tasty ways to slip walnuts into your diet…

1. When making a smoothie, toss in one-quarter cup of walnuts or two tablespoons of walnut butter.

2. Make a savory Walnut Crumble Topping to sprinkle on and season cooked vegetables. Mix one cup finely chopped, toasted walnuts, one cup whole wheat panko, one tablespoon minced fresh thyme, ⅛ teaspoon salt and one tablespoon extra virgin olive oil. Store in a sealed freezer bag in the freezer.

3. Sprinkle two tablespoons of finely chopped Maple Candied Walnuts over a dish of yogurt or fruit for a naturally sweet dessert, snack or breakfast.

4. Make this appetizer: Stuff one-half teaspoon of goat cheese into a date, then tuck in a walnut half.

5. Before roasting fish fillets, coat them with crushed walnuts.

6. Grill or roast peach or pear halves. Drizzle one teaspoon of honey into each half and add one tablespoon of walnuts.

7. Make a kale salad with diced fresh pears and walnuts. Toss with vinaigrette.

8. Toss shaved and blanched brussels sprouts with a walnut vinaigrette. Crush ¼ cup walnuts. Sauté one minced shallot in two teaspoons walnut or olive oil Add three tablespoons rice wine vinegar or Champagne vinegar and one teaspoon Dijon mustard in a small bowl. Stir in walnuts.

9. Add walnuts to brown rice to augment the protein in vegetarian main dishes.

10. For a heart-healthy dessert, dip walnut halves in melted dark chocolate and let it cool and harden.

11. Sprinkle crushed walnuts over mashed cauliflower. (No really—try it!)

12. Make a breakfast bowl of cooked oatmeal topped with chopped walnuts and vanilla yogurt.

13. Keep a jar of walnuts on your desk to snack on throughout the day.

14. Pack several single serving-size snack bags of walnuts mixed with dried cranberries (look for the kind that doesn't have added sugar) to keep handy for breakfast or lunch on the run.

15. Try walnut oil in salad dressings. It's made from nuts roasted before pressing, so it has a deep nutty flavor.

Stairway to Heaven?

People who live above the third floor in high-rise buildings are much less likely to survive a cardiac arrest than those who occupy lower floors—and the risk goes up with increasing height.

Reason: Higher floors slow emergency-response times.

To learn more about walnuts, visit *Bottom LineInc.com* for more articles about walnuts and nutrition, diabetes, stress and cancer. Interested in other healthy nuts too? See *Best Nuts for Your Health* at *bottomlineinc.com/best-nuts-for-your-health.*

Better Health with Texting

Clara Chow, MBBS, PhD, director, cardiovascular division, The George Institute for Global Health, Sydney, Australia.

Coronary heart disease patients who received four regular text message reminders each week to eat right, exercise and quit smoking made lasting lifestyle changes, new research has found.

Details: After six months, the participants getting text messages had lower levels of LDL "bad" cholesterol levels, lower blood pressure and more weight loss than those who didn't get these texts.

Bonus: About half of the smokers getting text messages quit smoking versus 20% who didn't get texts.

Helpful: If you have heart disease, ask a friend or relative to send you this type of text message regularly.

The Heart Health Workout

Barry A. Franklin, PhD, director of preventive cardiology/cardiac rehabilitation at William Beaumont Hospital in Royal Oak, Michigan. He is a past president of the American Association of Cardiovascular and Pulmonary Rehabilitation and the American College of Sports Medicine and coauthor of *One Heart, Two Feet.* CreativeWalking.com

What if there were a piece of exercise equipment that could cut your risk of dying from heart disease by nearly

half? This is actually possible by simply using a treadmill—in a strategic way. The approach is not complicated or even that difficult, but few people take advantage of it.

THE "MET" SECRET

We all know that walking is an excellent form of exercise. What makes a treadmill so efficient is that you can control your pace and/or incline so that you maintain your desired intensity and get the maximum benefit from your exercise routine.

The treadmill's winning secret is that it gives you the ability to monitor energy expenditure, also called a MET, which stands for metabolic equivalent. Every one MET increase in your fitness level cuts your risk for death from heart disease by 15%, so increasing METs by three, for example, will cut risk by 45%. Many treadmills display METs readings. You can also estimate METs with an app for your smartphone or tablet. The Exercise Calculator for the iPhone or iPad displays METs when you enter your weight, type of activity and length of time exercising.

Simply put, METs allow you to track the intensity of your workout by estimating the amount of oxygen your muscles are burning to fuel you through various activities. For example, sitting requires one MET…and normal walking requires two to three METs—that is, two to three times as much oxygen and calories as you'd burn while relaxing in a chair. Light jogging requires eight METs…and running at a 6 mph pace, 10 METs.

With immediate feedback from your METs reading, you can effectively gauge how hard you're working out…and receive the motivation to push yourself at the safest and most effective intensity levels.

Important: If you've been sedentary, start your treadmill walking at 2 mph to 3 mph with no incline. Gradually increase your speed over the next eight to 10 weeks, then progress to graded treadmill walking or slow jogging. If symptoms such as shortness of breath, dizzi-

Treadmill Safety

Treadmills are generally a safe way to exercise, but accidental falls can happen. *To stay safe...*

- **Always straddle the treadmill before turning it on,** and don't assume it will always start at a slow, comfortable speed.

- **Lightly hold the handrail for support while walking.**

- **Always warm up and cool down** before and after the aerobic phase of your workout. Never suddenly stop the treadmill.

ness and/or chest pain develop, stop and tell your doctor.

Here's how to most effectively use a treadmill for specific exercise goals…

•**Quick but effective workout.**

What to use: Incline and speed. When it comes to getting the most out of exercise, intensity and duration are inversely related. By combining higher treadmill inclines with increased speeds, you'll bolster your MET level and reach your target heart rate sooner. Working at your target heart rate helps improve fitness.

With fast, graded treadmill walking, you can get a great workout in just 20 to 30 minutes.

Example: Increase speed slightly (0.1 mph to 0.2 mph) every minute for five minutes. Then increase the incline setting, which is measured as a percentage, by 0.5% (for example, going from 1% to 1.5% incline) and walk for five minutes. Alternate this sequence once or twice (increasing speed and incline each time) until you feel you're working hard, but can still carry on a conversation.

•***Weight loss.***

What to use: Incline. With incline walking, more muscle mass—especially in the quadriceps and glutes—is activated with each stride. And the more treadmill incline you use, the more calories you'll burn.

A mere increase of just 1% on the incline setting (for example, going from 1% to 2%) at a comfortable walking speed (such as 1.5 mph to 2.5 mph) will boost your energy expenditure by about 10%, and I'll bet you won't even feel a difference. If you walk faster, you'll burn even more calories because you'll be working at a higher MET level.

Research shows that regular brisk walks of at least 30 minutes five or more days a week is the best approach to weight loss. Walking on level ground at 2 mph or 3 mph equates to about two or three METs. To help protect your knees, slow your pace as you gradually work up to higher levels of inclines.

Good news: At high inclines, walking may burn as many calories as jogging or running.

DON'T FORGET STRENGTH TRAINING

To get the most from your treadmill walking—or any cardio activity—be sure to add some resistance or strength training to further build your muscle strength. Strength training complements aerobic exercise, reducing your risk for heart disease. You'll also improve your insulin sensitivity (to help fight diabetes) and boost your bone mass (to guard against osteoporosis).

Best: Target various upper and lower body muscle groups, including the chest, back, shoulders, abdomen, quadriceps and hamstrings, using hand weights and/or weight machines. Some yoga poses can also increase muscle strength and endurance.

Aim for eight to 10 exercises...and do at least one set of 10 to 15 reps per set, at least twice a week.

BONUS TOOLS

You've probably seen people at the gym wearing ankle weights while walking on the treadmill. I'm not a fan. They can strain the lower extremities, increasing your risk for orthopedic or musculoskeletal problems.

Better approach: Try walking with a backpack carrying a comfortable amount of weight. You'll burn more calories than you would if you were walking without one. A snug fit will keep the weight close to your spine and hips—which may help you avoid balance problems and improve your bone density.

And don't forget your headphones. Music (whatever genre you like) can reduce perceived exertion and may make your workout seem easier. It can be more motivating than watching TV.

Better Beta-Blocker Treatment

Jeffrey Goldberger, MD, chief, cardiovascular division, University of Miami Miller School of Medicine.

Heart attack survivors given just one-fourth of the standard dose of a beta-blocker (commonly used to slow the heart rate) lived just as long, on average, as those on a full dose—and in some cases even longer, a new observational study of nearly 7,000 adults has found.

Reason: Beta-blocker dosage needs to be customized for heart attack survivors, taking into account other health conditions, heart attack severity and genetic factors.

Caution: Never change a medication dosage without consulting your doctor.

Omega-3 Supplements May Save Your Life After a Heart Attack

Study titled "Effect of purified omega-3 fatty acids on reducing left ventricular remodeling after acute myocardial infarction (OMEGA-REMODEL study): a double-blind randomized clinical trial" by researchers in the department of cardiovascular medicine, Harvard Medical School, and Brigham and Women's Hospital, both in Boston, presented at the American College of Cardiology's 64th Annual Scientific Session in San Diego.

You've survived a heart attack. But you're worried—could another one be waiting to happen? After all, it's a vulnerable time. As your surviving heart muscle works harder to compensate for damaged tissue, you can experience further scarring and inflammation that can weaken your heart even more. But there's a simple, safe, natural, food-based supplement that cardiologists now recommend that can greatly improve your odds of keeping your heart healthy. And while it's no surprise that omega-3s are linked with heart health, this is different—a particular kind and dose of omega-3 could literally keep you alive. *Here's how to save your heart in three seconds a day...*

OMEGA-3 FOR A BROKEN HEART

Omega-3 fatty acids, the kind primarily found in cold-water fish such as salmon, have had a heart-healthy reputation for a long time. It's good for your heart to eat fish twice a week or, if you don't eat fish, to add other omega-3-rich–foods to your diet. And omega-3 supplements have been shown to reduce the risk for

Sex and Your Heart

Contrary to commonly held beliefs, sex is not associated with heart attack. A 10-year study of more than 500 patients recovering from heart attacks found that less than 1% had their heart attack within an hour of having sex. Additionally, second heart attacks were not linked to sexual activity.

Explanation: Sexual intercourse generally involves physical activity no more strenuous than a brisk walk or climbing two flights of stairs.

Dietrich Rothenbacher, MD, MPH, professor of epidemiology, Ulm University, Germany.

irregular heartbeat (arrhythmia) and prevent related fatalities, as well as reduce high triglycerides and high blood pressure, although there isn't enough evidence to determine whether taking them helps healthy people prevent heart disease, according to NIH's National Center for Complementary and Integrative Health.

The latest research makes it clear that there is at least one group of people for whom the benefits of high doses of omega-3s are extraordinarily powerful—people who've had a heart attack.

EIGHT OUNCES OF SALMON IN A PILL

In this study, 358 patients who had had heart attacks were randomly assigned to take four grams of purified prescription-only omega-3 fatty acids (about the amount found in eight ounces of salmon) or a placebo (a capsule of corn oil) each day for six months. They started within one month of the heart attack. *The researchers wanted to know how omega-3 fatty acids affected...*

•**The left ventricle of the heart,** which usually deteriorates after a heart attack

•**The size of the area damaged by their heart attacks,** which can enlarge after a heart attack

•**Signs of inflammation.**

Results: Compared with placebo, the omega-3 fatty acids were a powerhouse of heart help. Patients taking omega-3 fatty acids were 39% less likely to show deterioration in heart function than those taking placebo. Their hearts also showed much less scarring—very important because the more scarred the heart tissue is, the less well it functions. The omega-3 fatty acids also had a powerful anti-inflammatory effect, with inflammatory enzymes being way down in patients in the omega-3 group compared with patients in the placebo group.

TAKE THESE RESULTS TO HEART

Four grams of omega-3 fatty acids is a high dose—for Americans. The study researchers noted that most Americans do not get the amount of omega-3 they need, in large part because we don't eat oily fish such as sardines, tuna, trout and salmon twice a week as recommended by the American College of Cardiology and the American Heart Association. In fact, in the study of heart attack survivors, omega-3 blood levels in patients in the high-dose omega-3 group increased quite a bit, but only up to the same levels generally seen among some populations in Japan whose diet is rich in fish—and who have lower risks for heart disease and sudden death from heart attack than Americans.

Nor did the researchers report any side effects, such as interference with blood clotting, which is a concern since omega-3s are natural anticoagulants. Still, check with your doctor before taking high-dose omega-3s, especially if you are on a blood thinner. These researchers used a prescription-only form of omega-3 supplement, Lovaza, which is FDA-approved for reducing high triglyceride levels. There are many good omega-3 supplements on the market, but you'll want to see what your insurance will cover.

All of us can safely benefit from improving our blood levels of omega-3s by eating fatty fish twice a week or by getting omega-3s from other foods. But if you've had a heart attack or know someone who has, a discussion with the cardiologist about taking four grams of omega-3s in a supplement might be a lifesaving conversation.

Drugs Better Than Stents for Most Angina Patients

Harmony R. Reynolds, MD, is a cardiologist and the Saul J. Farber assistant professor of medicine, Leon H. Charney Division of Cardiology, NYU Langone Medical Center, New York City.

People with partly blocked coronary arteries may feel chest pain (angina) when walking or having a cardiac stress test, but the pain goes away if they stop and rest. For these stable angina patients, drugs—particularly statins—often are better than surgical stent insertion.

Important: Some patients with stable angina do need stents or surgery—talk to your doctor.

A Lifesaving Option for People Too Weak for Heart Surgery

Study titled "5-year outcomes of transcatheter aortic valve replacement compared with standard treatment for patients with inoperable aortic stenosis (PARTNER 1): a randomized controlled trial," by researchers at 21 medical centers in the US, Canada and Germany, including Cleveland Clinic, Ohio, published in *The Lancet.*

Imagine this nightmare scenario—you are told that you have a major problem in your heart that, if left untreated, will definitely kill you. But you're also told that you're too sick and weak to survive surgery. So do you sit around waiting to die?

Up until about 10 years ago, that's exactly what happened to very sick people with aortic valve stenosis, a narrowing of the opening from the heart to the aorta. Then came a "Band-Aid fix" that stretches open the valve, but that works for only a little while. Now, a lifesaving valve replacement option that doesn't involve open-heart surgery is available—even your doctor may not yet know about it.

Gender and the Heart

In men, the muscle that wraps around the left ventricle gets thicker with age...in women, it stays the same or gets smaller.

Implication: Women with heart failure might get less benefit from drugs that reduce heart-muscle thickness.

Radiology

FIXING A FAULTY VALVE

In aortic valve stenosis, the valve becomes narrowed (usually because of a buildup of plaque). This causes the heart to work harder and harder to pump oxygen-rich blood out of the heart and to the rest of the body. All that extra effort leads to thickening of the walls of the heart, chest pain and reduced blood flow. Eventually, the heart simply fails to adequately pump blood and could actually just stop. Surgically replacing the faulty valve with an artificial one is the ideal solution, but about one-third of patients are too weak from the extent of their heart disease to survive open-heart surgery.

Standard treatment for these people has been either medical treatment to control high blood pressure that is caused by the heart having to work harder or balloon aortic valvuloplasty, which involves threading a small balloonlike device through an artery in the leg to fit in the aortic valve and widen it.

New approach: Transcatheter aortic valve replacement (TAVR for short) is proving to be safe and far more effective than standard treatment for people who can't have surgery. It involves inserting a new valve to replace the faulty valve via a technique similar to balloon aortic valvuloplasty—by passing the new valve through a catheter that has been threaded through an artery in the leg to the heart. Its lifesaving value was recently proven in a long-term, international study.

YOU ARE NEVER TOO OLD TO LIVE

Researchers from 21 medical centers in Canada, Germany and the United States compared standard treatment with TAVR in 358 patients with severe aortic stenosis who were not eligible for valve-replacement surgery. As mentioned, standard treatment consists of either balloon aortic valvuloplasty or blood pressure medication. (Of the patients receiving standard treatment in this study, 79% had balloon aortic valvuloplasty.) The patients were followed for five years or until they died.

By the end of the study, 28% of those in the TAVR group and 6% of those in the standard-treatment group were still alive. Participants in the TAVR group lived a median of 19 months longer than those who received standard treatment. You might think that the statistics still sound grim, but the fact is that the average age of the participants at the start of the study was 83. Those who had TAVR were less likely to die of cardiac causes than those in the standard-care group. They also felt better and were less likely to be hospitalized.

And the results for TAVR get even better. *Here's why…*

Of the people in the standard-treatment group who were alive at the end of the study period, all but one had actually gone on to get an artificial valve—two ended up getting TAVR on their own and the others became strong enough to undergo surgical valve replacement.

If you (or a loved one) are told you have aortic stenosis but you won't be able to withstand the operation to replace the valve, ask about TAVR. Don't settle for a temporary solution when a safer, better treatment is available.

Better Care After Heart Surgery

John Nabagiez, MD, director of cardiothoracic surgery research, Staten Island University Hospital, New York City.

House calls can prevent re-hospitalization within 30 days after being discharged following heart surgery. Having a physician's assistant (PA) make two home visits during the week after heart surgery reduced rehospitalization by 41%, compared with those who didn't get home visits, in a new study of nearly 1,200 heart patients.

Why: During home visits, cardiac PAs can quickly identify postsurgical complications before they become serious.

An Irregular Heartbeat Can Cause a Stroke: New AFib Guidelines

Hugh Calkins, MD, a professor of medicine and the Nicholas J. Fortuin M.D. Professor of Cardiology at The Johns Hopkins University School of Medicine, and director of Cardiac Arrhythmia Services and Electrophysiology Laboratory at The Johns Hopkins Hospital, both in Baltimore.

If you have a type of irregular heartbeat known as atrial fibrillation (or "A-fib"), your increased risk for stroke and other serious conditions can be a frightening prospect to live with.

Good news: New guidelines to improve treatment for people with A-fib—the first such recommendations in nearly 10 years—have recently been released by the American College of Cardiology, the American Heart Association and the Heart Rhythm Society. The guidelines are important because they help ensure that A-fib patients are receiving the highest standards of care.

New treatment approaches…

IS MEDICATION RIGHT FOR YOU?

Stroke is the number-one problem caused by A-fib—but prescribing a blood-thinning medication (anticoagulant) to prevent stroke isn't always straightforward—each drug has possible side effects that must be balanced against its benefits.

Fortunately, decision-making about drugs for A-fib just got a lot easier for doctors. Guidelines now endorse the use of a new medical calculator—the exact name is "CHA2DS2-VASc Score for Atrial Fibrillation Stroke Risk"—that includes several specific stroke risk factors, such as vascular disease and female gender, to more accurately predict who is likely to suffer a stroke and whether treatment with a blood thinner is right for the patient. Older risk calculators did not include these specific risk factors.

What to do: If you have been diagnosed with A-fib, tell your doctor that you want to check your stroke risk with the CHA2DS2-VASc Score to determine whether or not you should be on a blood-thinning medication to prevent a stroke. The calculator and instructions on how to use it are available online at many websites, including *ClinCalc.com/cardiology/stroke/CHADSVASC.aspx.*

THE BLOOD THINNER QUESTION

The new guidelines also recommend for the first time that doctors treating patients with A-fib consider prescribing one of three blood-thinning drugs that have entered the marketplace in the last five years—*dabigatran* (Pradaxa), *rivaroxaban* (Xarelto) and *apixaban* (Eliquis). A fourth new blood thinner called *edoxaban* (Savaysa) has been released since these guidelines were published and will be included in the next update. Although more expensive than *warfarin* (Coumadin), the standard blood thinner, these drugs may offer some advantages over it.

For more information on choosing the right blood thinner: See "The Truth About Blood Thinners" on page 293 in the Medications chapter.

BEYOND STROKE PREVENTION

The frequency of A-fib symptoms can be eliminated or reduced with antiarrhythmic medication, such as *flecainide* (Tambocor) or *propranolol* (Inderal), or catheter ablation. With this procedure, a catheter (thin, flexible tube) is inserted through a vein in the groin and snaked into the heart. Radiofrequency energy is used to destroy "aberrant pacemaker" cells that send out irregular impulses that trigger A-fib.

For best results: The most successful outcomes occur in medical centers where the procedure is performed regularly. Guidelines also recommend that an electrophysiologist (a cardiologist who specializes in treating electrical problems of the heart) perform a minimum of two A-fib ablation procedures each month to maintain competency. There is no substitute for experience, for both the physician and ablation center, when it comes to complex cardiac procedures.

AFib Patients Need This Test

Hiroshi Ashikaga, MD, PhD, is assistant professor of medicine and biomedical engineering at Johns Hopkins University School of Medicine, Baltimore.

Atrial-fibrillation patients at the highest risk for stroke can be identified with a cardiac MRI. People suffering from the common heart-rhythm disorder atrial fibrillation (A-fib) already have five times higher risk for stroke.

Recent finding: A-fib patients with a specific alteration in the function of the heart's left atrium have slower blood flow and are at even higher risk for blood clots and future stroke.

Weight Loss Helps A-Fib

Prashanthan Sanders, MBBS, PhD, director, Centre for Heart Rhythm Disorders, The University of Adelaide, Australia.

In a recent four-year study of overweight atrial fibrillation (a-fib) patients, 84% of those with a high level of cardiorespiratory fitness (a measure of how well the heart, lungs and muscles supply oxygen during workouts) had no arrhythmias, compared with 17% who had a low level of this type of fitness. *How does one improve cardiorespiratory fitness?* Work with your doctor to design an exercise program—and stick with it!

Some good options include: Cycling, brisk walking and swimming.

How to Survive the Worst Type of Stroke

Edward C. Jauch, MD, director of the division of emergency medicine at the Medical University of South Carolina in Charleston, where he is also a professor in the department of neurosciences, the associate vice-chair for research in the department of medicine and director of Acute Stroke Trials, ongoing clinical research into the optimal treatment approaches for stroke.

I f someone asked you for a quick definition of a stroke, you would probably say that it is caused by a blood clot…and requires quick treatment with a clot-dissolving drug. These points are true for the most common strokes, called ischemic strokes, but there's another type of stroke that doesn't get nearly as much attention.

The "other" stroke: A hemorrhagic, or bleeding, stroke is entirely different from an ischemic stroke—and usually more devastating. Fortunately, new research has uncovered potentially lifesaving advice for people who suffer this type of stroke. *The facts you (and your loved ones) need…*

THE GRIM STATISTICS

Up to 20% of the nearly 800,000 new or recurrent strokes that occur each year in the US are hemorrhagic strokes, but they account for 40% of stroke deaths.

What makes these strokes so dangerous? Hemorrhagic strokes result from bleeding into or around the brain, a catastrophic event that damages brain tissue. In addition, as the pooled blood degrades, it releases iron from red blood cells. Iron is toxic for brain tissue.

WORST HEADACHE OF YOUR LIFE

While most people can identify the main symptoms of an ischemic stroke (for example, facial drooping…numbness or weakness on one side of the body…and/or trouble speaking), the red flags for hemorrhagic stroke are not as well known.

With hemorrhagic strokes, a sudden, intense headache is usually the main symptom. Sometimes mild headaches can be a warning sign a few days or weeks before this type of stroke.

Important: Headache sometimes occurs with an ischemic stroke, but it's usually accompanied by other symptoms, such as those described above. With a hemorrhagic stroke, additional symptoms may include nausea, vomiting and/or loss of consciousness. Symptoms can overlap, however, with both types of stroke, and only an imaging test can tell the difference.

If you have a severe headache that's unusual for you: Call 911. This is particularly true if you have stroke risk factors such as smoking, high blood pressure or diabetes.

A lifesaving new finding: For people suffering a subarachnoid hemorrhage (a type of hemorrhagic stroke described below), treatment at a comprehensive stroke center was associated with a 27% reduced risk for death, compared with care at a hospital that did not provide specialized stroke care. Comprehensive stroke centers have specialists who are trained to deal with these strokes and 24-hour access to a neurosurgeon (if needed).

For the nearest comprehensive stroke center: Go to the National Stroke Association website, *Stroke.org/emergency-stroke-center-locations*. A family member can ask the ambulance driver to take you there.

HOW BLEEDING STROKES OCCUR

There are two main types of hemorrhagic stroke…

•**Subarachnoid hemorrhage.** About half of hemorrhagic strokes occur in the subarachnoid space, between the inner and middle layers of tissue that cover the brain.

What happens: Most subarachnoid hemorrhages are caused by a ruptured aneurysm, a bulge in an artery wall that tends to develop after age 40, due to years of high blood pressure. It can also be congenital (present at birth). An aneurysm that doesn't bleed isn't necessarily a problem—you can have one for decades and not know it unless it shows up during an imaging test for some other condition.

But once an aneurysm "bursts" and bleeds, you will likely have a "thunderclap" headache that gets progressively worse—and may be followed by a brief loss of consciousness. You may also have blurred vision or loss of vision and/

or pain behind and above one eye. Permanent brain damage or death can occur within hours or even minutes. Get to an ER.

Next steps: This type of stroke can be quickly identified with a CT scan or an MRI, and with magnetic resonance angiography (MRA) and/or cerebral angiography (a catheter is used to inject a dye, which illuminates blood vessels in the brain). Once the damaged artery is identified, there are two main choices…

•**Clipping, the traditional approach, is done under general anesthesia.** A surgeon creates an opening in the skull (craniotomy), locates the aneurysm and seals it off with a titanium clip that remains on the artery permanently.

•**Endovascular coiling is a newer approach.** With this minimally invasive technique, there is no incision in the skull. A tiny catheter is inserted into an artery in the groin, then threaded through the vascular system (with the aid of a special type of X-ray) until it's inside the aneurysm. Then, a flexible platinum coil is placed within the aneurysm to stop the bleeding.

Which technique is better? It depends on the location and size of the aneurysm, as well as the overall health of the patient. One large study found that the risk for disability or death in patients who were treated with coils was almost 27% lower than in those who were clipped. However, the study found a greater risk for the brain to bleed again with coils versus clipping.

•**Intracerebral hemorrhage.** Intracerebral hemorrhages cause bleeding within the brain. They're often caused by decades of high blood pressure, which can damage small blood vessels. They can also be caused by excessive doses of blood thinners taken for cardiovascular disease… or bleeding disorders (such as hemophilia).

Along with a severe headache, symptoms might include weakness, paralysis, a loss of speech or vision and sometimes mental confusion. Headache and high blood pressure are more common with this type of stroke than with ischemic stroke, but only a CT scan or MRI can provide an accurate diagnosis.

In some cases, surgery or endoscopic drainage may be helpful to remove blood that's causing excess pressure. *Next steps…*

•**Lower systolic (top number) blood pressure to below 140.** This will reduce brain bleeding.

•**Reverse the medication's effects in patients with strokes that are caused by blood thinners.** This can be done, for example, by giving an intravenous solution that contains clotting factors, platelets or other products that help blood clot.

Survivors of hemorrhagic stroke should receive rehabilitation care to aid their recovery.

Cold Weather and Stroke

A study of nearly 300,000 adults with atrial fibrillation (A-Fib) found that their risk for an ischemic stroke was nearly 20% higher in winter than in summer.

Theory: Cold weather promotes the formation of blood clots that can travel to the brain.

If you have A-Fib: Dress warmly and talk to your doctor about other ways to control your risk for stroke during the colder months, such as making sure that your dose of any medication you may be taking (for example, a blood thinner) is adequate.

Tze-Fan Chao, MD, cardiologist, Taipei Veterans General Hospital, Taiwan.

Skipping Meds Greatly Ups Heart Patients' Risk of Stroke

Kimmo Herttua, PhD, head researcher, Center of Maritime Health and Society, University of Southern Denmark.

Nieca Goldberg, MD., cardiologist and medical director, Joan H. Tisch Center for Women's Health, NYU Langone Medical Center, New York City.

Gayatri Devi, MD, neurologist and memory loss specialist, Lenox Hill Hospital, New York City.

Journal of the American College of Cardiology

People at risk for heart disease are much more likely to die from a stroke if they don't take cholesterol-lowering statin drugs and blood pressure medications as prescribed, a recent study reports.

Folks with high blood pressure and high cholesterol had a seven times greater risk of suffering a fatal stroke if they didn't follow their drug regimen to lower cholesterol and blood pressure.

The study findings were published online in the *Journal of the American College of Cardiology*.

Fatal stroke risk also increased if these patients stuck to one type of medication but not both, the researchers found.

For example, if patients kept taking blood pressure medication but dropped their statins, their risk of dying from a stroke increased by 82%. Turning the tables, they had a 30% added risk of stroke if they took their statins but didn't take their blood pressure medications.

"High blood pressure and high cholesterol concentration are key risk factors for stroke for which effective medication is available," said study lead author Kimmo Herttua, PhD, head researcher for the Center of Maritime Health and Society at the University of Southern Denmark. "A major obstacle for the full benefits of lipid-lowering and antihypertensive treatments is the non-adherence of patients to drug therapy."

STUDY DETAILS

In this study, Dr. Herttua and colleagues tracked data on more than 58,000 patients in Finland with high cholesterol levels. During an average 5.5 years of follow-up, 532 died of stroke.

The researchers used prescription records to track whether people were taking medications as their doctors ordered. They found that only six out of 10 people took statins as prescribed.

WHY DO PATIENTS SKIP THEIR MEDS?

Doctors struggle to get patients to stick to any sort of health-improving regimen, noted Nieca Goldberg, MD, a cardiologist and medical director of NYU Langone's Joan H. Tisch Center for Women's Health.

"One of the challenges in taking care of patients is getting them to start a program and get them to continue it, whether it's getting them to exercise, cut down on their sugar intake or take their medicine," she said.

Doctors may not be properly explaining the role of these drugs in their health, and the necessity of taking them as prescribed, both Dr. Goldberg and Dr. Herttua said.

"People need to understand the connection between taking those medicines and preventing a heart attack or stroke," Dr. Goldberg said. "Face-to-face time being limited in the doctor's office, that is kind of getting lost in the visit."

Patients also might be struggling to keep up with all of the medications they need to take in a day. "The more medication recommended, the less likely a patient is to remember to take them," Dr. Herttua said.

DRUG COSTS ALSO MIGHT PLAY A ROLE

"Generics aren't as cheap anymore. There are rising prices for generics," Dr. Goldberg said. "Sometimes instead of not taking the pill at all, a patient may cut the dose. It's important not to do that, because you want to make sure you have the most effective dose."

Finally, people might simply burn out, throwing up their hands in despair at all the steps they must take to maintain their health.

"It's a drag," Dr. Goldberg said. "People don't want to feel like a patient. They want to feel like themselves."

New technologies might help people stay on top of their medications, Dr. Herttua said. For example, daily text messages could remind patients to take their statins and blood pressure pills.

Medical science also could help by combining different medications into a single "polypill," cutting down on the number of prescriptions a patient has to manage, Dr. Herttua said.

Doctors also can help patients by emphasizing the importance of these medications to their brain health, said Gayatri Devi, MD, a neurologist and memory loss specialist at Lenox Hill Hospital in New York City.

info For more on stroke risk factors, visit the U.S. Centers for Disease Control and Prevention at *cdc.gov/stroke/conditions.htm*

Surgery, Stents Equally Effective for Opening Neck Arteries

Mayo Clinic, news release

Surgery to open narrowed neck arteries and stenting to keep the arteries open are equally safe and effective at reducing stroke risk, a recent study reveals.

About 5% to 10% of all strokes in the United States are caused by narrowing of the so-called carotid arteries—the major arteries in the neck, explained lead investigator Thomas Brott, MD. He is a neurologist and professor of neurosciences at the Mayo Clinic in Florida.

"Since there are about 800,000 strokes a year, we're talking about 40,000 to 50,000 strokes a year. If we can find the best way to prevent those strokes, then we will have provided a service to those patients," Dr. Brott said in a clinic news release.

Plaque buildup in the neck arteries can reduce blood flow and cause clotting, increasing the risk of stroke. Surgery removes the narrowed segment of the artery. Stenting involves placing a tiny tube, called a stent, in the narrowed area to open the artery wider.

The study included more than 2,500 people with an average age of 69. The researchers followed the patients' health for up to 10 years after undergoing either stenting or surgery. About 7% of patients in both groups had a stroke during the follow-up period, the investigators found.

Regardless of the procedure, re-narrowing of the neck artery occurred in about 1% of patients per year, the study revealed.

"This very low rate shows these two procedures are safe and are also very durable in preventing stroke," Dr. Brott said.

"Because Medicare-age patients with carotid narrowing are living longer, the durability of stenting and surgery will be reassuring to the patients and their families," he added.

The findings show that doctors and patients can choose either option based on the patient's medical condition and preferences, Dr. Brott concluded.

info The U.S. National Institute of Neurological Disorders and Stroke has more about stroke prevention at *ninds.nih.gov/disorders/stroke/preventing_stroke.htm*

Seizures Common in Stroke Survivors

Alexander Merkler, MD, fellow, neurocritical care, Weill Cornell Medical College, New York City.
Amy Guzik, MD, assistant professor, neurology, Wake Forest Baptist Medical Center, Winston-Salem, North Carolina.
American Stroke Association annual meeting, Los Angeles.

Seizures are common in the years following a stroke, a recent study found, with nearly one in six survivors requiring hospital care after a seizure.

Researchers noted that the seizure rate following stroke was more than double the rate compared to people who'd experienced traumatic brain injuries such as concussions.

The researchers also noted that people who had certain type of stroke had an even higher risk for seizure. "One in four patients with a hemorrhagic-type stroke [when a blood vessel in the brain bursts] will develop seizures," said study lead author Alexander Merkler, MD, a fellow in neurocritical care at Weill Cornell Medical College in New York City.

"Patients with stroke should be aware they may develop seizures and should be counseled on common symptoms or signs of seizures," Dr. Merkler added.

STUDY DETAILS

In the new study, researchers examined hospital visits from 2005–2013 in California, Florida and New York. They focused on more than 600,000 people with a first stroke and nearly 2 million people with traumatic brain injuries. The study authors wanted to compare seizures after stroke to those after traumatic injury to the brain, a known risk factor for seizures.

The researchers found that 15% of stroke patients had a seizure over an average of three years of follow-up, while nearly 6% of those who suffered traumatic brain injuries had a seizure. People who suffered strokes caused by bleeding in the brain had the highest risk of seizure, the study found.

SEIZURE MIGHT BE DIFFICULT TO SPOT

A seizure can include more symptoms than people might assume, Dr. Merkler said.

"Seizures are episodes of excessive electrical activity in the brain that often cause patients to have convulsions or abnormal behavior," he said. "The typical conception of a seizure is a patient shaking uncontrollably, but seizures can be more subtle than that: Patients may only have a subtle twitch in the face, trouble speaking or even just stare into space."

Seizures tend to be brief, at less than one minute, but patients may lose consciousness or not breathe correctly. This puts them at serious risk if they're driving, swimming or operating machinery, Dr. Merkler said. Rare kinds of seizures known as status epilepticus last more than five minutes and may lead to brain injury when oxygen doesn't travel to the brain, he said.

"It's unknown whether ordering preventive anti-seizure medication for every patient with a stroke is beneficial and cost-effective," Dr. Merkler said. "Further research will be needed."

Amy Guzik, MD, an assistant professor of neurology at Wake Forest Baptist Medical Center in North Carolina, praised the study, although she pointed out that it was limited because it only looked at patients who were treated for seizures at hospitals. As a result, she said, it may underestimate the prevalence of post-stroke seizures.

"We need to let our patients know that seizure is a risk after stroke," she said. "If you have any new symptoms, call 911 or your doctor."

Vitamin C May Prevent Stroke

Study of 65 people by researchers at Pontchaillou University Hospital and University of Rennes, France, presented at the American Academy of Neurology's 66th annual meeting in Philadelphia.

According to a recent finding, people who had a stroke were more likely to have low blood levels of vitamin C than people who had not had a stroke. A deficiency of vitamin C may raise blood pressure, a risk factor for stroke. Also, vitamin C helps your body build collagen, which is important for blood vessel health.

Best: Get at least 75 milligrams (mg) of vitamin C a day.

Best sources of vitamin C: Red peppers (118 mg per cup)…broccoli (78 mg per cup)…oranges (63 mg per fruit).

"Stroke Camp" Seems to Help Caregivers Cope

Michele Gribko, MS, RN, stroke coordinator, North Shore University Hospital, Manhasset, New York. American Stroke Association, news release.

Caring for a loved one who's suffered a stroke can be stressful, to say the least. Now, a specially designed "stroke camp" may provide caregivers with support, relief and education, researchers say.

Family and friends who care for stroke survivors often experience loneliness and depression, experts noted.

"There are over 6 million stroke survivors in the United States—stroke can be life-changing and isolating for both the survivor and caregiver," said Michele Gribko, MS, RN, a nurse and stroke coordinator at North Shore University Hospital in Manhasset, New York.

The new study was led by Maureen Mathews of OSF Healthcare, in Peoria, Illinois. Her team focused on a two-and-a-half day camp for stroke survivors and their caregivers, staffed by health care providers and therapists. The camp provides caregivers with an emotional and physical break, support from others in the same situation and learning sessions.

Sixty-seven caregivers who attended the Retreat and Refresh Stroke Camp from 2009 to 2015 completed surveys afterwards. Eighty percent said their role as a stroke patient caregiver affected their life and work.

For example, 75% cited loss of time and freedom; 64% cited the strain of being forced to change personal plans; 43% said they felt confined to home; and 40% mentioned money worries.

Major strains noted by the caregivers included the survivor's inability to communicate (50%) and the loss of companionship (45%).

Half of the caregivers said they had felt overwhelmed, stressed or depressed when the stroke survivor first returned home from the hospital.

However, after attending the stroke camp, 79% of the caregivers said they felt less alone, 77% said it "recharged" them, and 58% said they learned new things, according to the study. The findings were presented at the annual meeting of the American Stroke Association, in Los Angeles.

Gribko believes that these types of programs bring real benefit.

"The study shows a need for a respite for stroke survivors and caregivers to bond with each other, share their experiences and learn about stroke," she said. "Providing a camp in which everyone who attends can relate to each other is a great way in which people can bond and create support and friendship that they normally might not have had the opportunity to do. "

Not only the caregiver benefits, Gribko added. "Stroke survivor's mental and physical recovery is better when their caregiver is well-educated and supported," she said.

info The American Academy of Family Physicians has more about caregiver health and wellness at AAFP.org. Search "caregiver health".

New Device Reduces Stroke Risk

William Maisel, MD, MPH, acting director, Office of Device Evaluation, Center for Device and Radiological Health, US Food and Drug Administration, Silver Spring, Maryland.

The Enroute Transcarotid Neuroprotection System (TNS) provides a way for doctors to access neck arteries through an incision in the neck, rather than through the groin. The system is for patients with narrowed carotid arteries who have twisted blood vessels that don't allow access via the groin. Enroute TNS has been approved by the FDA for people undergoing procedures to restore normal blood flow in neck arteries.

Stroke Link with Cancer

Study of 3,247 ischemic stroke survivors by researchers at Zeenat Qureshi Stroke Institute, St. Cloud, Minnesota, presented at a meeting of the American Stroke Association's International Stroke Conference 2015.

Stroke survivors may have higher risk for cancer. Among 3,247 ischemic stroke survivors who started out cancer-free, 2% were diagnosed with cancer within two years—a 40% higher rate than the norm for older US adults.

Possible reasons: The same risk factors that lead to stroke may also make cancer more likely—for example, smoking or unhealthful eating habits. Or an underlying condition such as chronic low-grade inflammation may make both stroke and cancer more likely.

CHAPTER 13

Infectious Diseases

A Hidden Cause of Chronic Disease

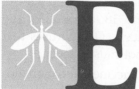

Everyone gets infections from time to time—a swollen cut...a tooth abscess...or simply a common cold. Most infections come on quickly, cause a brief period of discomfort and then disappear, either on their own or with medication.

What research is now finding: The acute illnesses that we get from infections might be just the tip of the iceberg. Experts now believe that some of the most serious chronic diseases are actually old infections in disguise.

SIMMERING DAMAGE

If you're struck with a nasty infection, you probably assume that once you start feeling better, everything is fine. But that may not be true. Even after your symptoms are gone, some bacteria and viruses have the ability to linger almost indefinitely—you can have a subclinical infection that persists months or even years after the initial illness is gone.

WHEN INFECTION LINGERS

Some infections, such as those caused by the human papillomavirus (discussed on next page), have a proven link to chronic diseases. Others may be part of a constellation of risk factors that may also include genetics or immune system vulnerabilities. *Examples...*

•**Atherosclerosis.** Up to half of those with atherosclerosis (the accumulation of cholesterol and other fats on artery walls) have none of the usual risk factors, such as smoking or high blood pressure. Yet something causes the fats to accumulate.

Arterial inflammation is a known trigger for atherosclerosis—and inflammation is often due

Bennett Lorber, MD, a professor of microbiology and immunology and the Thomas M. Durant Professor of Medicine at Temple University School of Medicine in Philadelphia, where he specializes in anaerobic infections, the interaction of society and infectious diseases and the infectious causes of "noninfectious" diseases.

to infection. When researchers examined the blood vessels of patients with atherosclerosis, they repeatedly discovered *Chlamydophila pneumoniae* (a bacterium that causes pneumonia and bronchitis), *Helicobacter pylori* (a bacterium that causes ulcers) and other infection-causing organisms. This doesn't prove that the organisms were responsible for the atherosclerosis. Some bacteria or viruses may have been innocent bystanders that just happened to be there.

What's more, if the microbes caused atherosclerosis, eliminating them should have been helpful—but heart attack patients who were treated with antibiotics were just as likely to have a second heart attack as those who weren't given the drugs. It's possible, however, that the bacteria were eliminated after the arterial damage was done.

What is known: It's been proven that patients with periodontal disease (a gum infection) are more likely to get heart disease. So are people with high levels of C-reactive protein (CRP), an inflammatory "marker" that may be elevated by any type of infection.

My advice: Since CRP is a heart disease risk factor—one that may be caused by infection—it's worth getting it checked. Ask your doctor for advice on the frequency of CRP testing. People who test high might be motivated to take better care of themselves—stopping smoking, eating a healthier diet, lowering blood pressure, etc. Be sure to get regular dental checkups, too.

Also helpful: If you have been diagnosed at any time with C. pneumoniae, H. pylori or another serious infection, tell your doctor so that he/she can consider this as a potential risk factor for atherosclerosis.

•**Rheumatoid arthritis.** It occurs when the immune system attacks the membrane that lines the joints, usually in the hands and feet. Periodontal disease appears to increase risk for rheumatoid arthritis.

What may happen: One of the bacteria (Porphyromonas gingivalis) that causes virtually all periodontal disease produces enzymes that allow the infection to survive in crevices between the teeth and gums. These enzymes then trigger a chemical reaction that produces immunogens, molecules that activate an immune response in the body's joints.

Scientific evidence: A study of more than 6,600 men and women found that those with moderate-to-severe periodontitis were more than twice as likely to have rheumatoid arthritis as those with no or only mild periodontitis.

Even though not everyone with periodontal disease will develop rheumatoid arthritis (or have worse symptoms if they've already been diagnosed), there's strong evidence that the two are related.

My advice: In addition to daily brushing and flossing, get your teeth checked at least once a year. Periodontal disease can be treated with professional care. It will help you save your teeth—and possibly your joints as well.

•**Cervical and anal cancers.** Virtually all of these malignancies—along with many cancers of the oral cavity—are caused by the human papillomavirus (HPV), the most common sexually transmitted infection in the US.

HPV is so common that most sexually active men and women will get at least one form of the virus. Most people will never know they're infected (your immune system usually eliminates the virus with time), and there's no blood test to detect it. Most HPV viruses have oncogenic (cancer-causing) potential. Two of the highest-risk strains, types 16 and 18, account for the majority of cervical cancers. (The viruses that cause genital warts do not cause cancer.)

My advice: The HPV vaccine is recommended for young men and women before they start having sex, but it's effective for anyone who hasn't yet been exposed. Even if you've already been infected with HPV, the vaccine may protect you against a strain that you haven't yet been exposed to. Talk to your doctor for advice.

Also important: Women between the ages of 21 and 29 should have a Pap test every three years, and starting at age 30, they should have a Pap and HPV test at least every five years until age 65. (The HPV test may detect the virus before cell changes can be seen with the Pap test.) A form of the Pap test can also be done for men and women who engage in anal sex.

Fight the Flu!

Marc Siegel, MD, an internist and clinical professor of medicine at NYU Langone Medical Center in New York City. He is a medical correspondent for Fox News and is the medical director of Doctor Radio on SiriusXM Satellite Radio. He is also the author of *The Inner Pulse: Unlocking the Secret Code of Sickness and Health.* DoctorSiegel.com

Getting a flu shot seems fairly straightforward. But these days, there may be more to it than simply rolling up your sleeve and getting a jab in the arm. There are multiple flu vaccines to choose from (including some that aren't injected), but your doctor may not offer enough guidance. *The facts you need to know…*

A DEADLY ILLNESS

People who have never had the flu may think that it's easy to manage, like a common cold. Those who have had it know better. The flu can leave you bedridden, achy and feverish—sometimes for weeks.

The CDC recommends that everyone six months and older get vaccinated. That's because every year, an average of more than 30,000 Americans die from flu-related complications. Older adults and those with other health problems, such as diabetes, asthma, heart disease or cancer, are at highest risk for flu and its complications.

GETTING THE RIGHT VACCINE

Flu season in the US can begin as early as October and last until May.

My advice: Get vaccinated as soon as the vaccine becomes available (ideally by October), so you don't forget. It takes about two weeks for the body to develop flu-fighting antibodies. *The main options—all are usually covered by insurance…*

•**High dose.** Because older adults are more likely to get seriously ill from the flu, and their immune response is often weaker than a younger person's after being vaccinated, they face a double risk. Fluzone High-Dose is a trivalent vaccine, meaning that it protects against three types of flu—two strains of Type A and one strain of Type B. The high-dose vaccine has four times more of the active ingredient than is used in regular flu shots. Studies have shown that people age 65 or older who get the high-dose vaccine have a stronger immune response, but experts aren't completely sure if this vaccine gives greater flu protection than the standard flu shot.

My advice: Since the high-dose vaccine appears to be just as safe as standard flu shots, it's a good choice for older patients.

An alternative: A vaccine booster. It's an effective way to increase immunity in older adults. I administer one dose of a standard vaccine early in the season, then give another dose about four months later.

•**Four-way protection.** Even though trivalent vaccines that protect against three flu strains have long been the standard, there are now quadrivalent vaccines, which add an additional B strain. However, the quadrivalent vaccine may not be available from your doctor or pharmacy.

My advice: If a quadrivalent vaccine is not available, get the trivalent vaccine. Both vaccines should protect against the most common flu strains. People over age 65 should ask their doctor whether the high-dose or quadrivalent vaccine is right for them based on their level of immunity and the circulating Type B strains.

•**Nasal spray.** FluMist is a nasal spray that is an effective alternative to shots—with no pain or crying children. A quick spritz and you are done.

However: It's not for everyone. FluMist is a quadrivalent vaccine that isn't approved for children under age two or for adults age 50 and older. Unlike the killed-virus vaccines that are used in injections, the spray contains a live, attenuated (weakened) form of the flu virus. For this reason, it shouldn't be used by those with an impaired immune system or chronic lung disease, such as asthma.

•**Ouchless.** What if you do not want a shot, but you have a health condition that prevents you from using the nasal vaccine? You can now opt for an intradermal quadrivalent shot, which is less painful because it uses a needle that is 90% smaller than those used for regular flu shots. It is injected into the skin, unlike other flu shots, which are injected deep into muscle.

Also: In 2014, the FDA approved Afluria, a trivalent vaccine that's administered via "jet injection"—a device is used to shoot a high-pressure stream of liquid through the skin. (It feels like the snap of a rubber band.)

The downside: Both intradermal and jet injections may be more likely to cause redness, swelling and itching than standard shots.

On the other hand, they are believed to provide the same level of protection as standard injections…and are less upsetting for those who don't like shots.

•**Egg-free.** Traditional vaccines are made by culturing viruses in chicken eggs—a potential problem for those with severe egg allergies. Now there are two options (Flucelvax and Flublok) that rely on cell-based technology instead of using the flu virus and eggs in the manufacturing process. The egg-free vaccines are just as effective as the standard flu vaccines and can be produced more rapidly in a sudden flu outbreak.

However: In my experience, most people with mild egg allergies can tolerate the older, egg-based vaccines—a cell-based vaccine might be helpful, though, if your allergies are unusually severe. Ask your doctor for advice.

THE TRUTH ABOUT TWO FLU SHOT "DANGERS"

Anyone who has ever gotten a flu shot knows that some arm soreness, swelling and/or redness may occur for a day or so around the injection site. But what are the recent reports of SIRVA (it stands for shoulder injury related to vaccine administration) all about? This condition, marked by severe pain, limited flexibility and/or weakness in the shoulder, is actually quite rare and occurs only when an injection of any kind in the shoulder's deltoid muscle is given too deep or too high. If you're concerned about injection site side effects, including SIRVA, consider getting your flu shot from a trained professional who can provide follow-up care…or ask for a flu vaccine that doesn't require an injection.

And what about the mercury-based preservative known as thimerosal? No link has ever been found to autism. Very credible research has repeatedly shown that the low doses used in vaccines do not cause harm.

However: You can ask for a single-dose vial. Unlike the multidose vials, which contain thimerosal to avoid possible contamination, single-dose units are free of the preservative.

Beat the Flu…Naturally

Jamison Starbuck, ND, is a naturopathic physician in family practice and a guest lecturer at the University of Montana, both in Missoula. She is a past president of the American Association of Naturopathic Physicians and a contributing editor to *The Alternative Advisor: The Complete Guide to Natural Therapies and Alternative Treatments.*

You got a flu shot, wash your hands frequently and eat a nutritious diet. There's no way you'll get the flu, right? Despite your best efforts, it still can happen. You'll know soon enough when you're overcome with those all-too-familiar body aches and are beset with fever or chills…a runny nose…headache…tickly cough…and fatigue. As soon as these symptoms strike, it's time to try my "accelerated flu recovery" protocol, which can also be used if you're taking a conventional flu medication such as Tamiflu. *My advice…*

•**Start an antiviral tincture.** Research shows that botanical medicines with antiviral properties stimulate our immune defenses, in part by increasing white blood cell activity. I like herbs in tincture form because they are easily absorbed by the body.

My favorite antiflu formula: Mix equal parts echinacea, osha, lomatium and Oregon grape root (or find a product that contains at least two of these herbs).

Typical adult dose: For three to five days, take 60 drops every four waking hours in two ounces of water 30 minutes before or after eating. (Check with your doctor first if you take medication or are allergic to plants in the daisy family, since some of the herbs could cause a reaction.)

•**Use a face pack.** To speed your flu recovery, it helps to use a "face pack" to get rid of virus-laden mucus from your nose and sinuses.

What to do: Apply one drop of an essential oil—eucalyptus, lavender, sage or thyme, for example, work well for flu—directly to your face at six sinus points (blend with a little baby oil if your skin is sensitive). The sinus points are located on each side of the middle of your nose, about one inch away from the edge…and about one-quarter inch under the inside curve of each eyebrow and above the center of each eyebrow. When you have congestion or the flu, these points may be tender to the touch. Gently rub the essential oil into each spot for 30 seconds (be careful not to get the oil in your eye). Then cover the top of your nose and forehead with a hot, moist towel. Place a dry towel on top of the moist one and lie down with your head slightly elevated for 15 minutes. Breathe deeply, and blow your nose from time to time as needed.

•**Take an Epsom salts bath.** Epsom salts help relieve the body aches that accompany acute flu.

What to do: Put two cups of Epsom salts directly into a hot bath and soak for about 20 minutes once daily. Drink plenty of water before you get into the bath to avoid getting dehydrated and feeling light-headed from the heat. After soaking, drain the water while you remain seated in the tub. Immerse a facecloth in cool water, wring it out and briskly rub the cool, moist cloth all over your arms, legs and trunk before leaving the tub. Take about 45 seconds to do this cooldown—it stimulates blood flow, which promotes healing. Then towel off and lie down, well covered, for at least an hour's rest.

•**Avoid "immunity busters."** When you have the flu, you need to avoid anything that taxes your immune system—for example, ex-

One-Minute Immunity Boost

Take a one-minute cold shower to ward off illness. Research at the Thrombosis Research Institute in London has found that cold water stimulates immune cell production.

Theory: The body tries to warm itself during and after a cold shower, which speeds up the metabolic rate, activating the immune system.

DailyMail.com

ercise, work, stress and technology (computers and cell phones). Your body will heal most quickly if you get a jump-start on healing during the first three days of the flu—before your immune system gets overwhelmed.

Important: See your doctor if you have a fever for more than two days, chest pain, difficulty breathing and/or severe pain—these symptoms could signal a serious condition such as pneumonia.

Statins Can Reduce Flu Vaccine's Effectiveness

Robert L. Atmar, MD, is clinical research professor and interim chief of infectious diseases at Baylor College of Medicine, Houston, and coauthor of a commentary on flu-vaccine effectiveness, published in *Journal of Infectious Diseases*.

People over age 65 who are taking statins should talk with their doctors about getting a high-dose flu vaccine rather than the standard dose. The high-dose form may offer some extra protection.

Flu Shot May Guard Against Irregular Heart Rate

HeartRhythm, news release.

Along with reducing your flu risk, a flu shot may protect you from a common heart rhythm disorder that significantly increases stroke risk, researchers report.

The study of about 57,000 people in Taiwan found a significant association between the flu and new cases of atrial fibrillation, a condition that causes an irregular and often abnormally fast heart rate. The condition has been linked to a fivefold increased risk of stroke, according to researchers.

Among people who had not received a flu shot, those who got the flu were 18% more likely to develop atrial fibrillation than those who did not get the flu. The risk among vaccinated people who got the flu was about the same as unvaccinated people who did not get the flu, the study authors said.

Flu vaccination was consistently associated with a lower risk of atrial fibrillation (AF) in different groups of patients, according to the study published online recently in the journal *HeartRhythm*.

"According to the findings presented here, the possibility of AF should be kept in mind when patients with influenza infection complain of palpitations or experience ischemic stroke," lead investigators Tze-Fan Chao, MD, and Su-Jung Chen, MD, of Taipei Veterans General Hospital, and colleagues wrote.

"Influenza vaccination should be encouraged for patients, especially those who have a high risk of atrial fibrillation, to try to prevent the occurrence of atrial fibrillation and subsequent stroke. However, a further prospective study is necessary to confirm our findings," they added.

In an accompanying editorial, two cardiologists from Northwestern University in Chicago said the study suggests the flu vaccine has broader potential public health benefits.

"The results of this study beg the question as to whether the acute treatment of the influenza infection itself, or addressing the inflammatory response associated with infection, may help prevent secondary episodes of AF," Nishant Verma, MD, and Bradley Knight, MD, wrote, "Beyond the prospective trial mentioned by the authors, we look forward to future studies into

Blood Test Reveals All

Every virus you have been exposed to can be identified in a drop of blood. A new experimental blood test can detect exposure to more than 1,000 strains of viruses from 206 species—virtually all the viruses known to affect humans.

Study of 569 people by researchers at Harvard Medical School and Brigham and Women's Hospital, both in Boston, published in *Science*.

these and other areas that may help confirm and validate the observed findings."

The U.S. National Heart, Lung, and Blood Institute has more about atrial fibrillation at *NHLBI.nih.gov/health/health-topics/topics/af.*

Zika Warning Goes Beyond Pregnant Women

Phyllis Kozarsky, MD, is professor of medicine at Emory University School of Medicine, Atlanta.

People who are immunocompromised should stay away from Puerto Rico, the US Virgin Islands, Mexico and other Zika-affected areas, warns Phyllis Kozarsky, MD. The Zika virus, now rampant in Central and South America and the Caribbean, is transmitted by mosquitoes. Most media reports have focused on its danger to pregnant women—it is linked to birth defects. However, people whose immune systems are compromised, including those taking high-dose steroids or undergoing chemotherapy, are at risk for serious illness from Zika. If you do go to (or live in) an infected area, wear insect-repellent all the time—the Aedes mosquito, which carries Zika, bites at any time of day.

More information: *CDC.gov/zika/geo.*

The Blood Supply and Zika

Susan Stramer, PhD, vice president of scientific affairs, American Red Cross, Washington, DC.

The Red Cross has implemented the FDA's updated blood donation guidelines to help reduce risk of transmission of the Zika virus through blood transfusions. As a precaution, people who have traveled to Mexico, the Caribbean, or Central or South America within the past 28 days should not donate blood.

Donors who have traveled to these countries and developed Zika symptoms (such as fever, rash, joint pain and conjunctivitis) within 14 days after donation, or have been diagnosed with a Zika infection, should immediately notify the Red Cross so that their donation can be quarantined.

The Red Cross screens all blood donors and accepts donations only from those who are healthy and feeling well. Anyone with Zika symptoms, even though they have not traveled to an area with the outbreak, should not donate blood.

What's Causing Your Tongue Problems?

Jordan S. Josephson, MD, an endoscopic sinus surgeon and director of the New York Nasal and Sinus Center in New York City. He is also an attending otolaryngologist specializing in sinus problems at Mount Sinai St. Luke's Hospital, Manhattan Eye, Ear and Throat Hospital and Lenox Hill Hospital. Dr. Josephson is the author of *Sinus Relief Now*. SinusReliefNow.com

I t's easy to assume that if your tongue is sore, discolored or causing some other symptom, it signals an oral health problem. While that is sometimes true, it's often just the tip of the iceberg.

What most people don't realize: Your tongue gives important clues to your overall health and can actually help predict health problems elsewhere in your body.

Beware: New research shows that certain tongue problems, including those associated with cancerous tumors, are on the rise. *What you need to know…*

TRICKY TONGUE PROBLEMS

It's a good idea to examine your tongue at least once a week.

What to do: When you first wake up, stand in front of a mirror close to a window with natural light shining into your mouth. Do not brush your teeth or tongue first, since doing so may remove signs of problems.

Important: If you notice that your tongue has a new or unusual coating, color or texture or you have an unexplained taste in your mouth, see an otolaryngologist—an ear, nose and throat (ENT) doctor—for an evaluation.

Common tongue problems that can signal health issues elsewhere in the body…

No Lyme Disease in Your Area?

Don't count on it. The black-legged tick that transmits Lyme has now been reported in more than 45% of US counties, up from 30% in 1998.

Journal of Medical Entomology.

•**Slimy or patchy white tongue.** Surprisingly, this condition, commonly known as thrush, could be a red flag for a sinus infection or gastroesophageal reflux disease (GERD). Thrush, which is typically caused by a fungal infection, can be a tip-off that a patient's sinuses are inflamed or infected or that stomach acid is flowing back into the mouth and/or sinuses—this causes irritation and increases risk for infection.

While most sinus infections are caused by viruses or bacteria, fungi (especially mold) can also lead to inflammation/infection in the nose and sinuses.

Recent finding: The number of cases of fungal sinusitis has significantly increased over the past three decades, due in part to inappropriate use of antibiotics and the use of new immunosuppressive drugs, such as those prescribed to treat rheumatoid arthritis and given after organ transplant.

Treatment for thrush needs to be aggressive, including prescription topical antifungal medications (swishes and lozenges). Treating fungal sinusitis or GERD will also help thrush. Reducing alcohol and sugar intake may help starve the fungi, which feed on sugar and yeast.

•**White or red sores.** If you have a stubborn white or red sore or patch (or a lump, bump or an ulcer) on or under your tongue that doesn't go away within a week or two, be sure to see your dentist or doctor.

There could be several possible causes for such sores or patches—the most serious being tongue cancer. Other symptoms of this type of malignancy may include chronic tongue pain, a sore throat and trouble swallowing, chewing or moving your tongue. If your dentist or doctor is concerned, he/she should refer you to an otolaryngologist who will perform a biopsy. You may need surgery to remove a tumor (minimally invasive techniques are used whenever possible, especially if diagnosed early), along with radiation and/or chemotherapy for larger and more advanced tumors.

Recent research: Oropharyngeal cancers (affecting the back of the tongue, throat, soft palate and/or tonsils) are on the rise in both men and women in the US—largely due to the increasing prevalence of human papillomavirus (HPV), which can be spread through oral sex. Researchers think that an increase in people having oral sex, especially with many partners, could be behind the rise in oropharyngeal cancers. Smoking and alcohol consumption are also risk factors.

•**Burning mouth.** A fiery sensation in the tongue (and sometimes lips, gums and throat), known as burning mouth syndrome, typically occurs out of the blue, but upper respiratory tract infections, sinus infections, dental work and stress have been known to trigger it. For unknown reasons, postmenopausal women are also at increased risk.

Other culprits: Too little vitamin B-12, riboflavin, folate, zinc or iron.

What helps: The first step is a complete physical examination that includes blood tests and a comprehensive medical history. You'll likely also need a consult with a nutritionist or integrative health practitioner who can help assess you for nutritional deficiencies and work with you to improve your diet and recommend supplements.

Flu Medication That Increases Flu Cases

Report by researchers at McMaster University, Hamilton, Ontario, Canada, reported in *Proceedings of the Royal Society B.*

Flu sufferers who take antifever medications are more likely to share the flu with others. The use of antifever medications, known as antipyretics, increases the number of flu cases by about 1% a year in the US.

Reason: Flu victims who take the medications may feel better and go to work or school, spreading the virus.

MRSA Lesson from the NFL

William Schaffner, MD, an infectious disease specialist.

It's hard to imagine how a small cut could lead to a deadly infection. But that's what happens to thousands of Americans who are infected each year with methicillin-resistant *Staphylococcus aureus* (MRSA). One recent high-profile victim is New York Giants tight end Daniel Fells, who spent several days in the ICU and may never play professional football again.

No one knows how Fells contracted MRSA, but his case is especially tragic because the infection can usually be cured by draining the area and/or giving powerful antibiotics—when it's caught early enough.

It's possible that a cortisone shot Fell received for an ankle injury temporarily masked the signs of his MRSA infection. Other anti-inflammatory drugs, including ibuprofen and aspirin, may also have this effect.

The vast majority of MRSA cases occur in hospitals, but your odds of becoming infected are higher anytime you're in a crowded setting, such as gyms and schools. MRSA is usually contracted during skin-to-skin contact, but you can also become infected if you have an open wound and touch a contaminated surface.

What to look for: Redness, swelling and pain that seem unusually severe—especially if accompanied by fever or chills.

Beware: The irritation is often mistaken for a spider bite.

If you have any of the red flags above, see a doctor immediately. A MRSA infection can become life-threatening within hours.

To protect yourself: Be sure to always keep cuts and wounds clean and covered until healed.

You Can Cure Hepatitis C...the Trick Is Paying for It

Paul J. Thuluvath, MD, a gastroenterologist, chief of the division of gastroenterology at Mercy Medical Center in Baltimore and the medical director of Mercy's Melissa L. Posner Institute for Digestive Health & Liver Disease. A clinical professor of medicine and surgery at the University of Maryland School of Medicine, also in Baltimore, he is the author of *Hepatitis C: A Complete Guide for Patients and Families.*

Think that you'd never be affected by hepatitis C? That could be a dangerous assumption. Most of the roughly four million Americans who carry this virus don't realize that they have it.

For those with hepatitis C, the good news is that the FDA recently approved new medications that eliminate the virus in nearly 100% of those who take them. That's roughly double the cure rate of older hepatitis C medications—and without the dreaded side effects, such as debilitating fatigue, nausea, skin rashes, anemia and depression, commonly caused by ribavirin and interferon, long used as the standard treatments.

Here's the catch: Many people can't afford to take these powerful new drugs, which can cost more than $100,000 for a recommended course of treatment. *What you need to know about hepatitis C and the new—but costly—medications...*

GETTING TESTED

Up to 75% of the people infected with hepatitis C are baby boomers (those born between 1945 and 1965). For this reason, the Centers for Disease Control and Prevention recommends that all people in this age group get tested for the virus.

Remember: Many people with hepatitis C have no symptoms—jaundice (yellowing of the skin and eyes), dark-colored urine, fatigue and loss of appetite are among the red flags that can (but don't always) occur during the acute (initial) or chronic (more than six months after infection) phase of hepatitis C infection. The only way to know if you carry the hepatitis C virus is to receive a blood test.

Typical cost: Up to $150, which is usually covered by insurance.

Because it is a blood-borne virus, some Americans were infected with hepatitis C during blood transfusions or organ transplants that were done before the blood supply was screened for the virus. Others were infected by contaminated needles (from drug use—the most common cause—or tattoos) or, less commonly, from unprotected sex with an infected partner.

BEST TREATMENT OPTIONS

If you test positive for hepatitis C, you should talk to your doctor about getting treated. When choosing a drug, doctors look at viral genotypes (the specific type of virus that's causing infection), along with the severity of liver disease and other factors, such as viral counts. *New treatments...*

•**Harvoni.** This drug, a once-daily combination pill that includes the antiviral drugs *sofosbuvir* and *ledipasvir,* is for people with hepatitis C genotype 1, which affects up to 75% of those who carry the virus. Depending on the severity of the patient's liver damage, the medication costs about $63,000 (for an eight-week course) to $94,000 (for a three-month course). Side effects include fatigue, headache and insomnia, but they're usually tolerable.

•**Viekira Pak.** This "pak" contains two different pills—one combines the antiviral drugs *ombitasvir, paritaprevir* and *ritonavir...*the second pill is *dasabuvir,* another antiviral. Viekira Pak is prescribed for patients with or without cirrhosis who are infected with genotype 1. The cure rate for this medication is close to 100% for genotype 1b and about 95% for genotype 1a.

Typical cost: About $83,000 to $168,000. Viekira Pak causes some of the same side effects as Harvoni.

Note: Viekira Pak has been linked to liver failure, so the FDA has recently warned that it may not be appropriate for patients with advanced liver damage.

•***Sofosbuvir* (Sovaldi) plus ribavirin.** This drug combination is mainly used for patients with genotype 2 or genotype 3 infections, which

---

*Caution: All of the direct-acting antiviral drugs can interact with other medications and supplements—tell your doctor about all the drugs/supplements that you're using.

account for about 20% of all hepatitis C patients. The cure rate is about 80% to 90%. Side effects are similar to those linked to Harvoni, plus possible anemia caused by ribavirin.

Typical cost: $84,000.

COPING WITH COSTS

Most people who are exposed to hepatitis C develop a chronic infection that slowly (over decades) causes liver damage, so early treatment is preferable to avoid permanent liver damage. But for now, most insurers will approve treatment only for patients who already have advanced scarring or cirrhosis. Since cirrhosis increases the risk for liver cancer, it is better to get treated before cirrhosis develops.

Note: Even though up to 80% of people who are prescribed one of the costly hepatitis C drugs are initially denied coverage, some of them may get the medication after repeated appeals. *If you have hepatitis C…*

•**Get tested for liver damage.** Your insurer won't pay for the new treatments until you get a needle liver biopsy (a small piece of liver is removed with a needle) to determine the extent and severity of liver damage. If a biopsy shows that you have some liver damage but not enough to get insurance coverage, you'll have to make some hard choices—get another biopsy and subject yourself to a repeated invasive procedure or wait until symptoms develop, which indicates irreversible and advanced liver disease.

What helps: Even though health insurers require a biopsy, you can get some information about liver damage with a blood test or Fibro-Scan, which is similar to an ultrasound. These tests aren't as accurate as biopsies but can help your doctor decide if you need the more invasive procedure.

•**Ask about clinical trials.** If you are denied insurance coverage and can't afford to pay out of pocket, you might qualify to participate in a study that will provide the new drugs at no cost to you. Most hepatitis C clinical trials are done without a placebo group, so everyone participating gets medication. For drugs that have already been approved, sometimes the FDA will request Phase 4 trials to gather information

on any side effects with long-term use. Consult your doctor or check *ClinicalTrials.gov.*

•**Look into PAPs.** Pharmaceutical companies and other organizations sponsor patient-assistance programs (PAPs) that offer discounted drug prices for people without health insurance, or for those with insurance who can't afford prohibitively expensive co-payments. Your doctor will have information. Other resources—*GoodRx.com…HelpRx.info…*and *NeedyMeds.org.*

The Dark Side of the Hepatitis Cure

US Food and Drug Administration safety alert announcement titled "FDA Drug Safety Communication: FDA warns of serious liver injury risk with hepatitis C treatments Viekira Pak and Technivie."

The FDA is warning of potentially life-threatening complications from some of the drugs that treat hepatitis C—at least 26 people taking either Viekira Pak or Technivie, both made by AbbVie, have had a severe, atypical worsening of their already existing liver disease. In some cases, the damage led to the need for liver transplantation or to death. If you're taking one of these medications—or know someone who is—talk to your doctor right away.

Most of the patients affected already had advanced cirrhosis (scarring of the liver), and several people had other medical conditions that were contraindications—meaning that they shouldn't have been taking the medications in the first place.

But the terrible results for these patients raises serious doubt about a common insurance practice—denying these expensive medications to people with hepatitis C that hasn't yet caused liver disease. Waiting until people with hepatitis C actually have advanced liver damage before agreeing to pay for these drugs is a penny-pinching policy that may be putting patients in harm's way.

New Hepatitis C Drug Is a Game-Changer

Sammy Saab, MD, MPH, is professor of medicine and surgery, David Geffen School of Medicine, and head of Outcomes Research in Hepatology, Pfleger Liver Institute, University of California-Los Angeles.

Zepatier combines two enzyme inhibitors—*grazoprevir* and *elbasvir*—that attack the disease in two different ways. It is the first oral medicine approved for hepatitis treatment of people on dialysis. The list price of Zepatier, about $54,000 for a 12-week course, is well below the $83,000 or more for competing drugs...and the lower price may make physicians more willing to battle insurers to get the cost covered.

Caution: Doctors must check patients for drug resistance before starting therapy and must do liver-function tests during treatment.

Nasty Germs Are Lurking in Your "Clean" Home: What You Need to Do Now

Lisa Yakas, MS, a microbiologist and senior certification project manager, food equipment, for NSF International (formerly National Sanitation Foundation), based in Ann Arbor, Michigan. NSF.org
Charles Peter Gerba, PhD, professor of microbiology and environmental sciences who specializes in virology, parasitology and risk assessment at University of Arizona College of Agriculture and Life Sciences, Tucson. He is coauthor, with Allison Janse, of *The Germ Freak's Guide to Outwitting Colds and Flu*.

A clean house feels great! But germs are wily and can thrive even in sparkling "clean" homes—particularly in areas that people don't realize are microbial hot spots. Research shows that about 12% of foodborne diseases in the US actually start in the home.

Shocking statistics: Coliform bacteria (a family of organisms that includes Salmonella and E. coli) were present in 81% of tested households...nearly one-third of the homes tested positive for yeast and molds...and more than 5% harbored Staph, a bacterium that can cause serious—sometimes antibiotic-resistant—diseases and infections, such as abscesses, pneumonia and food poisoning, according to the NSF International Household Germ Study. These germs can make anyone sick—especially people who are immunocompromised, young children and the elderly.

WHERE GERMS HIDE OUT

Most people know that doorknobs are often teeming with germs, and the kitchen sink, even a shiny one, can harbor more bacteria than the average toilet seat.

Smart ideas: Use disinfectant wipes to clean high-touch areas, such as doorknobs and kitchen door handles.

But throughout the home, there are other areas that people simply don't think to disinfect. *Where you're vulnerable...* *

IN THE BATHROOM

•**Toothbrush holders.** You probably know to store toothbrushes upright to air-dry between uses—it helps prevent the growth of microorganisms that could cause oral or systemic infection. This is good advice, but it doesn't address the holders themselves.

What most people ignore is the significant amount of "drippage" from multihole toothbrush holders. This provides a perfect germ environment. We found that 64% were contaminated with yeast or molds...27% had coliform bacteria...and 14% tested positive for Staph.

What to do: Clean the holders at least once a week with warm, soapy water. (If you can't reach inside, fill the holder with soapy water and give a vigorous shake...rinse...and repeat until the water runs clean.) If the holder is dishwasher-safe, run it through a hot cycle.

Also: There are no regulations that brand-new toothbrushes must be sterile, so give yours an overnight soak in antimicrobial mouth rinse before the first use.

•**Bathroom towels are loaded with germs.** That's partly because people don't wash their hands thoroughly enough. A scant 16% follow the CDC's advice to lather the fronts and backs of the

*Use dishwashing liquid whenever soapy water is mentioned.

hands, between the fingers and under the nails, taking a full 20 seconds to do a thorough job.

And people who wash their hands well after "Number 2" often give them just a ritual rinse after urinating because they believe that urine doesn't contain germs. Not true. Urine can be loaded with viruses, including adenoviruses (which cause colds, sore throats and other symptoms) and even the virus that causes encephalitis. I'd estimate that up to 70% of the population is excreting viruses in urine at any given time.

Also, every time you flush the toilet with an open lid, bacteria spray as far as six feet into the air around the toilet and can migrate to your towels. And because towels tend to stay moist, they harbor large populations of pathogens. Studies have shown that hand towels can have more E. coli than a toilet bowl after the toilet is flushed.

What to do: Wash bathroom towels every two to three days. Close the toilet lid before you flush. Thoroughly wash your hands or use hand sanitizer after every trip to the bathroom.

•**Bars of soap.** Germs can live quite comfortably in the "slime" on any bar of soap, even antibacterial soap. This can be risky for people with compromised immune systems—the elderly…transplant patients…and those with serious underlying diseases, such as diabetes.

Expert advice: Use an alcohol-based hand sanitizer, even when you are at home, whenever you would wash your hands (unless your hands are very dirty—then wash them first). People who use a hand sanitizer daily can reduce their risk for infection by 70% to 80%. If you prefer not to use a hand sanitizer, at least switch from bar soaps to liquids.

IN THE KITCHEN

•**Kitchen sponge.** It's the dirtiest thing in the house. When we tested sponges, we found that 15% tested positive for Salmonella. Sponges often are contaminated with E.coli as well. The more you use the sponge—such as for wiping counters and cleaning the microwave—the farther germs will spread.

What to do: Disinfect your wet sponge by zapping it for 30 seconds in the microwave, running it through a dishwasher cycle or soaking it

in a bleach-water solution at least once a week. The kitchen sink should be washed and disinfected on the sides and bottom once or twice each week with a disinfecting cleanser.

•**Cutting boards.** We found that the average cutting board had 200 times more fecal bacteria than toilets. You're safer making a sandwich on a typical toilet seat than on a typical cutting board!

What to do: After cutting meats or uncooked produce, wipe a wooden board generously with a sponge that has been soaked in a solution of two tablespoons of bleach to one gallon of water. Let it sit for a few minutes, then wipe off the excess. You can clean plastic cutting boards by running them through the dishwasher. Some cutting boards are impregnated with triclosan, an antimicrobial product. But there's no good evidence that it makes a difference.

•**Kitchen towels.** In a recent study, researchers observed 132 people preparing meals from raw chicken or ground beef. The participants were frequently seen touching their kitchen towels after handling the raw meats and before washing their hands. When they did wash their hands, they used the contaminated towels to dry them.

What to do: Don't wipe your hands on towels after handling raw meat. Wash your hands first or use paper towels.

•**Can openers.** How often do you clean yours? Once a week? Never? Can openers are actually among the most germ-laden objects in the entire house. E. coli and/or Salmonella were found on can openers in 36% of the households we studied.

What to do: Wash the can opener every time you use it. If it's dishwasher safe, place it in the dishwasher after every use. If you are hand-washing it, wash the can opener in hot, soapy water and rinse thoroughly before air-drying. Be sure all food residue is removed from the area around cutting blades. Use an old toothbrush to scrub hard-to-reach crannies.

•**Refrigerator door seals.** Research we conducted has found that refrigerator door seals (along with refrigerator vegetable compartments) often are contaminated with Listeria, a bacterium that can cause serious illness such as sepsis or meningitis.

What to do: Run a damp, soapy cloth across the surface of the door seal and through the inner channel once a week. Pay particular attention to areas where crumbs or drippings are most likely to accumulate.

•**Blenders.** They're among the "dirtiest" items in the kitchen. Many people, inspired by the smoothie craze, use their blenders daily. To save time, they just give the blender a quick rinse. Not good enough.

The rubber gasket at the base of the pitcher is often contaminated with mold, yeast, E. coli and/or Salmonella. Washing the pitcher will clean only the outer edge of the gasket and won't touch the "sealed" part that can come in contact with the food.

What to do: You have to disassemble the blender to get it really clean. After every use, remove the screw-on bottom, the gasket and the top components. Clean each item separately in warm, soapy water, then let everything dry completely before putting it back together.

•**Pet bowls.** Not surprisingly, the food/water bowls used by your dogs and/or cats are often contaminated with Staph, E. coli and other germs.

What you may not realize: When you pick up your pet's bowl, bacteria from the rim/sides can be transferred to your hands—and from there to counters, kitchen knives, cutting boards, etc.

What to do: Pet bowls should be washed daily either in a sanitizing dishwasher (with the family's dishes if you like)...or scrubbed by hand in hot, soapy water, then rinsed. Once a week, soak pet bowls in a bleach rinse (one tablespoon of bleach per one gallon of water) for 10 minutes. Rinse well and allow to dry.

ELSEWHERE IN THE HOME

•**Phones, remotes, computer keyboards.** When was the last time you wiped down your cell phone, computer keyboard or mouse or TV remote control? When someone in your family has the flu or a cold, about 60% to 80% of household gadgets are probably contaminated with the virus.

Don't assume that germs can't survive on inanimate objects. In fact, they may live longer on your cell phone than on your skin (which has anti-microbial properties). And because we use phones frequently, they're a common source of reinfection.

Example: Suppose that while working in the kitchen, you touch raw chicken that has Salmonella. Your phone rings. When you take the call, the germs will be transferred to your cell phone.

Later, after you have washed your hands, you'll pick up the same germs when you use the phone again.

What to do: If you use your phone after touching raw meat, use a disinfecting wipe to clean your phone immediately after washing your hands. At least once a week, wipe down your devices (including computer keyboards) with an alcohol sanitizer. Do it daily during cold and flu season.

•**Dirty laundry.** It's not surprising that germs love dirty laundry. Clothes that you've worn have skin cells, bodily secretions and plenty of moisture—all the things that germs need to survive. And the fecal material that's always present on used underwear is a common cause of infections.

What to do: Use the "hot" setting when washing underwear. The water should be 140°F to 150°F. If you're buying a new washer/dryer, look for one that's NSF certified. To earn certification, the machine must be able to reduce microbe populations by 99.9%.

Killer Mosquitoes

Kelly Middleton, director of community affairs, Greater Los Angeles County Vector Control District, quoted in *The Los Angeles Times*.

Aggressive mosquitoes in California can transmit dengue fever, chikungunya and yellow fever, though the chance of being infected in this manner is small. The nonnative

Asian tiger mosquitoes and yellow fever mosquitoes are spreading across southern California because of the extended drought. They are half the size of normal mosquitoes and have black-and-white stripes. They bite during the daytime as well as evening and are known to follow people into cars and buildings.

Many Travelers Fail to Get Needed Vaccinations

Study of more than 40,000 US travelers by researchers at Harvard Medical School and Massachusetts General Hospital, both in Boston, reported at a recent meeting of specialists in infectious illness during Infectious Diseases Week in San Diego.

Many US travelers fail to get vaccinations before going overseas. Outbreaks of infections such as measles and hepatitis A could be prevented if more people were vaccinated against the diseases. Many people do not realize how prevalent these diseases are outside the US. Measles outbreaks occur in developed countries, including Europe, and while hepatitis A is rare in the US, it is common in places with poor sanitation and limited access to clean water.

Self-defense: Visit a travel clinic four to six weeks before an international trip, or see your doctor to get recommended shots.

Adults Don't Need Tetanus Shot Every Decade: Study

Oregon Health & Science University, news release.

Adults can get tetanus and diphtheria vaccine boosters every 30 years instead of the recommended 10 years, a new study suggests.

Reusable Grocery Bags Can Make You Sick

A recent study found that 97% of people never clean their bags—and most were crawling with bacteria, such as Escherichia coli, that can cause gastrointestinal ailments. Bags may collect pathogens from, say, a package of meat or raw produce, and then spread them to other foods.

Self-defense: Don't carry meat in reusable bags…and keep meat, as well as produce, separate from other foods. Wipe bags with bleach or machine-wash them after every use.

Charles Gerba, PhD, professor of microbiology and environmental sciences, The University of Arizona, Tucson.

"We have always been told to get a tetanus shot every 10 years, but actually, there is very little data to prove or disprove that timeline," said researcher Mark Slifka, PhD. He is a professor at the Oregon National Primate Research Center at Oregon Health & Science University.

Revising that vaccination schedule could also save the U.S. health care system hundreds of millions of dollars a year, the researchers added in a university news release.

For the study, the investigators examined immunity levels in over 500 adults. The researchers found that after completing the standard five-dose childhood vaccine series, adults remain protected against tetanus and diphtheria for at least 30 years without the need for further booster shots.

"If you ask around, you often find that it is hard for people to remember if they had their last tetanus shot eight years ago or even 11 years ago," Dr. Slifka said. "If we were to use a simple age-based system, people would only have to remember to get their shots when they turn 30 and again when they turn 60."

The study authors noted that the World Health Organization recommends only a single adult booster vaccination during military service or when a woman becomes pregnant for the first time. The United Kingdom and some other countries recommend no adult booster shots at all.

Ticks Carry More Than Lyme Disease

Study of 7,643 ticks by researchers at Bard College, Annandale-on-Hudson, New York, published in *PLOS One*.

One tick can cause two infections. Deer ticks that carry Lyme disease bacteria can also be infected with *babesiosis*, a less common disease that infects red blood cells. A single bite from a doubly infected tick can cause a person to develop both diseases. In an area of New York State where tick-borne disease is common, nearly one-third of ticks were found to be infected with the bacteria that cause Lyme disease...and one-third of the infected ticks—or about 7% of all the ticks studied—also carried a second disease. Most people bitten by ticks do not develop Lyme or other tick-borne diseases.

Shocking Danger for Contact Lens Wearers

Jennifer Cope, MD, MPH, a medical epidemiologist with the Centers for Disease Control and Prevention's Division of Foodborne, Waterborne and Environmental Diseases in Atlanta. CDC.gov

There has been an increase in recent years in the number of eye infections caused by the rare but dangerous Acanthamoeba parasite. These infections can be very difficult to treat and sometimes lead to blindness.

Contact lens wearers usually are the victims, because Acanthamoeba can attach itself to the surface of a contact lens and then enter the eye through tiny cuts in the cornea. Contact lenses can cause some of these tiny cuts (microtrauma).

Three things contact lens wearers can do to stay safe...

•**Remove your lenses before showering, bathing and swimming.** Acanthamoeba can live in tap water...swimming pool water...hot tub water...and even in natural bodies of water, both fresh and salt. This danger exists even if the water has been treated by a local water district and is perfectly safe to drink...and even if swimming pool water has been chlorinated. Acanthamoeba can survive these treatments, and infections have been increasing since 2004. Previously there were one to two cases per million American contact lens wearers. Now there are about 15 cases per million. It is not clear what is causing the increase.

•**Remove and thoroughly disinfect** your lenses as soon as possible if they are exposed to water. Peroxide cleaning systems are the only type that have been shown to kill Acanthamoeba.

•**Never use tap water to rinse off lenses or lens cases.**

Plague Is On the Rise

Natalie Kwit, DVM, MPH, is an epidemic intelligence service officer at National Center for Emerging and Zoonotic Infectious Diseases, Centers for Disease Control and Prevention, Atlanta.

Plague cases in humans have been reported in Arizona, California, Colorado, Georgia, Michigan, New Mexico, Oregon and Utah. Plague is a bacterial infection carried by a rodent flea.

Self-defense: Wear insect repellent. Use flea-control products on pets. If you develop fever, chills, weakness and swollen lymph nodes—and have been in areas where plague is a concern—see your doctor immediately. Plague is treatable with antibiotics.

New Lyme Disease Bacteria Discovered

U.S. Centers for Disease Control and Prevention, news release.

A new Lyme disease-causing bacteria has been identified in the United States, and it may bring even worse symptoms, health officials said.

Borrelia burgdorferi was the only bacteria species believed to cause Lyme disease in North America—until this new discovery, the researchers said. The newly-identified bacteria, called *Borrelia mayonii*, appears closely related to B. burgdorferi, say a team from the U.S. Centers for Disease Control and Prevention.

The first indication there might be a new species of Lyme disease-causing bacteria was unusual lab test results from six samples from people suspected to have the illness. Further genetic testing at the CDC and the Mayo Clinic in Rochester, Minnesota, pinpointed the new species of bacteria.

So far, it has only been found in the upper Midwest, the study said.

Preliminary findings suggest that illness caused by the new bacteria is similar. But, there may be some differences. Both cause fever, headache, rash, and neck pain in the first days after infection, and arthritis weeks after infection.

But the new bacteria also seems to cause nausea and vomiting, diffuse rashes rather than a single so-called "bull's-eye" rash, and a higher concentration of bacteria in the blood, the CDC said.

Both types of bacteria are transmitted to people through the bite of an infected black-legged, or deer, tick, the CDC said. The new bacteria has been found in ticks gathered from at least two counties in northwestern Wisconsin, the CDC noted.

The first patients found to have B. mayonii-linked Lyme disease were likely bitten by ticks in north-central Minnesota and western Wisconsin. But it's very likely that ticks infected with the bacteria are found throughout both states, the CDC said.

In order to get a better understanding of tick-borne diseases in general, the CDC funded a three-year effort to collect up to 30,000 specimens from people with suspected tick-borne illness.

"Coupling technology with teamwork between federal, state, and private entities will help improve early and accurate diagnosis of tick-borne diseases," Ben Beard, PhD, chief of CDC's Bacterial Diseases Branch, said in the news release.

Newly Designed Endoscope Reduces Risk of Bacterial Infections

U.S. Food and Drug Administration, news release.

A newly designed Olympus duodenoscope was recently approved by the U.S. Food and Drug Administration.

The new device has modifications to reduce the risk of bacterial infections, the FDA said. The original model will be recalled and repaired by Olympus, according to the FDA.

Duodenoscopes are flexible, lighted tubes. During a procedure, the device is threaded through the mouth, throat and stomach to the small intestine. They're used to diagnose and treat problems in the liver, pancreas and gallbladder, the FDA explained.

Early in 2014, the FDA issued a warning that duodenoscopes are hard to clean. And, the FDA noted that even when health care workers follow manufacturers' directions, patients were still at risk for infection. The warning came after a number of patients who had duodenoscope procedures were infected with drug-resistant "superbugs."

The FDA issued recommendations for the cleaning and sterilization of duodenoscopes. The agency has also been working with three makers of the devices to improve their safety.

Along with design modifications to its device, Olympus also made labeling changes. The company also said it will conduct annual inspections of each scope in use to ensure their safety.

The design modifications were to a part of the device known as the elevator channel. Leakage into the elevator channel posed an infection risk to patients because this sealed area cannot be cleaned and disinfected between use in different patients.

The Olympus TJF-Q180V's new design, as well as the new annual inspection program, is intended to reduce the risk of fluid leakage into the elevator channel, which in turn can reduce patient exposure to bacteria and other potential infections.

Blood Test Might Predict When Antibiotics Won't Help

Ephraim Tsalik, MD, PhD, emergency medicine physician, Durham VA Medical Center, and assistant professor, medicine, Duke University School of Medicine, Durham, North Carolina.

Dominik Mertz, MD, MSc, assistant professor, division of infectious diseases, department of medicine, and medical director, infection control, Hamilton Health Sciences, McMaster University, Hamilton, Ontario, Canada.

Science Translational Medicine.

Researchers say they're closer to developing a blood test that distinguishes between viral and bacterial respiratory infections. This would help doctors predict when antibiotics will and will not work.

Such a test, done right in the doctor's office, might also help curb overuse of antibiotics—a practice that has led to drug-resistant bacteria, experts suggest.

IS A BLOOD TEST NECESSARY?

When diagnosing respiratory infections—such as colds, pneumonia and bronchitis—it helps to know whether the illness is caused by a virus or bacteria, explained study lead author Ephraim Tsalik, MD, PhD. He is assistant professor of medicine at Duke University School of Medicine in Durham, North Carolina.

"Antibiotics treat bacteria, but they do not treat viruses. That's why distinguishing between these various causes of illness is very important to get the right treatment to the right patient, and to offer a prognosis for how the patient is likely to do," Dr. Tsalik said.

Respiratory infections are one of the most common reasons for doctor visits. And about three-quarters of patients get bacteria-fighting antibiotics even though most have viral infections, Dr. Tsalik said. "Viruses, for the most part, get better on their own," he said.

Patients sometimes demand antibiotics even if the illness appears to be a virus, and doctors sometimes prescribe them in order to be "better safe than sorry," he explained. Both cases can expose patients unnecessarily to potential side effects, Dr. Tsalik said.

Equally concerning is that unnecessary use of antibiotics raises the risk that bacteria will figure out how to resist the medications, Dr. Tsalik said. Awareness has grown worldwide in recent years over bacterial germs that are no longer easily killed off with antibiotics.

A quick and affordable test could provide important information about sick patients, said Dominik Mertz, MD, an assistant professor of infectious diseases at Canada's McMaster University. Dr. Mertz wasn't involved in the new research.

While the new test isn't ready yet, Dr. Mertz said, "it might be a new approach that could eventually get there. The test results could be used to reassure yourself as a physician as well as the patient."

STUDY DETAILS

In the current study, Dr. Tsalik and colleagues developed a test to distinguish viruses from bacterial infections by analyzing the workings of genes in the blood. The investigators tried the test out on 273 people with respiratory infections and 44 healthy people.

Overall, the test was accurate 87% of the time in distinguishing between bacterial and viral infections, and infections caused by something else. This is better than the 78% accuracy rate of an existing test that analyzes inflammation linked to illness, the researchers said.

"Even with that imperfect test, other studies showed that using it can reduce antibiotic use by about 40 to 50% compared to no testing at all," Dr. Tsalik said.

The new test works by detecting how genes "turn off and on in a particular pattern" in response to bacteria, a virus or another cause, he said. Dr. Tsalik added that it's unique because of its speed and simplicity. There are no details yet about price, but he said researchers want to make it affordable.

What's next? Dr. Tsalik said researchers want to evaluate the test using people of various ages and ethnicities. They are also exploring whether similar tests can detect other types of bacterial and viral infections and fungal infections.

The study is published in *Science Translational Medicine.*

ℹ️ **info** Duke Medicine has more about viral and bacterial infections at *dukemedicine.org/blog/it-bacterial-infection-or-virus*

Seniors Often Bring Drug-Resistant Germs to Rehab Centers

Lona Mody, MD, MSc, professor of internal medicine, University of Michigan, and associate division chief, division of geriatric and palliative care medicine, and associate director, clinical and translational research, Geriatrics Center, University of Michigan Medical School, Ann Arbor, Michigan.

Philip Tierno, MD, PhD, professor, microbiology and pathology, NYU School of Medicine, NYU Langone Medical Center, New York City.

JAMA Internal Medicine, online.

Seniors transferred from a hospital to a rehabilitation facility often bring dangerous germs with them, a new study suggests.

The finding stems from an investigation that looked at resistant germ rates in the kind of post-hospital recovery centers that seniors often spend time in before returning home.

"Hand hygiene is considered to be the most important strategy to prevent infections and spread of drug-resistant organisms," explained study lead author Lona Mody, MD.

The problem is that most of the current focus is placed on ensuring caregiver hand hygiene, not patient hand hygiene, noted Dr. Mody, who is a professor of internal medicine. A focus on patient hand hygiene is going to be increasingly important, because "we are now facing a tsunami of an aging population in our hospitals, post-acute care facilities and long-term care facilities," according to Dr. Mody.

Every year, about 2 million Americans become infected with antibiotic-resistant bacteria, and about 23,000 die as a result, according to the U.S. Centers for Disease Control and Prevention.

RESEARCH DETAILS

To assess hand-related germ risk, the investigators tallied the presence of multidrug-resistant germs among more than 350 seniors, with an average age of 76. The study participants were being temporarily cared for in six different rehabilitation/assisted-living centers in Michigan, directly after being hospitalized for a short time.

Following germ testing on admission, the investigators continued to track three common resistant germs, including the potentially serious staph infection known as MRSA. Tracking continued on a monthly basis until discharge from the facility or for up to six months.

Almost one-quarter of the patients had at least one such germ on their hands at admission, including MRSA, the researchers reported.

In addition, about 10% then went on to newly acquire at least one type of resistant germ on their hands, and about two-thirds of carriers still had the germs at discharge, the study revealed.

What's more, the team suggested their findings may underestimate the gravity of the situation, given their focus on new incoming patients, rather than long-term residents.

HANDWASHING IS KEY

The researchers said that they suspect the main culprit is a lack of routine hand washing.

Going forward, Dr. Mody said it will be important to combat the risk from these bacteria by developing new programs "that reinforce patient hand hygiene."

"Today, patient hands come in contact with environmental surfaces, rehabilitation equipment, health care worker hands, and other patients," she said, a risky fact of life that will require a concerted response on the part of both patient advocates and hospitals.

EXPERT COMMENT

But Philip Tierno, MD, a professor of microbiology and pathology with the NYU School of Medicine at NYU Langone Medical Center in New York City, suggested that it's important to place the findings in context.

"Germ transmission by hand is certainly a big problem," he said. "And clearly hand washing is very important. But it should be understood that this study did not prove, for example, that the patients picked up their germs in the hospitals they came from. In fact, it's very likely they brought germs with them into the hospital, and still had them when they came out."

Why? "Because it's the 'Wild West' out there," said Dr. Tierno. "Resistant germs are not just in hospitals. They're everywhere."

The two main reasons Dr. Tierno offered: Inappropriate prescribing of antibiotics, and the widespread use of antibiotics in industrial animal feed.

"So, certainly hospitals and care facilities are a hotbed of resistant germs. And yes, what I call 'great hygiene' is very important—meaning washing your hands prior to eating or drinking," he explained.

But if we're going to make any headway against resistant germs, everyone needs to heed that advice, not just patients, he said. "Because resistant germs come from the everyday handling of meat and raw vegetables. From simply picking up flora as you walk through life and interface with people. From touching doorknobs, elevator buttons, and stair rails. These germs come from the world in which we all live," Dr. Tierno said.

Resistance to HIV Drug Growing, Study Finds

University College London, news release.

HIV resistance to the antiretroviral drug *tenofovir* (Viread) is increasingly common, a new study finds.

The researchers said their finding is surprising and alarming because the drug plays a major role in treating and preventing infection with HIV, the virus that causes AIDS.

"Tenofovir is a critical part of our armamentarium against HIV, so it is extremely concerning to see such a high level of resistance to this drug," study author Ravi Gupta, BM, BChir, MPH, from the department of infection and immunity at University College London in England, said in a university news release.

"It is very potent drug with few side effects, and there aren't any good alternatives that can be deployed using a public health approach.

Tenofovir is used not only to treat HIV but also to prevent it in high-risk groups, so we urgently need to do more to combat the problem of emerging resistance," Dr. Gupta said.

Resistance often occurs when patients don't take their drugs as directed. To prevent resistance, people need to take the drugs correctly about 85% to 90% of the time, the researchers said.

STUDY DETAILS

For the study, the investigators looked at more than 1,900 HIV patients worldwide who had uncontrolled HIV despite taking antiretroviral drugs. Tenofovir-resistant HIV strains were found in 60% of patients in sub-Sahara Africa, the researchers found. That compares to just 20% of patients in Europe with tenofovir-resistant strains, the researchers said.

About-two thirds of patients with tenofovir-resistant HIV also had resistance to both other drugs used in their therapy. This suggests that their treatment was totally compromised, the study authors said.

In sub-Sahara Africa, up to 15% of HIV patients treated with tenofovir-based drug combinations will develop resistance to tenofovir in the first year of treatment, and this rate is likely to rise over time, the researchers estimated.

They added that tenofovir-resistant HIV strains could be passed on to other people and become more widespread, potentially weakening global efforts to control HIV.

It's not clear how likely drug-resistant strains of HIV are to spread. If these strains were less effective at spreading, Dr. Gupta said, the researchers should've seen lower levels of the HIV virus in people with the resistant strain. But, that wasn't the case.

"We found that virus levels were no lower in individuals with the resistant strain and were high enough to be fully infectious. We certainly cannot dismiss the possibility that resistant strains can spread between people and should not be complacent. We are now conducting further studies to get a more detailed picture of how tenofovir resistant viruses develop and spread," he concluded.

CHAPTER 14

Longevity and Optimum Aging

How to Live to 100

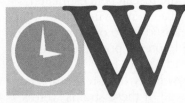

Will you live to 100 and beyond? Certainly genetics is a key factor, but the number of years that you actually accrue—and how healthy you are during those years—often are within your control.

Consider: The number of centenarians—people who live to the ripe old age of 100 or beyond—increased by 51% between 1990 and 2000. The average life expectancy in the US is now 78.8 years, a record high.

Improvements in health care deserve some of the credit, but personal choice is a strong predictor of how long you'll live. About 70% of "normal," age-related declines—including those caused by heart disease, diabetes and other chronic diseases—are mainly due to lifestyle factors.

But which factors are the most important? Not smoking is one. But there are four other lifestyle changes that make the biggest difference when it comes to living a healthier, longer life. They'll also improve your life right now by boosting your mood, energy and cognitive focus.

EXERCISE MORE AS YOU GET OLDER

Some exercise is better than none, but it's a myth that just a little exercise is enough. Walking to the mailbox or enjoying the occasional game of golf isn't enough.

Everyone should exercise hard at least five days a week. Make it six days if you're 50 or older. Tough workouts stress muscles, bones and blood vessels and cause adaptive microtrauma, small injuries that trigger the body's self-repair mechanisms.

Result: Healthier and stronger tissues.

Henry S. Lodge, MD, FACP, an internist and the Robert Burch Family Professor of Medicine at Columbia University Medical Center, New York City. He heads a private practice in New York City and is ranked one of the Best Doctors in America by Castle Connolly. Dr. Lodge is author, with Chris Crowley, of *Younger Next Year* and *Younger Next Year Exercise Program*.

A study that looked at 10,000 middle-aged men over a five-year period found that those who were fittest were three times less likely to die than those who were the least fit. Even more encouraging, men who were largely sedentary at the start of the study but who boosted their exercise levels reduced their mortality by half.

Suppose that you're 30 pounds overweight and a smoker, but you exercise every day. You'll still live longer than someone who is thin and doesn't smoke but does not exercise. (Obviously, you'll do even better if you give up the smokes and lose a few pounds.)

My advice: Lift weights a few days a week, and do serious aerobic exercise four days a week. You can vary your routine with other types of exercise such as yoga. Ideally, you'll exercise for about 60 minutes each time. During the aerobic workouts, keep your heart beating at approximately 60% to 65% of your maximum heart rate—and faster as you get in better shape.

I also advise patients to join a gym, even if they would rather not. Many people think that they'll get all of the exercise that they need by working out "informally"—by using a home treadmill, for example, or by going for runs or bike rides in the neighborhood. But most people don't stick with it.

In my experience, a gym membership is a good investment. Once you've written a check, you're already invested in making it work. Once you make it to the gym, you're going to exercise—and it's more fun to do it with others than alone.

Helpful: Sign up for classes or other group activities such as spin classes, aerobics sessions and Zumba that require you to be there at certain times. Or hire a personal trainer on a regular basis to give you a routine to follow.

GIVE UP WHITE FOODS

Sure, you've heard this before, but it bears repeating because it's crucial to living longer. Give up or strictly limit white potatoes, white rice, white bread and white pasta. Even though "simple" carbohydrates have only about half the calories of fat, they're more likely to cause weight gain because they act like pure sugar in the body. They cause surges in insulin that trig-

ger inflammation and increase the risk for heart disease, diabetes and other chronic diseases.

Important: I don't recommend formal diets for weight loss. Calorie control obviously is important, but strict dieting rarely works. Most people will lose weight just by giving up junk food—and white, starchy foods are junk. Replace junk food with natural foods that haven't been processed or refined such as fruits, vegetables, whole grains, fish, etc.

Studies have shown that eating a Mediterranean-style diet (which actually is high in fat but includes the healthy foods above) is probably ideal for health as well as longevity. For more information on healthier eating, read Dr. Walter Willett's book *Eat, Drink and Be Healthy.*

LOG YOUR LIFE

Can you live longer just by writing down, every day, what you ate and how much you exercised? Surprisingly, the answer is yes.

Even though it's a bit of a hassle, keeping a daily diary of health-related details is a sign that you care. It's also a good form of accountability. You might be less likely to skip a day's exercise or chug down a supersized soft drink when you know that you'll have to confess it (if only to yourself).

The health software that now is standard issue on some smartphones makes it particularly easy to track your habits. The iPhone Health app, for example, automatically counts the number of steps you take and how far you have walked or run. You can use other features to track your weight and what you eat. I also like the apps MapMyRide (for cycling) and MapMyRun (for running).

STAY CONNECTED

People who have close friends and are engaged in their communities tend to live a lot longer than those who are loners. It makes sense because humans, like wolves, evolved as pack animals. We need people around us.

Single men, for example, have higher rates of heart disease and cancer than married men—and they tend to die years sooner. People who go home to an empty house after a heart attack are twice as likely to have a second heart attack within a few months. Those who are angry and

245

isolated have four times the mortality rate of those who are happier.

My advice: Do whatever you can to connect with other people. Make plans with friends even when you would really rather be alone. Get involved in charities and other altruistic activities. Attend religious services. Take advantage of Meetup and other web-based social groups.

Obviously, someone who's naturally solitary will never want to become the life of the party. That's fine because what matters is the aggregate of your social connections. A few truly caring relationships can expand your life (and your life span) just as much as a wide social network.

Also, consider adopting a dog—or a cat, rabbit or bird. The emotional connections that we form with animals can rival, in terms of health benefits, those that we form with fellow humans.

One study, for example, looked at dog ownership in heart attack patients. People who didn't have a dog were six to eight times more likely to die of a second heart attack than those who did.

Not a dog lover? That's OK because any pet that you truly love and care for can offer the same benefits.

Moderate Drinking May Not Lengthen Life, Study Suggests

Tanya Chikritzhs, PhD, professor and director, Alcohol Policy Research team, National Drug Research Institute, Curtin University, Perth, Australia.

R. Curtis Ellison, MD, scientific co-director, International Scientific Forum on Alcohol Research.

Jurgen Rehm, PhD, professor and chair, Addiction Policy, Dalla Lana School of Public Health, University of Toronto, and director, Social and Epidemiological Research department, Center for Addiction and Mental Health, Toronto, Canada.

Journal of Studies on Alcohol and Drugs

Despite previous studies suggesting a bevy of health benefits, a new analysis challenges the idea that drinking alcohol in moderation might prolong your life.

After reviewing nearly 90 previously completed studies, researchers said that moderate drinkers may not have a survival benefit compared to people who don't drink at all.

"So-called 'moderate' drinkers do not live longer than nondrinkers," said review co-author Tanya Chikritzhs, PhD. She is a professor and director of the Alcohol Policy Research team at Australia's National Drug Research Institute.

Not everyone agrees with that conclusion, but some health experts do.

"Scientific data continue to support the premise that small to moderate amounts of alcohol on a regular basis are consistent with a healthy lifestyle for middle-aged and older adults," said R. Curtis Ellison, MD, professor of medicine and public health at Boston University School of Medicine.

Dr. Chikritzhs and her colleagues contend that previous reviews missed an important limitation: People who abstain from drinking often do so because they're ill. As a result, the researchers said, abstainers are more likely to die earlier, a fact that can throw off findings about the influence of alcohol consumption on life span.

REVIEW OF ALCOHOL STUDIES

In the new review, the researchers examined 87 studies and removed those that didn't take into account the fact that abstainers may avoid drinking due to illness. After the study authors "corrected" this issue, Dr. Chikritzhs said, they found no sign of a life span benefit from moderate drinking.

In addition, she said, "among people who drink, it was actually the 'occasional' drinkers—those who drank less than a drink every 10 days or so—who did the best." But, she added, this finding appears to be a statistical fluke because that isn't enough alcohol to influence health.

In addition, she said, "It is becoming clearer that it is much more likely to be the case that being a low or moderate drinker in middle age or older is a marker of good health, not a cause of it."

In the big picture, Dr. Chikritzhs said, "alcohol is a legal substance that many people enjoy, and that's fine. But when it comes to health or thinking of alcohol as some sort of 'medicine,' even low doses are unlikely to prevent death."

And, she said, when you consider its potential for addiction and negative effects when used to excess, "for most folks, when it comes to health, drinking less is better."

EXPERT COMMENTARY

Dr. Ellison said the new review was biased and "does not stand up" to the vast research in this area. "Anytime you have to rely on humans to tell you what they actually drink, there is always the chance that there will be mistakes in their reporting," he said.

Experiments involving people and animals show that "small amounts of an alcoholic beverage, especially wine, are associated with less atherosclerosis [clogged arteries] and coronary heart disease—even in rats, mice and pigeons," he said.

Jurgen Rehm, PhD, professor and chair of Addiction Policy with the University of Toronto's Dalla Lana School of Public Health, agreed that experiments show beneficial effects from alcohol. However, he said, even a single drink can boost some risks, such as that of breast cancer—thus, canceling out the benefit.

"If people drink only one drink a day," he said, "it is a wash. There are much better ways to get health benefits."

info For more about the health effects of alcohol, try the U.S. National Institute on Alcohol Abuse and Alcoholism at *NIAAA.nih. gov.*

Beware Unexpected Causes of Falls

James L. Weiss, MD, professor of cardiology and director of the Heart Station, Johns Hopkins University School of Medicine, Baltimore, reported in *Health After 50.*

Avoid sudden drops in blood pressure... Postprandial hypotension can cause a sudden drop in blood pressure within two hours of eating, resulting in light-headedness that makes older people more likely to fall.

Best: Eat smaller, low-carbohydrate meals and drink lots of water...consume a caffeinated beverage or take a caffeine tablet before meals (caffeine causes blood vessels to constrict and therefore increases blood volume)...limit alcohol consumption...don't stand up suddenly after eating...and don't take antihypertensive drugs right before meals.

Infections Can Make You Fall...

Farrin A. Manian, MD, MPH, core faculty educator, Massachusetts General Hospital, Boston.

Blood, urinary and respiratory infections may cause up to 45% of falls, especially among older adults. A recent study reported that many patients had no (or only vague) symptoms of illness, so their falls instead were blamed on frailty, balance problems and other age-related conditions.

What frequently gets overlooked: Infections may cause weakness and can trigger low blood pressure, leading to dizziness, confusion—and falls.

Eat More Protein, But Do It Right to Avoid Muscle Loss

Douglas Paddon-Jones, PhD, professor, department of nutrition and metabolism, The University of Texas Medical Branch, Galveston.

Are you young at heart? What about "young at body"? We go crazy trying to maintain that goal, but the truth of the matter is that most of us lose 0.5% to 1% of muscle mass per year starting at age 40. So by the time we hit 60, this gradual loss has really added up. Age-related muscle loss increases the risk of falling. It also can cause you to gain or lose too much weight either because of muscle wasting or because you don't have the energy to stay in shape. And not only will you feel old, you'll likely look old. There's an easy way, through diet, to help prevent loss of muscle mass, but there is some controversy about how to do it right.

THE TRUTH ABOUT PROTEIN

As we age, we experience anabolic resistance. This means that the body does not turn the protein we consume into muscle as efficiently as it once did. Researchers at the University of Arkansas for Medical Sciences have come up with a solution. They say to eat a lot of protein—much more than the USDA recommended daily allowance (RDA) of 0.8 grams per two pounds of body weight, which amounts to about 48 grams per day for a 120-pound woman and 68 grams for a 170-pound man. They recommend doubling that amount. These researchers found that it was OK to protein-load at dinner, as most adults do, as opposed to worrying about getting equal amounts of protein at every meal. You'll still reap the benefits of increased protein intake, they said.

They conducted a study in which they divided 20 adults, ages 52 to 75, into four groups. Two groups were assigned a diet that matched the USDA RDA standard, with one group consuming protein in equal portions throughout the day and the other consuming the majority of it at dinner. The other two groups consumed twice the USDA RDA standard, following the same even and uneven protein-distribution patterns.

The results: After just four days, regardless of the distribution of protein, those who consumed the higher amount of it had higher whole-body net protein gains with higher rates of protein synthesis—the ability to turn protein into muscle—compared with those who ate less of it.

EAT PROTEIN RIGHT

But hold off on packing in the protein at dinner. Douglas Paddon-Jones, PhD, professor of nutrition and metabolism at The University of Texas Medical Branch, Galveston, challenges the study findings and says that we should think in terms of maximum protein consumption per

meal and not focus on the total protein consumption per day.

Like most researchers, Dr. Paddon-Jones agrees that increasing protein consumption over the RDA is important when it comes to building and maintaining muscle mass and function, especially for older adults. But protein-loading at dinner or at any meal will not produce the same protein synthesis as eating adequate amounts of protein throughout the day.

Through his research efforts, Dr. Paddon-Jones found that somewhere around 30 grams of protein, which equals about four ounces of lean meat, is close to the maximum amount of protein our bodies can use at one time to build and repair muscle. Although there is no harm and potentially some benefits to consuming additional protein at each meal if your energy demands are high, excess consumption of any macronutrient is increasingly likely to be turned into glucose and eventually fat. Our bodies don't have the temporary storage capacity for excess protein to be used later or the next day in the same way carbohydrates and fat are used.

Between 25 grams and 30 grams of protein is all most of us need per meal.

TREAT MEALS RIGHT

Breakfast is the low hanging fruit when it comes to improving your protein intake per meal because it's the meal that people most often skip or the one that is usually virtually devoid of any protein. Getting at least 25 grams of protein at breakfast might seem daunting to many. Adults should forgo bagels, croissants and sugary cereals and consider eggs (two scrambled equals 14 grams of protein), yogurt (20 grams per seven-ounce container of 2% fat Greek yogurt) and oatmeal (6 grams per one-cup serving of regular cooked, not instant). Add nuts (6 grams per ounce of almonds), whole-wheat toast (7 grams per two slices) and a latte (8 grams per cup of milk) and you'll be up to 25 grams of protein quicker than you can say mocha cappuccino.

On the flip side, while many people skip breakfast, they overeat protein at dinner, often eating a steak the length of their forearm or a chicken breast the size of their face. OK, maybe we are exaggerating just a bit—but you get the picture. Most lean meats have about 30 grams of protein per four-ounce serving. Anything over that amount is probably not doing you a lot of good even if it's the only protein you've eaten all day.

For vegetarians or vegans, soy, legumes, quinoa, nuts and mushrooms are protein-rich foods and all vegetables have some sort of protein in them. Spinach, for example, has five grams per cup.

If you're too busy to get your protein from food at any given meal, protein powders or bars can be an alternative—but read labels carefully. The 20 to 30 grams of protein that come in a serving of whey protein powder, for example, won't do you as much good if the product is laden with sugar and fat.

BUILD MUSCLE THROUGH DIET

As we all know, diet and exercise are both important when it comes to health, regardless of age. But focus first on nutrition in preparation for exercise, because diet is the fundamental to getting the most benefit from fitness routines. Consuming the optimal amount of protein per meal will maximize your body's ability to use that protein efficiently.

Are Your Bones as Healthy as You Think?

Lani Simpson, DC, CCD, a chiropractic doctor and certified clinical (bone) densitometrist specializing in osteoporosis and hormone balancing. She is the author of *Dr. Lani's No-Nonsense Bone Health Guide* and host of the PBS show "Stronger Bones, Longer Life," airing nationally. She also cofounded the Osteoporosis Diagnostic Center in Oakland, California, and has a private practice in Berkeley.

You might think that a bone fracture is a relatively minor health problem. But if you are a woman or a man over age 50, it means that you should get a bone density test if you've never had one before.

An often-overlooked problem: Most primary care doctors are good at reviewing their patients' overall well-being, but bone health is frequently given short shrift. Discussing the strength of your bones—and the possible need for bone density testing—should always be part of your regular checkup.

Remember: Men get osteoporosis (thinning of the bones), too. In fact, complications following hip fracture are a leading cause of death in older women and men.

Mistakes to avoid…

MISTAKE #1: Not discussing bone density testing. Your age will help determine whether you need bone density testing. The National Osteoporosis Foundation recommends it—even in the absence of osteoporosis risk factors—for all women age 65 and older…and all men age 70 and older.

Testing is also advisable for postmenopausal women under age 65, menopausal women and men age 50 to 69 if they have risk factors. There is a long list of risk factors that includes medical conditions such as liver disease, kidney disease, thyroid problems and diabetes…the use of certain medications that can cause bone loss, such as steroids…being Caucasian or Asian…and having a family history of osteoporosis. Frequency of the testing varies—check with your doctor.

Note: I also recommend a baseline test prior to menopause in women who have risk factors.

Good news: Especially for women with risk factors, bone density testing is usually covered by insurance. If your insurer does not cover it, it's a test worth paying for (it usually costs $150 to $250).

MISTAKE #2: Seeing a technician—or radiologist—who isn't properly credentialed. Only some states require bone density technicians to be trained in densitometry (the measurement of bone density), and no states require this training of the physicians who interpret the test results. This lack of professional training is responsible for most testing errors.

What you can do: It's not enough to ask your technician if he/she has been trained—he may say "yes" (and believe it), even though the person who did the "teaching" was not properly trained. When scheduling your test, make sure the doctor who will be interpreting your results is a clinical densitometrist. To find a list of certified clinical densitometrists (CCDs) in your state, check The International Society for Clinical Densitometry's website, *ISCD.org.*

MISTAKE #3: Not being positioned properly during the scan. Bone density is measured with a type of scan that uses technology known as dual-energy X-ray absorptiometry (DXA). For details on the test, see "Bone-Testing Basics" below.

It's an excellent test—when it's performed correctly. One of the most common errors is improper positioning when checking the bone density of the hip. During this part of the test, your technician should use a small device that fits between your feet to cause a 15- to 20-degree internal hip rotation.

In that position, the neck of the femur measures at its lowest bone density level…any other positioning could falsely inflate your score by up to 10%—an amount that can be the difference between whether or not a doctor diagnoses a troubling level of bone loss.

What you can do: Prior to your DXA, discuss the proper positioning with your doctor. When you are at the test, you can say to the technician, "My doctor really stressed to me the importance of getting the proper hip rotation." That will alert your technician that you know about this element of the test…and encourage him to do it correctly.

If you're not sure whether the device was used with earlier testing, ask the technician to check your previous scan so that he can make sure your hip is rotated to the same degree it was previously.

MISTAKE #4: Skipping important lab tests. Your DXA results are only one piece of your bone health puzzle. Laboratory tests are just as essential in forming a complete picture of your bone health. When it comes to diagnosing and treating osteoporosis, lab tests are mainly used to rule out potential secondary causes, such as low vitamin D levels, thyroid or parathyroid problems, or digestive disorders.

However, it's also critical that your doctor assess your sex hormone levels, which have a direct impact on your bone health. For women, perimenopause- and menopause-induced low estrogen can cause a 1% to 3% loss of bone mass annually for five to 10 years. In men, hypo-

Extra Calcium May Not Protect Aging Bones

Current guidelines recommend that people over age 50 consume at least 1,000 milligrams (mg) to 1,200 mg of calcium a day.

But: Recent research found no proof that boosting calcium intake strengthens older bones or prevents fractures. Moreover, excess calcium supplementation raises risk for constipation, kidney stones and possibly heart attack.

Meta-analysis of more than 100 investigations of calcium supplements by researchers at University of Auckland, New Zealand, published in *BMJ.*

gonadism (low testosterone) is a leading cause of osteoporosis.

What you can do: In addition to a complete blood count (that includes white and red blood cell counts) and a comprehensive metabolic panel (that checks kidney and liver function and electrolyte levels, etc.), ask for a vitamin D test and a thyroid stimulating hormone (TSH) test. Vitamin D increases calcium absorption by 50%, so you need adequate levels to maintain healthy bone. Untreated thyroid disease can result in bone loss.

Depending on your personal history, your doctor may also want tests to measure your calcium, phosphorus and magnesium levels…parathyroid functioning…cortisol levels…and more.

BONE-TESTING BASICS

A dual-energy X-ray absorptiometry (DXA) scan is simple, painless, requires no injections and exposes you to very little radiation (a small fraction of that used for a chest X-ray).

What happens: While lying on your back in your clothes, with your arms at your sides, you'll be asked to hold your breath and not move for a few seconds while the machine passes over you. The complete test takes about 20 minutes.

Important: You should avoid taking calcium supplements for 24 hours before the test—an undigested pill could lodge in an area and falsely bolster your results.

Calcium Linked to Vision Loss

Caitlin Kakigi, BA, medical student, department of ophthalmology, University of California, San Francisco, and coauthor of a study of 3,191 national health survey participants, published in *JAMA Ophthalmology*.

Taking more than 800 mg/day of calcium was associated with nearly twice the risk of being diagnosed with age-related macular degeneration (AMD), which can cause severe vision loss.

Important: Calcium has important benefits for many medical conditions, including osteoporosis and high blood pressure. Do not reduce or discontinue use of calcium supplements without speaking to your doctor.

High-Dose Statins May Ease Macular Degeneration for Some

Mark Fromer, MD, ophthalmologist, Lenox Hill Hospital, New York City.

Nazanin Barzideh, MD, chief, vitreoretinal surgery, division of ophthalmology, Winthrop-University Hospital, Mineola, New York.

Massachusetts Eye and Ear Infirmary, news release.

High doses of cholesterol-lowering statin drugs—medicines such as Lipitor, Crestor and Zocor—may help people with a common eye disease called macular degeneration, a small study suggests.

In the early stage clinical trial, a team from Harvard Medical School assessed the effects of statin treatment in people with the dry form of age-related macular degeneration (AMD).

AMD affects more than 150 million people worldwide. The dry form is much more common and accounts for about 85% of cases, according to the researchers.

Effective treatments are available for the wet form of AMD, but not the dry form, so dry-form AMD remains the leading cause of blindness in the developed world.

In AMD, fat deposits form under the retina, so that patients develop blurring or blindness in the center of their vision.

STUDY DETAILS

In the study, 23 patients with dry-form AMD were given a high dose (80 milligrams) of *atorvastatin* (Lipitor).

In 10 of the patients, the fat deposits under the retina disappeared and they had a slight improvement in vision clarity, according to the study published online in the *Journal EBioMedicine*.

It typically took a year to 18 months of treatment for these positive results to arise, the researchers reported.

They noted that prior attempts to find ways to eliminate the fat deposits under the retina have failed.

However, "we found that intensive doses of statins carry the potential for clearing up the lipid [fat] debris that can lead to vision impairment in a subset of patients with macular degeneration," said study co-author Joan Miller, MD. She is chair of ophthalmology at Harvard Medical School and chief of ophthalmology at Massachusetts Eye and Ear Infirmary and Massachusetts General Hospital, both in Boston.

STUDY IMPLICATIONS

"We hope that this promising preliminary clinical trial will be the foundation for an effective treatment for millions of patients afflicted with AMD," she said in an infirmary news release.

Study co-author Demetrios Vavvas, MD, PhD, clinician scientist at Massachusetts Eye and Ear Infirmary, said in the news release, "Not all cases of dry AMD are the exactly the same, and our findings suggest that if statins are going to help, they will be most effective when prescribed at high dosages in patients with an accumulation of soft, lipid material."

However, he believes that, based on the new findings, "it may be possible to eventually have a treatment that not only arrests the disease but also reverses its damage and improves the visual acuity in some patients."

The next step is to conduct a larger study of statin treatment in patients with dry AMD.

"This is a very accessible, FDA-approved drug that we have tremendous experience with," Dr. Vavvas said. "Millions of patients take it for high cholesterol and heart disease, and based on our early results, we believe it offers the potential to halt progression of this disease, but possibly even to restore function in some patients with dry AMD."

EXPERT REACTION

Two eye experts were cautiously optimistic about the new findings.

"Although the study is relatively small, the positive outcomes certainly warrant a larger clinical trial," said Mark Fromer, MD, an ophthalmologist at Lenox Hill Hospital in New York City. "This may benefit millions of patients with macular degeneration and slow their progression to more serious disease."

Nazanin Barzideh, MD, chief of vitreoretinal surgery at Winthrop-University Hospital in Mineola, New York, called the research "exciting," and noted that heart disease treatments have long shown some secondary effects in easing AMD.

info The U.S. National Eye Institute has more about age-related macular degeneration at *NEI.nih.gov/health/maculardegen.*

Eat Your Vitamin C!

Christopher Hammond, MD, is Frost Chair of Ophthalmology at King's College London, UK, and leader of a study of 2,054 twins, published online in *Ophthalmology.*

Vitamin C may reduce cataract risk, we hear from Christopher Hammond, MD. But the vitamin is most protective when it comes from food—not supplements.

Recent finding: Study participants with a higher dietary intake of vitamin C had one-third lower risk for cataracts than people who consumed the least vitamin C. Those who took vitamin C supplements showed no significant risk reduction.

Spinach Improves Sight

Juan (Joanne) Wu, MS, doctoral candidate in nutrition epidemiology, department of nutrition, Harvard T.H. Chan School of Public Health, Boston, and leader of a study of more than 102,000 people, published in *JAMA Ophthalmology.*

People who consumed the highest levels of the carotenoids lutein and zeaxanthin, present in dark, leafy greens and other vegetables and fruits, had a 40% lower likelihood of advanced age-related macular degeneration (AMD) than those who ate the very lowest amounts.

Study participants with the highest levels of lutein and zeaxanthin consumed six or more daily servings of fruits and vegetables. The foods richest in lutein and zeaxanthin include cooked spinach, kale, collards and turnip greens. [*Editor's note*: Eat no more than one cup a day because oxalate-rich foods such as spinach are linked to kidney stones.]

You Don't Have to Give Up Those Car Keys

Patrick Baker, an occupational therapist, certified low-vision therapist and certified driver-rehabilitation specialist at the Cleveland Clinic in Cleveland, Ohio.

Driving may be the most hazardous thing that most of us do each day, but simply growing older—or having a chronic medical condition, no matter what your age, that affects your vision, thought process or physical abilities—doesn't mean that you can't continue to be independent.

To drive safely as long as possible: It's crucial to proactively avoid problems that can limit your car-handling competence. *Here's how…*

PREEMPT PROBLEMS

Beyond commonsense imperatives such as getting regular medical, vision and hearing checkups, a few simple steps will help ensure that your driving abilities are intact.

At your checkup with your primary care doctor, have a candid talk to discuss any medical conditions you may have that could affect your driving now or in the future.

For example, a stroke may result in lingering visual or movement problems...diabetes might be causing neuropathy in your feet, making it difficult to feel the gas or brake pedals...and cataracts, macular degeneration or glaucoma may limit vision if it's not carefully treated. A conversation with your doctor can help you minimize these issues and prevent them from becoming a bigger problem down the road. *Also...*

MANAGE YOUR MEDS

Some prescription or over-the-counter medications can impair your ability to drive by triggering drowsiness, cutting concentration, inducing shakiness or uncoordinated movements, or increasing your reaction time. Taking multiple drugs—a common practice among older adults and those coping with chronic medical problems—can make matters even worse by amplifying medication side effects. Certain dietary supplements, such as melatonin or valerian, may also have an effect.

What to find out: Show your doctor or pharmacist a list of all the medications (prescription and over-the-counter) and dietary supplements you take and ask how they interact and may affect your driving abilities.

Also: Ask if the timing of when you take any drugs or supplements that may affect cognition or coordination can be altered—for example, taken before bedtime instead of in the morning.

Important: If you are on painkillers or narcotics, also ask your spouse or a trusted friend if the medication makes you "loopy"—an effect that you may not notice but is perhaps obvious to another person.

CUSTOMIZE YOUR CAR

Age can compromise your eyesight and bring physical changes that make it more difficult to see the road while driving—for example, many people lose one to three inches of height due to bone loss and spinal compression. Or a stroke or eye condition (such as cataracts) may affect your peripheral vision, interfering with your ability to spot traffic alongside your car. To address these changes, it helps to customize your car. *Here's how...*

•**Set power seats at the highest level.** Also, consider adding a firm cushion (such as the durable type used for outdoor furniture) to the driver's seat so that your chin is at least three inches higher than the top of the steering wheel.

•**Use extra (or bigger) mirrors inside and/or outside your car to increase your field of vision.** For example, you can get a mirror that attaches to your rearview mirror to expand your view to the rear. Or you can get bigger mirrors or extra mirrors that can be bolted onto existing side mirrors or the side of the car itself. Check with your car dealer for details for your make and model.

•**Keep your headlights clean.** Also, consider replacing the bulbs—even before they burn out. The bulbs get dimmer before they've completely burned out.

•**Opt for automatic.** If you're buying a new car, be sure to get one with automatic transmission, power steering and power brakes, which don't require as much strength to operate. Also, consider a car with backup alert sensors, which detect objects in your blind spots.

SPRUCE UP YOUR SKILLS

A driving refresher course (ideally taken every three to five years) will keep you up to date on the newest traffic rules and can reduce road mishaps.

Good news: Some car insurance companies even lower premium rates if you take one of these courses, which usually lasts four to eight hours.

Good choice: A course such as those offered by AAA or AARP is likely to have an instructor who is well versed in issues facing older adults—as well as classmates who are true peers. If you are interested in taking a driver course because of a medical condition, consult The Association for Driver Rehabilitation Specialists (*ADED.net* and search "CDRS provider") to find a program near you.

FOCUS ON FOOTWEAR

When it comes to hitting the gas and brake, what's on our feet can be just as important as our ability to see and react. *Consider these important footwear-related issues...*

253

• **Choose the right sneaker.** Running-style sneakers with soles that are thick, chunky and/ or beveled can catch on pedals as you move your foot, so opt for a flat sole, such as a tennis-style or walking sneaker.

• **Go for thin soles.** People with diabetic neuropathy or limited foot sensation should wear thinner-soled shoes while driving. Thin soles, which don't have much padding between the bottom of the feet and the car pedals, give you a better sense of how hard you are pushing the brake and accelerator.

Important: Be sure to choose a car that "fits" you well—with good sight lines to the sides and rear...controls that are easy to reach...and a model that is easy for you to get in and out of.

Hearing: The Crucial Test Missing from Most Checkups

Katherine Bouton, author of *Living Better with Hearing Loss: A Guide to Health, Happiness, Love, Sex, Work, Friends...and Hearing Aids* as well as *Shouting Won't Help.* She is a member of the board of trustees of the Hearing Loss Association of America, HearingLoss.org, and has had progressive bilateral hearing loss since she was 30.

I f you get an annual checkup, you probably assume that you're doing everything you need to do to take good care of your health. But chances are your physicals have not included a test that's crucial to your physical and mental well-being.

Shocking fact: Only about 30% of primary care physicians do a basic screening of their patients' hearing. In fact, most adults haven't had their hearing tested since they were in grade school! For most people with hearing loss, this means their problem (or the severity of their deficiency) goes undetected.

And don't assume that only the oldest adults are affected. More than half of the 48 million Americans who have trouble hearing are under age 55, and most of them aren't getting treatment.

Ignoring hearing loss is dangerous: In addition to the social isolation and depression that sometimes occur when people have trouble hearing, the condition has been linked to an increased risk for dementia. While there is more research to be done, many neuroscientists believe that if you are working hard to comprehend what's being said, you are using up the brain's stores of "cognitive reserve," which would instead be devoted to analytical thinking or memory.

That's not all. Because most age-related hearing loss occurs in the inner ear, which regulates balance, ignoring the problem increases one's risk of falling by threefold. Hearing loss also makes driving and walking on the streets less safe because you don't hear car horns and other traffic noises.

My story: My hearing loss began suddenly when I was 30. Like many people, I resisted getting help and didn't get hearing aids for 20 years. That was a mistake!

KEEPING IT SIMPLE

Testing for hearing loss is painless and easy. *My advice...*

• **Start now!** No matter what your age, ask your primary care physician to do a hearing screening during your annual physical. Professional guidelines vary on the frequency for such testing, but I believe that it's important enough to get screened every year—subtle changes can easily go unnoticed if you wait too long between testing.

As an initial screening, your primary care doctor will likely ask you a series of questions such as: "Does your spouse complain that the TV is too loud?" and "Do you find that people often say, 'Oh, never mind. It's not important.'?" The doctor may also snap his/her fingers behind your head or rub his fingers together next to your ear. If you seem to be having trouble hearing, he'll refer you to an audiologist for diagnostic testing. (An otolaryngologist, or ear, nose and throat specialist, may also employ an audiologist who gives hearing tests.)

• **Go to a true professional.** Try to stick to your doctor's referral. Lots of hearing-aid shops employ people who may not have adequate training to accurately diagnose hearing loss. You want to be sure to see an audiologist. They're trained to diagnose, manage and treat hearing and/or balance problems. An audiologist can also fit you with hearing aids.

THE BEST TESTING

When you go to an audiologist, you'll be asked about your general health history, work history, exposure to noise and use of certain medications—drugs such as nonsteroidal anti-inflammatory drugs (NSAIDs), certain antibiotics and loop diuretics (commonly used to treat heart failure) can cause temporary hearing loss...and repeated doses of other drugs, including the cancer drug *cisplatin* (Platinol), can cause permanent hearing loss. *The audiologist will then take you to a soundproof room for the following tests...*

•**Pure-tone test.** This test provides a baseline of the softest level at which you can hear sounds.

What happens: You put on headphones, and the audiologist activates tones at different pitches and loudness. You respond by raising a finger or pressing a button when the tone is heard. The test is given in one ear at a time. If the test is normal, the audiologist will probably send you home. If not, other tests follow.

•**Bone-conduction test.** This test helps identify whether hearing loss originates from the inner, middle or outer ear.

What happens: You will be fit with a headset that has a vibrator placed on the bone behind the ear. This bypasses the ear canal (outer and middle ear) and sends vibrations directly to the cochlea (inner ear). Again, the audiologist will activate tones at different intervals.

If the result is normal or better than the pure-tone test, it suggests the problem is in the middle or outer ear—sound is not getting through to the cochlea. If the result is worse than the pure-tone test, it points to a problem in the cochlea.

•**Speech perception test.**

What happens: While hiding his mouth (so there's no cheating by lipreading), the audiologist reads a list of common two-syllable words (or a recording is played) to determine the lowest level at which you can correctly identify 50% of the words spoken. If you cannot hear 50% of the sounds, the volume is turned up until you can. The test is given in quiet or with noisy background sounds. It helps to determine the extent of hearing loss and the need for a hearing aid.

•**Tympanometry test.** This test helps detect problems in the middle ear. It can reveal tumors, fluid buildup, impacted earwax or a perforated eardrum—all of which can lead to hearing loss.

What happens: The audiologist uses a probe that changes the air pressure in the ear canal and causes a healthy eardrum to easily move back and forth.

Important: While you're being tested, stay still and do not speak or swallow to make sure your results are accurate.

WHAT'S NEXT?

If your audiologist recommends hearing aids, don't panic. Unlike the bulky devices you may have seen in the past, today's hearing aids are comfortable, highly effective—and most are small enough to not be seen when looking at the wearer's face. But they are also expensive—up to $4,000 per aid—and are not covered by insurance.

For people with mild-to-moderate hearing loss, personal sound amplification products (PSAPs) are a less expensive option (up to $700 a pair). They help in specific situations, such as a noisy restaurant, crowded airport or large lecture hall.

Ear Implant Helps More Than Hearing

Study led by researchers at Assistance Publique-Hôpitaux de Paris, France, published in *JAMA Otolaryngology–Head & Neck Surgery*.

Cochlear implants help more than hearing. A cochlear implant is a small electronic device that boosts hearing in someone who is deaf or severely hard of hearing. Seniors with the implants reported better quality of life, lower rates of depression and improved thinking skills. The number of patients free of depression was 59% before receiving a cochlear implant and 76% one year after receiving the device.

Decline in Senses Affects Nearly All Seniors

University of Chicago Medical Center, news release

Nearly all older US adults have an age-related decline in at least one of their senses, a recent study finds.

Researchers checked more than 3,000 people between the ages of 57 and 85. The investigators found that 94% had a problem with at least one of their five senses: taste, smell, hearing, sight or touch.

Almost 40% had problems with two senses, and 28% had problems with three or more of their senses, the study found.

"We know that sensory impairment is common and is often a harbinger of serious health problems, such as cognitive [mental] decline or falls, as well as more subtle ones like burns, caused by loss of touch sensitivity, food poisoning that goes undetected because of loss of smell and taste, and smoke inhalation, from loss of smell," said study author Jayant Pinto, MD.

"Our findings here give us a better appreciation of the prevalence of multi-sensory loss, a first step toward learning more about what causes the senses to decline," Dr. Pinto, an associate professor of surgery at the University of Chicago, said in a university news release.

The most common problem was a decrease in the sense of taste. Nearly three-quarters of those in the study had a decline in taste. For about one-quarter of the study volunteers, their sense of taste was rated only fair, and for almost half, it was poor.

Declines in the sense of touch were also common. The researchers found that 38% of the study participants had only a fair sense of touch, while 32% had a poor sense of touch.

About 64% of the study group had a major decline in at least one sense, and 22% had major declines in two or more senses, according to the study.

Decreases in numerous senses were strongly associated with age, gender and race, the study authors reported in the *Journal of the American Geriatrics Society.*

As expected, the oldest people had the most sensory deficits. Men tended to have worse hearing, smell and taste problems, but better vision than women. Blacks scored lower than other races on all senses, except hearing. Hispanics had worse vision, touch and smell, but their sense of taste was better, the study findings indicated.

Possible causes of age-related declines in the senses include nerve degeneration, environmental factors or genetic susceptibility, the researchers suggested.

"We need to understand the biology behind the links between age and sensory loss, and design better ways to prevent its decline," Dr. Pinto said. "People caring for older adults—including family members, caregivers and physicians—should pay close attention to impairments in vision, hearing, and smell."

info The U.S. National Institute on Aging offers healthy aging advice at *nihsenior health.gov.*

Voice Problems with Age

Susan A. Eicher, MD, associate professor of otolaryngology, Baylor College of Medicine, Houston.

As we age, our muscles and other soft tissues atrophy to some degree, including those in our vocal cords and throat. Older adults may experience a reduction in vocal pitch, volume and endurance. In addition, mucous membranes in the throat thin and dry out during the aging process, which can result in hoarseness.

Talk to your doctor about ways to ease these age-related changes, such as drinking plenty of water (half your body weight in fluid ounces) each day and avoiding alcohol and caffeine. Many medications, such as some blood pressure drugs and antihistamines, can also cause dehydration.

What helps: You can strengthen your voice by reading or singing out loud for 10 or 15 minutes two or three times a day. You may also want to consult a speech-language pathologist, who can devise a program of vocal exercises to specifically address your concerns.

But keep in mind that changes in your voice can also be caused by many medical conditions, including gastroesophageal reflux disease (GERD), allergies, upper-respiratory infection, and in some cases, cancer or Parkinson's disease. If your vocal changes are accompanied by other symptoms, such as pain, coughing up blood, difficulty swallowing, a lump in the neck or hoarseness (possible signs of cancer or other conditions) lasting longer than three weeks, consult an otolaryngologist.

Sounding "Old" Is Not Always About Age

Study titled "Voice Changes in Elderly Adults: Prevalence and the Effect of Social, Behavioral, and Health Status on Voice Quality" National Cancer Center, Gyeonggi, and University of Ulsan, Seoul, both in South Korea, published in *Journal of the American Geriatric Society*.

If you read Little Red Riding Hood aloud to a child, you probably make Grandma's voice weak and quavering to sound "old." But the truth is you can have a strong voice at any age—unless you have a specific health problem...one that affects your whole health, not just your vocal chords.

In a recent study of 420 seniors (average age 72) with dysphonia, the medical term for decreased ability to produce a normal voice, South Korean researchers found that, compared to statistical averages, they were 300% more likely to have a particular medical condition—low thyroid function.

The condition, called hypothyroidism, is easy to overlook because many of the symptoms—constipation, fatigue and sensitivity to cold—are also symptoms associated with aging. While the new study doesn't prove causation, it does

suggest that in an otherwise apparently healthy 60-plus person, a weakening voice could be a clue—perhaps the only clue—to this health-compromising condition.

So if you have a "grandmotherly" or "grandfatherly" voice or know someone who does, speak up—to a doctor. Ask him or her to test your thyroid function.

Headstand for Health?

Rammohan Rao, PhD, associate research professor, Buck Institute for Research on Aging, Novato, California.

A headstand, or the sirsasana pose as it is known in yoga, can provide many health benefits, such as improved muscle strength, circulation and balance. Performing a headstand requires upper-body and abdominal strength, so overall physical fitness is important when trying to master this pose. Older adults can get the same benefits by taking brisk walks, swimming or doing other forms of exercise every day. Even working out as little as one hour a week can cut dementia risk, recent research has found. If you want to do headstands, check with your doctor first. They should not be done by anyone with neck or back problems, osteoporosis, high blood pressure or glaucoma.

Surprise! Retirement Is Good for Your Health

Paper titled "Does Retirement Improve Health and Life Satisfaction?" by Aspen Gorry, PhD, Utah State University, Devon Gorry, PhD, Utah State University, and Sita Slavov, PhD, George Mason University, published in *National Bureau of Economic Research*.
Study titled "Retirement—A Transition to a Healthier Lifestyle? Evidence From a Large Australian Study" by researchers at University of Sydney, Australia, published in *American Journal of Preventive Medicine*.

For years, we've heard dismal statistics about retirement and health. Keep working as long as you can, we're told, because people who retire tend to see their health status plummet in the years to follow. The purported increased risks included poor heart health and increased risk for depression.

Fortunately, we now know that for most people, the opposite is true. People who retire tend to be healthier—and happier—after they take the plunge.

Why did earlier studies get it so wrong? One reason is that many lumped data from all retirees together. Some people have to retire because of failing health, so not accounting for this fact made it seem that retirees overall were less healthy than their peers who continued to work. Once the less-healthy must-retire folks were not driving the results, a rosier picture emerged.

When researchers from the National Bureau of Economic Research, for example, analyzed data on around 6,000 Americans over age 50, they found that health status got better after retirement for those who retired simply because they became eligible for Social Security or pension benefits. Since many people, even those in good health, retire when they become eligible for benefits, they were able to measure the impact of retiring for reasons unrelated to health. Even more promising—health status continued to improve, so it was better four years later compared to the first year of retirement.

Life satisfaction improved, too.

A TIME TO GET HEALTHIER

A new Australian study sheds light on how retirement may improve health. Researchers followed 27,000 Australians over age 45, tracking their lifestyle habits over about three years, during which time about 11% retired. *Compared to those who kept working, the retirees…*

• **Got about 52 minutes more physical activity a week.**

• **Spent about 40 minutes less in sedentary pursuits.**

• **Slept about 15 minutes more a night.**

These stats include everyone who retired. But when the researchers looked closer, they found that those who retired for health reasons still improved their health habits a bit—but not nearly as robustly as those whose health was not the prime reason for quitting work.

IF YOU CAN AFFORD TO RETIRE, WHY WAIT?

Some people love working and never want to quit. Others think they'll love retirement but end up finding themselves bored stiff—or lonely and depressed. Some take to drink. In short, just quitting work won't make you healthier and happier, and it's not the best choice for everyone—even if you can afford it.

But the new research does suggest that retiring when you can best enjoy the time will likely lead to a healthier and happier time of your life.

To paraphrase the old song, it's nice not-work if you can get it.

Dating: The Fun Way to Boost Your Health

Judith Sills, PhD, a Philadelphia-based clinical psychologist. A three-year National Science Foundation fellow, she is a contributing editor at *Psychology Today*. She is also the author of *Getting Naked Again: Dating, Romance, Sex, and Love When You've Been Divorced, Widowed, Dumped, or Distracted*.

If you're not in a committed relationship, maybe it's time to consider dating again. And if you're age 50 or older—the point at which most of us become much more focused on staying healthy—then it's an especially good time to give dating a chance.

While the prospect of dating as a mature adult can seem overwhelming or downright scary, here's some compelling motivation—the latest research indicates that being in a relationship can improve your health in a variety of ways.

And take heart: There are specific tips for daters who are 50+ that can make getting out there again much easier.

HEALTH BENEFITS GALORE

Plenty of singles age 50 or older say they don't need a relationship to be happy. But those who are in committed relationships seem to have significant health advantages over those who fly solo.

Case in point: An analysis of data from more than 300,000 adults found that those without strong relationships were 50% more likely to die from all causes over a seven-year period—a risk that's the equivalent to daily smoking! Additionally, men and women who live alone and have a heart attack are twice as likely to have a second heart attack within a few months.

The list goes on. Married people are less likely to get pneumonia than singles, and those who are married or live together in midlife are less likely to develop dementia.

HOW TO GET BACK OUT THERE

If you have been out of the single world for a long time, you might not be sure that you want to get back in the dating game.

But one thing is certain: Humans have a deep need for intimacy and companionship.

And while some people are perfectly satisfied with their close friends and family, a healthy committed relationship generally offers a greater level of stability and support. After all, if your best friend moved to a different state, you wouldn't follow that person, but you likely would if it were your partner.

The advantage of later-life dating is that you've been through it all before. And you probably have some idea of what you're looking for. Also, while you may be a bit insecure in how you look as you age, you may have more confidence in your personality and social skills.

Advice for dating after age 50…

•**Get online.** The Internet is a fantastic way to meet people. The number of potential partners vastly exceeds those you'll meet any other way. If you're willing to put in the time—writing an interesting profile, putting up an attractive photo and wading through the possibilities—you will get dates. (They won't all be fabulous, but many will be fun and you'll start to meet people.)

There are hundreds of dating websites to choose from. The most popular sites, such as Match ($35/one month) and eHarmony ($59.95/one month), have the most members (and potential partners), but they tend to attract younger users.

Helpful: Try sites that target older adults, such as OurTime ($20/one month) or Senior-

PeopleMeet ($20/one month). Monthly prices are lower if you sign up for a longer time. Plenty of Fish is a free dating site for all age groups.

•**Don't waste time.** A survey by the Pew Research Center found that one-third of those who connect online never take the next step and meet face-to-face. Unless your only goal is Internet flirting, pin down a time to meet. You don't want to rush it, of course, but don't wait too long. If you like the person after exchanging three or four e-mails, it's time for a phone call or a meeting (in a low-key public place like a coffee shop). If someone you're interested in doesn't ask you out first, take the plunge and do it yourself.

•**Set aside your preconceptions.** Dating sites have analyzed what their members want—or think they want. Women, for example, tend to respond to men of certain ages, or with particular jobs or education levels. Men tend to reach out to women who are blond. Give other types of people a chance!

•**Give yourself (and your date) some slack.** When dating, you will no doubt have some anxious and awkward moments. What do you do when every attempt at conversation withers and dies? Or when your date doesn't laugh at any of your jokes? Give yourself and your companion a break. First dates are hard, but it does get easier with practice.

Helpful: Forget the traditional dinner date. It's too much for a first meeting, particularly if the chemistry isn't there—or when you discover between the first and second courses that you do not seem to have a whole lot in common. Meeting for coffee, a drink or lunch is easier and less expensive—and you can quickly cut your losses when it just isn't clicking.

•**Keep your insecurities in check.** No, you're not the same person you were 30 years ago. You might have a few extra pounds or a little less hair. Just don't let the nagging negative voice in your head—"I'm not good enough"… "She is way out of my league"…or "What if he doesn't ask me out again"—ruin what could be a perfectly pleasant time.

Your date saw something in you before you met. Relax and enjoy yourself. Besides, everyone is insecure on first dates. The person sitting across from you is probably having his/her own insecure thoughts.

•It's not a job interview. An unfortunate first-date strategy is to ask a lot of questions. Granted, asking questions and showing interest will keep the conversation going. But it can also be intimidating—or simply off-putting.

Some women tell me that they "interview" potential partners to save time. They ask things like, "Are you looking for something serious?" "Do you own or rent?" "What kind of relationship do you have with your ex?" Men do their own interviewing but tend to take their cue from the workplace, posing questions such as, "So tell me…where would you like to be in five years?" None of this is friendly give-and-take—it feels more like interrogation.

My advice: Be a little less efficient. A date is a chance to get to know someone…to reveal a little about yourself…and have some fun. Keep it light.

•Aim for a full stomach. Think it's time to take a new relationship to the next level? A dinner date with great food could be the best way to do it. There may be some truth to the old cliché—the way to a man's (or woman's) heart is through the stomach. A study in the journal *Appetite* found that women who were shown romantic pictures after they'd eaten had more brain activation than women who looked at the same pictures on an empty stomach!

Easy Ways to Memory Fitness

Janina Krell-Roesch, PhD, is a research fellow in the Translational Neuroscience and Aging Program, Mayo Clinic, Scottsdale, Arizona.

Seniors who used computers at least once a week had a 42% decreased risk for onset of mild cognitive impairment (MCI) over a four-year period, reports Janina Krell-Roesch, PhD. Other mentally stimulating activities that reduced risk for MCI included magazine reading, 30%…participating in social activities, 23%…doing crafts, 16%…and playing games such as cards, 14%.

Could Dementia Villages Come to the US?

Dayne DuVall, LMT, CAEd, CRTS, certified Alzheimer educator and chief operating officer, National Certification Board for Alzheimer Care, Chicago.

Amazing things happen when people with dementia have the freedom to do things they enjoy, in familiar environments, surrounded by people who watch out for them and help them feel accepted.

In the Netherlands, a dementia village has become an international model of what can happen when people with dementia are given extraordinary freedom in a safe, structured environment. Meanwhile, in England and now in the US, many communities are exploring ways to become dementia-friendly so that people at earlier stages of memory-robbing conditions can remain actively involved in social and cultural activities.

Contrast that to what typically happens: We care for loved ones at home for as long as possible, and then the alternative is often an assisted-living facility or a nursing home. But when loved ones get there, they are often isolated, lonely, scared and oversedated—all of which accelerates their cognitive and physical decline. Assisted-living facilities are now what nursing homes used to be, and nursing homes are really hospitals.

There are better ways. *Here are some of them that you can take advantage of or adapt to your loved one's particular needs…*

A NEW MODEL: A VILLAGE BUILT FOR PEOPLE WITH DEMENTIA

Imagine an environment where someone with dementia can leave his house and take a walk whenever he wants, shop, take in a movie and eat with neighbors in a family-style dining room. The town looks like the kind of place he may have once lived in.

That's the experience in Hogewey in the Netherlands, a residential facility outside Amsterdam where elderly people with dementia live in a seemingly normal community, complete with parks, a grocery store, a restaurant, a theatre, post office, barbershop and other amenities. The residents are generally people with "moderate-stage" dementia.

Although they are restricted to the facility's grounds, the 152 residents are free to roam around the community, which has on-site geriatric nurses and caregivers dressed in street clothes who provide around-the-clock care. The residents live in groups of six to eight to a home, with one or two caretakers on site. Residents also manage their own homes, including cooking, cleaning and laundry—with some help. For safety's sake, cameras monitor the residents 24/7, and there's only one door in and out of "town," so there's little risk that residents will wander off the premises.

To some, it's a little disquieting to have a community where residents are essentially deceived into believing that they are living in a normal community—a real-life version of The Truman Show, as it were. But the benefits are that residents can maintain social engagement and much more independence. "There has to be some oversight—somebody has to be monitoring what's going on," says DuVall. "To me, the simulation connotes safety."

The benefits are many. Research shows that putting people with dementia into environments that mimic their familiar, formative experiences helps them cope better. So Hogeway mimics traditional towns from 50 or so years ago. There are even living clusters for different lifestyles such as urban, homemaker, trade/craft, upper class…and Indonesian.

According to CNN's chief medical correspondent Sanjay Gupta, MD, whose reporting helped create international interest in the Hogewey model, the residents take fewer medications and eat better than others of the same age and condition—and live longer, too. "On a mental level, they also seem to have more joy," he reported. "It's a difficult thing to measure, but that is the most important thing here at Hogewey."

WHAT WE CAN LEARN FROM HOGEWEY

The Hogewey model has inspired international interest. There are dementia villages being planned in Switzerland, England and Canada—and in Florida, where the Miami Jewish Health Systems is actively planning a Hogeway-like expansion of their dementia care facilities called EmpathiCare.

There are obstacles to widespread adoption of the model here, however. The primary one is cost. It's very expensive. In the Netherlands, Hogewey is heavily subsidized by the government, which covered almost all of the nearly $25 million dollars it cost to build and subsidizes operating expenses, too. Even then, the families of residents need to pay as much as $3,600 a month. In the US, a dementia village on that scale may be affordable only for the rich.

But sometimes, great ideas create change in surprising ways. The example of a more humane way to treat people with dementia, one that gives them more freedom and dignity than was thought possible, is inspiring. And it's just one example…many communities in the US are striving to find better ways to provide care. There may be elements of the Hogewey model—environments that mimic an earlier time, professionally staffed movie theaters that look like the real thing—that assisted-living facilities may adopt.

We can also change our communities so that it is easier for people with dementia to stay in their own homes longer, while remaining socially active. All over the US, people with early-stage dementia, who are largely still aware and functioning, are establishing "memory cafes" where they can come together to socialize and share resources. Entire states are trying to figure out how they can be "dementia-friendly"—safer and more accepting of residents with memory impairments.

Whether we build entirely new communities, or work to make our existing communities embrace people with dementia, the concept is the same—people with memory-robbing diseases who can stay social, engaged in meaningful activities and treated with respect, live better lives until the very end.

Sleep in Retirement Out of Whack...

Michael Breus, PhD, a sleep specialist in private practice in Los Angeles. He is the author of *Good Night: The Sleep Doctor's 4-Week Program to Better Sleep and Better Health.* TheSleepDoctor.com

It's very common for people to get "off schedule" when they begin retirement, but this can have some significant effects on their quality of sleep and overall health. So it's good to pay attention if you feel "out of whack."

Restorative sleep can help ward off anxiety, depression, weakened immunity, weight gain and even diabetes and heart disease.

In general, the most restorative overnight sleep begins before midnight. During sleep, 90-minute cycles of light, deep and dreaming sleep repeat four to six times overnight. The amount of time you spend in each stage of sleep changes as the night progresses. You spend more time in the lighter stages as the night begins and more time in the deep, restorative stages before awakening in the morning. People who go to bed very late may not spend enough time in the deeper sleep stages.

The best thing a retiree can do is go to bed and wake up at the same time every day. Since you no longer have to wake up to get to work, you could create a new morning routine, such as a morning swim or brisk walk. Or you could meet friends at the gym or a local coffee shop.

If you have trouble sticking to a sleep schedule, consult a sleep specialist. Some adults and teens who are unable to fall asleep until the wee hours of the morning suffer from a sleep disorder known as delayed sleep phase syndrome. A sleep specialist can help the patient reset his/her circadian rhythm with treatments such as light therapy and the hormone melatonin.

Many Older Americans May Get Unneeded Breast, Prostate Cancer Screenings

Firas Abdollah, MD, Henry Ford Health System, Detroit.
Robert Smith, PhD, vice president, cancer screening, American Cancer Society.
JAMA Oncology, online

Many older Americans are unnecessarily screened for breast and prostate cancer, which can lead to treatments they don't need, a new study contends.

The practice may also be costing the U.S. health care system $1.2 billion a year, the researchers added.

Almost 16% of those 65 and older are being screened for breast or prostate cancer even though they may have less than 10 years to live, the study found. A 10-year life expectancy is a benchmark for deciding whether to screen or not. And guidelines recommend against screening for these cancers in people with a life expectancy less than 10 years, the researchers said.

"Physicians, as well as patients, should consider life expectancy when deciding the necessity of prostate cancer or breast cancer screening," said lead researcher Firas Abdollah, MD, of the Henry Ford Health System in Detroit.

"To achieve this goal, we need to overcome many hurdles," he said, which include the lack of easy-to-use and accurate life expectancy calculators to guide doctors in making screening recommendations.

Also, busy doctors may find it hard to explain the concept of life expectancy and why screening is not recommended for certain individuals, he added.

Robert Smith, PhD, vice president for cancer screening at the American Cancer Society, said: "This can be a hard conversation for doctors to have with patients. If a patient shows some enthusiasm for getting these tests, it's just easier to do the test than it is to have that conversation, especially if you're not that good at doing it."

In addition, it's difficult to estimate whether somebody has 10 years to live, Dr. Smith said.

The report was published online in the journal *JAMA Oncology*.

Dr. Smith said that the U.S. Preventive Services Task Force recommends mammograms for women up to age 74. The task force does not recommend screening for prostate cancer at all, he said.

Using 10-year longevity as a benchmark for screening is the American Cancer Society's guideline, Dr. Smith said.

"We recommend that men should not be offered prostate cancer screening if they don't have 10 years of life left," he said. "Our breast cancer guideline is the same."

Dr. Abdollah said cancer screening aims to detect tumors early, before symptoms appear. "Evidence suggests that detection and treatment of early stage tumors may reduce cancer mortality among screened individuals," he said.

Despite this benefit, screening may also cause harm, he said. Screening may identify low-risk tumors that would never become life-threatening, but subject patients to the harms of unnecessary treatment, such as side effects of therapy and a reduced quality of life, he added.

RESEARCH DETAILS

For the report, Dr. Abdollah and his colleagues collected data on nearly 150,000 people 65 and older who responded to the Behavioral Risk Factors Surveillance System survey in 2012.

Among these people, 51% had had a prostate-specific antigen (PSA) test or mammography in the past year. Of those who were screened, al-most 31% had a life expectancy of less than 10 years. The rate of non-recommended screening was 15.7%, Dr. Abdollah said.

This rate varied across the country, from 11.6% in Colorado to just over 20% in Georgia, the researchers found. States with a high rate of non-recommended screening for prostate cancer also had a high rate of non-recommended screening for breast cancer.

Dr. Smith said the other side of the coin is that many doctors fail to recommend screening for patients who clearly have 10 years to live or more.

About one-third of women who die from breast cancer each year are over 70, Dr. Smith said. "That means there is a significant fraction of these deaths that could be avoided if women had been screened," he said.

Dr. Smith added that many doctors aren't aware of the tools available to predict longevity and many who are aware don't use them. "Doctors need to be better prepared to estimate longevity, and have conversations with patients about cancer screening," he said.

Dr. Smith did note that as patients get older they tend to lose interest in screening.

"There is a natural attrition as you get older—patients lose interest in prevention and doctors become preoccupied with managing life-limiting conditions," he explained.

info Visit the American Cancer Society at *cancer.org* for more on cancer screening.

CHAPTER 15

Medical Newsmakers

Living to 100—and Beyond

W̲hen we hear about people who live to age 100 or beyond, it may seem like a relatively rare occurrence. But in fact, the number of those "super agers" is dramatically increasing—in 1980, 15,000 Americans had reached the centenarian milestone…by 2014, their numbers had increased to more than 72,000. Overall, the life span of the average American has increased by more than 60% in the last century. Some experts believe that's just the beginning.

To learn more, we spoke with Michael Fossel, MD, PhD, a leading expert on aging who believes that both aging and chronic diseases can be slowed by "switching on" a gene that controls cellular health.

Are medical and social improvements responsible for longer average life spans in the US? They've certainly helped. We can now cure many childhood leukemias and treat diabetes and most infections. We are now less likely to experience malnutrition or hygiene-related diseases than we were a century ago—due, for example, to better agriculture and safer water supplies.

But these factors mainly affect the risk of dying young (or younger than you'd like). They don't guarantee that you'll live an extra-long life.

How much does one's lifestyle affect life span? Less than you'd think. Consider diet. Most people assume that a good diet is the secret to a long and healthy life. But research has failed to find a consistent link. When scientists interview centenarians, they find that their dietary habits are all over the map.

I'm not suggesting that diet doesn't matter. Many well-regarded studies—such as the Fram-

Michael Fossel, MD, PhD, a leading expert on the use of telomerase for age-related diseases. He is the founder and president of Telocyte, a company that is investigating telomerase therapy for Alzheimer's disease. He is the author of The Telomerase Revolution: The Enzyme That Holds the Key to Human Aging and Will Soon Lead to Longer, Healthier Lives. MichaelFossel.com

ingham Heart Study and the Nurses' Health Study—have shown that diet makes some difference. People who eat a lot of saturated and trans fats tend to get more heart disease and die younger...and those who sip a little red wine tend to be healthier.

But there's a ceiling effect. People who eat a reasonably good diet are more likely to live longer than those who eat poorly. There's just no definitive evidence that going from a reasonably healthful diet to a great diet will help you slow the aging process or stop age-related disease.

Don't people who exercise live longer? Yes. Studies show that people who exercise tend to live longer. But does the exercise itself get the credit? Or do these people simply have "healthy" genes that make them feel good and want to exercise? Correlation is not necessarily causation. While proving that exercise is good for you isn't as easy as you might think, it is certainly hard to argue against its value. I definitely encourage exercise.

But all our habits are mediated, in part, by how our bodies respond. The cells of young people generally have robust repair mechanisms that can mitigate damage caused by unhealthy behaviors. In older adults, the cells are less capable of self-repair—and that's when diseases get serious. While genes, diet and exercise play a small role, the major factor is still cellular aging.

Does cellular self-repair—or the lack of it—affect aging? Generally speaking, genetic damage occurs when cells divide. With each division, for example, telomeres (caps on the tips of each strand of DNA on your chromosomes—often compared to plastic tips on the ends of shoelaces) get slightly shorter.

Why it matters: Every shortening of the telomeres changes gene expression, the ability of genes to produce the proteins and other substances that maintain life—and that allow cells to repair themselves.

How does this affect life span? Every disease is caused in part by cellular breakdowns. Why do young people get fewer chronic diseases? Because their cells can readily recover from infections, inflammation and other "insults." Older cells, with their shortened telomeres and altered gene expression, aren't as resilient, and DNA repair, for example, slows down. This is why the risk for cancer, for instance, goes up exponentially with age.

Is it possible to prevent telomere shortening? In lab and animal studies, scientists have already found ways to "reset" telomeres to their original length. The evidence suggests that doing so could help people live longer, healthier lives.

The key to this process: Every cell in the body contains a gene for telomerase, an enzyme that lengthens telomeres. However, the gene only "turns on" in germ and stem cells (which can repair/divide indefinitely). Activating this gene in other cells could possibly do the same thing.

In studies, lengthening telomeres has been shown to improve immune function, blood pressure, bone density and other "biomarkers" for aging and age-related diseases. Now we need a mechanism to reliably use this process in humans.

CAN WE SLOW AGING?

Over-the-counter supplements known as telomerase activators are designed to help maintain and rebuild telomeres (caps at the end of each strand of DNA in our chromosomes, which help prevent deterioration of these gene-encoded structures). The supplements, available online, seem to improve some biomarkers of disease (such as cholesterol). Will this type of supplement help people live longer? There's no proof yet. Many experts on aging believe that the supplements may be somewhat helpful—although likely much less effective as they would need to be to prevent/cure age-related diseases. And they're expensive, costing several hundred dollars a month.

In the future: It may be possible to deliver an "active" telomerase gene directly to the body's cells. In theory, this could potentially prevent and even cure many—if not most—age-related diseases. While you could still die of trauma, infections, inherited genetic problems and other causes, we could essentially halt most "age-related" diseases, such as atherosclerosis, Alzheimer's, osteoarthritis, etc. You might have the health of a 30- or 40-year-old and could easily live to twice the current healthy life span.

Program Your Genes to Fight Genetic Disease Risks

The late Mitchell Gaynor, MD, founder of Gaynor Integrative Oncology and Gaynor Wellness, New York City. He is author of *The Gene Therapy Plan: Taking Control of Your Genetic Destiny with Diet and Lifestyle.* GeneChanger.com

Your body is a war zone, especially in this day and age, with your immune system battling the effects of processed foods that are laced with refined sugar and dangerous fats...plus exposure to pesticide residues, heavy metals and other environmental pollutants. Mix these perils with your genetic makeup, and your risk of cancer, cardiovascular disease, obesity or diabetes can multiply.

But you don't have to think of your genes as time bombs waiting for the perfect storm of environmental factors to light their fuses. Instead, you can turn the genes that promote aging, cancer, heart disease, obesity and diabetes on or off through lifestyle choices—especially nutrition.

We're all born with the genes we received from our mother and father...that part is fixed. But what is not fixed is gene expression, which can change throughout your life for good or bad, depending on what you're putting into your body.

Generally speaking, gene expression is a process whereby genetic information is copied in a cell and used to create protein molecules that perform specific functions in the body. For example, gene expression can protect the body against cancer growth (via tumor suppressor genes) or cause it (via tumor promoter genes). Environmental pollutants or an unhealthy diet can rally less-than-favorable gene expression.

Another example: if you're consuming a lot of refined sugar and flour because your diet is heavy in fast foods and processed foods, you're turning on a lot of inflammatory genes. Those inflammatory genes are making you gain weight, in part, by causing a hormone called leptin to go into overdrive. Leptin is responsible for regulation of appetite, food intake and metabolism. With leptin impaired, your cells'

ability to properly respond to insulin also becomes impaired. In response, your body produces more insulin, your blood sugar drops and you feel hungry—and eat—all the time, setting yourself up for diabetes and heart disease.

The antidote is to apply nutrigenetics. You have to strengthen your detoxifying genes through nutrition. We're talking about nutrients that literally turn on genes that code for detoxifying enzymes. But first, you need to know where your genetic vulnerabilities lie.

THE VALUE OF GENETIC TESTING

To learn about your genetic vulnerability, simply give thought to the health conditions your closest relatives are dealing with or have faced. Better, you may want to consider genetic testing, especially if you have a number of first-degree relatives (parents and siblings in particular, but grandparents, too) who have had breast, ovarian, uterine or colon cancer. Most health insurers will pay for these tests if there is a strong family history.

Don't wait for your doctor to suggest genetic testing—actively open up a discussion with him/her. A recent survey of breast cancer patients showed that one-third expressed a strong desire for genetic testing. They were worried about being vulnerable to other cancers and worried for their relatives—but 43% of these women had not had a meaningful discussion about it with a health-care professional, either because they did not know how to address the topic or because their doctors never brought up the subject. The more you know about your risk of specific diseases, the easier it is to design a lifestyle and diet regimen to counter your genetic vulnerabilities.

BEAT DISEASE AT THE GENETIC LEVEL

To help avoid buildup of environmental toxins, eat organic foods and use nontoxic detergents, bath products and other household items as much as possible.

Ecogenetics and nutrigenetics, are relatively new concepts not yet embraced by conventional Western medicine. But the number of hospitals and doctors embracing integrative medicine (combining alternative and standard Western medicine) to treat the individual rather than just the disease is rapidly on the rise. If you would like guidance in working to optimize nutrition and well-being on the genetic level, work with a specialist in integrative medicine. You can find such a professional near you through the Academy of Integrative Health & Medicine. (AIHM.org).

New Life for a Damaged Heart

Joel K. Kahn, MD, a clinical professor of medicine at Wayne State University School of Medicine and founder of the Kahn Center for Cardiac Longevity in Bloomfield Hills, Michigan. He is also an associate professor at Oakland University William Beaumont School of Medicine. Dr. Kahn is the author of *The Whole Heart Solution: Halt Heart Disease Now with the Best Alternative and Traditional Medicine.* DrJoelKahn.com

Even though medical advances have made it possible for people who suffer from heart attacks or other serious forms of heart disease to live longer than ever before, these patients face a lifetime of tests, daily medications and frequent doctor visits to keep their hearts working and to prevent subsequent damage.

But what if it were possible to go a step further—to actually replace damaged heart tissue with new, fully functioning cells…in essence, to rebuild a healthy heart? It sounds like science fiction, but the advances being made are promising. In laboratories and hospitals around the world, heart researchers are making remarkable strides in developing stem cell therapy for serious heart conditions.

A groundbreaking study: In research published in *The Lancet*, patients with heart scarring from previous heart attacks were given stem cells in their coronary arteries that were extracted from healthy tissue in their own hearts. Within 12 months, the amount of scar tissue was reduced by about 50%. (Patients in a control group given standard treatments had no improvement.)

Here's what you need to know about the exciting possibilities—and challenges—for the use of stem cell therapy in heart patients…

THE BODY'S TRANSFORMERS

So how exactly does stem cell therapy work? Think of stem cells as the key "blanks" that hardware stores use to copy a key. These blanks all look the same until the edges are cut and polished. Once a key is cut, it will open only a particular lock.

Stem cells are like key blanks (except that they also have the ability to divide and create exact copies of themselves). They're undifferentiated cells that can eventually turn into specialized, functioning cells.

While embryonic stem cells, which exist only briefly at the earliest stages of human development, can be developed in the lab, the stem cells that are used in today's treatments are usually taken from a donor's blood or bone marrow or from the patient's own bone marrow or heart—a process that usually involves an outpatient aspiration procedure.

REMARKABLE DISCOVERIES

Heart failure, the ineffective pumping of the heart that is usually caused by a heart attack, coronary artery disease or high blood pressure, has been a main focus of stem cell therapy. Nearly 5 million Americans have it, and more than half will die within five years after being diagnosed. No current treatments can repair damaged heart-muscle cells.

New approach: Patients with heart failure can be infused (often via a catheter that's threaded through the coronary artery into the damaged area of the heart) with millions of stem cells. The onetime treatment can potentially regenerate healthy heart cells. In theory, this approach could completely reverse heart failure—but the research is still in the early stages. *Among the important findings…*

•**In animal studies conducted at Johns Hopkins University and Cedars-Sinai Medical Center,** stem cells from the injured hearts of animals were extracted and cultured in a laboratory, then reinjected back into animals' damaged hearts. They quickly began to form new heart and blood vessel cells. Treated animals had about a 25% reduction in the size of damaged areas, or infarcts.

•**The landmark BOOST study,** led by German researchers at Hannover Medical School randomly assigned 60 patients with heart damage to receive either standard treatments or an infusion of autologous (their own) bone marrow stem cells. Six months later, patients given the stem cells showed an increase in left-ventricular ejection fraction (a measure of the heart's pumping ability) of 6.7%. In the control group, the improvement was just 0.7%.

While these and other studies are promising, overall results have been mixed. A large study conducted at Jamia Hamdard University in India, for example, found that heart attack patients given stem cell therapy showed no measurable increase in heart strength.

IS IT FOR YOU?

If you're a heart patient, don't expect your doctor to recommend stem cell therapy. It's an exciting development because we now know that it's possible to repair heart damage, but important questions remain.

Will the "replacement" cells function indefinitely? Will the results from animal studies apply to humans? Are stem cells derived from heart tissue more effective than those extracted from bone marrow?

Caution: Some cardiologists in the Bahamas and elsewhere have begun offering stem cell therapy for heart patients. At this time, however, there's more we need to know before stem cell therapy is ready for prime time—and the procedures aren't risk free.

Some early studies have found that stem cell treatments might cause an increase in heartbeat irregularities. Experts are also concerned that there might be an increase in atherosclerosis. One way to minimize these potential complications is to enroll in a formal study with careful observation (see below).

GETTING STEM CELL THERAPY NOW

If you've had a heart attack or been diagnosed with heart failure, you might want to participate in a clinical trial looking at stem cell therapy. To find a study in your area, go to *ClinicalTrials. gov*. In the search box, type in your city and the type of study you're looking for (for example, "New York," "heart failure" and "stem cells").

Important: Don't rule out such a study because you assume that there is always a placebo group. Some studies don't use placebos (everyone gets different forms of the new treatment), and other trials provide the best available standard treatment to those who don't receive the treatment being studied. You'll also get extensive and careful monitoring in either case. Ask your doctor for advice.

Scientists Create Bacteria in Lab With "Minimal" Genes Needed for Life

J. Craig Venter, PhD, founder, chairman and CEO, J. Craig Venter Institute.
Valda Vinson, PhD, deputy editor of research, *Science*.
Daniel Gibson, PhD, associate professor, J. Craig Venter Institute's Synthetic Biology group.
Science.

Scientists are closer than ever to cracking the hidden code of life itself, having engineered a synthetic bacteria with a "minimum" number of genes needed to support its existence.

The lab-created bacteria—called Mycoplasma mycoides JCVI-syn3.0—contains only 473 genes. That's fewer than any other healthy, replicating cell currently found in nature.

By stripping an artificial cell down to the bare necessities, researchers hope to learn more about how life began on Earth and evolved over time, the study authors said.

"We view life as DNA software-driven and we're showing that by trying to understand that software, we're going to get a better understanding of life," said senior author J. Craig Venter, PhD. He's a renowned genetics researcher and founder, chairman and CEO of the J. Craig Venter Institute, a non-profit genomics research group.

However, the most important lesson from this "minimal cell" experiment involves how much scientists don't know about the role that genes play in sustaining life, Dr. Venter and his colleagues said.

The study was released online in the journal *Science*.

RESEARCH DETAILS

Most of the genes in this synthetic bacteria have a specific job to do. Some play a role in reproduction, others sustain cellular structure and some are needed to maintain the cell's metabolism, the researchers said.

But the scientists couldn't determine a specific biological function for one-third of the genes they needed to keep in the bacteria for it to thrive. These 149 genes needed to be there. But no one knows why.

"The precise biological functions of roughly 31% of the genes remain undiscovered, which is, to me at least, a surprisingly high number," said Valda Vinson, PhD. She's the deputy editor of research for *Science*.

The mystery of these necessary but little-understood genes should provide some comfort to people worried about the implications of genetic engineering in humans, Dr. Venter said.

"When you can see that we only understand two-thirds of the most fundamental cell that we can compile right now, we're probably at about the 1% level in understanding of the human genome," he said.

There are about 21,000 genes contained in the human genome, the U.S. National Human Genome Research Institute says.

In 2010, researchers at the Venter Institute created the world's first self-replicating synthetic bacterial cell. It was a lab-produced copy of Mycoplasma mycoides. Normally, these bacteria cause a contagious lung disease of cattle, according to the World Organization for Animal Health. The lab-produced copy contained 901 genes, the study authors said.

That initial experiment showed that they could design a genetic structure in a computer, chemically produce it in a lab, and then create a synthetic cell by transplanting the lab-created genes into a "blank" cell.

For their next step, the researchers began to whittle away genes from the synthetic bacteria. They wanted to learn how many genes are absolutely needed for a cell to survive and replicate.

Earlier studies had predicted a set of between 256 and 375 essential genes, but genetic designs based on those numbers failed, Dr. Venter said.

So the researchers reverted to a trial-and-error approach. They removed different sets of genes to see how each contributed to the life of the synthetic bacteria.

Dr. Venter compared paring down non-essential genes to reverse-engineering a 777 aircraft.

"If you're just trying to find out functions of parts by removing them and you remove the engine from the right wing, the airplane can still fly and land, so you might say that's a non-essential component," he said. "You don't really discover the essentiality until you remove the second (engine)."

The researchers found that they needed to include many cells with no clear purpose to produce a bacterium that could both survive and replicate itself.

IMPLICATIONS

The ultimate goal of this research is to be able to build synthetic organisms on demand, said study co-author Daniel Gibson, PhD, an associate professor in the Venter Institute's Synthetic Biology group.

These cells could be used to produce antibiotics and other medications, biofuels, industrial materials and agricultural products, Dr. Gibson said. Other research efforts hope to use synthetic genes to create genetically engineered pigs that would have organs that could be transplanted into human beings.

"There's about a million people that die in the U.S. each year due to the lack of availability of organs for transplantation," Dr. Venter said. "There's lots of groups trying to isolate antibiotics from marine organisms. But, because we sequence literally tens of thousands of these, there's a lot of pathways that could be readily placed into synthetic cells for trying to produce new novel compounds."

The Venter researchers said they plan to make this synthetic cell available to other scientists relatively soon. They're considering a contest to see each year who can add the most important step in evolution to the cell.

"So we're hoping it becomes a widely used research and teaching tool," Dr. Venter said.

info For more on genetic engineering, visit the U.S. Food and Drug Administration website, *FDA.gov*, and search "genetic engineering".

A New Incision-Free Surgery

Flemming Forsberg, PhD, an ultrasound physicist and associate professor of radiology at the Sidney Kimmel Medical College of Thomas Jefferson University in Philadelphia. His research and clinical interests include ultrasound contrast imaging.

Imagine having a major surgery in which the surgeon uses a light beam to remove a tumor without a single incision. To some, this might sound like science fiction, but believe it or not, this type of surgery has now become a reality.

With high-intensity focused ultrasound, doctors can reach tissues deep within the body—in the bones, brain, blood vessels, etc.—without making a single cut...and often with minimal discomfort.

Focused ultrasound in action: The FDA has currently approved high-intensity focused ultrasound for treating uterine fibroids, prostate problems (cancer or prostate enlargement) and cancer that has spread to the bones.

Focused ultrasound differs from other scalpel-free technologies, such as Gamma Knife, because no radiation is involved and imaging feedback is in real time.

INTO THE FUTURE

Many additional uses for focused ultrasound are being studied. *Those that show tremendous promise...*

•**Deep-vein thrombosis (DVT).** Many blood clots that form in the deep veins in the legs dissolve on their own, but others keep growing and are often life-threatening when a part of the clot breaks off and travels to the lungs. The standard treatment is a lengthy course of *warfarin* (Coumadin) or some other blood thinner. A tissue plasminogen activator (tPA) that breaks down the clot is given if the clot is very large and/or life-threatening. Both of these treatments have a high risk for dangerous side effects. Clots can also be removed with a catheter, which is used to guide a balloon or to inject tPA. But this carries risks as well.

Ultrasound breakthrough: Early research suggests that ultrasound vibrations can break up clots and also make them more susceptible to tPA.

•**Drug delivery.** There are few drugs for Parkinson's or Alzheimer's disease—now or in development—that can help these conditions.

Reason: It's very difficult for drugs to pass through the blood-brain barrier, a protective layer of tightly joined cells that line the blood vessels in the brain.

Ultrasound breakthrough: High-intensity focused ultrasound temporarily causes the cell junctions to open, which allows drugs to pass into the brain. This could give Alzheimer's or Parkinson's drugs easier access to affected brain regions and help chemotherapy drugs reach hard-to-treat brain tumors.

•**Brain tumors.** Ultrasound energy can pass through the skull and burn away a tumor without affecting healthy parts of the brain. The focused beam can target an area as small as a grain of rice. This could be an important breakthrough because conventional surgery and/or radiation can cause unintended brain damage, resulting in a loss of mental or physical function.

Ultrasound breakthrough: In 2014, focused ultrasound was used for the first time to successfully treat a recurrent brain tumor. The patient, who was treated in Zurich, was awake during the procedure and experienced no side effects or complications.

However, ultrasound for brain tumors still presents technical challenges.

Example: Irregularities in skull thickness and the high speed of sound passing through bone can cause overheating in the brain.

One possible solution: Circulating chilled water around the scalp.

•**Essential tremor.** *The New England Journal of Medicine* recently published the results of a small exploratory study that used focused ultrasound for essential tremor, a neurological disorder that causes involuntary shaking. The study looked at 15 patients who had a poor response to medication. Doctors used ultrasound to perform unilateral thalamotomy, a procedure that destroys cells in the thalamus, an area of the brain involved in sensory and motor signal relay.

Results: After one year, tremors in the dominant hand had improved by 75%, and patients showed an 85% improvement in the ability to perform daily functions. The complications (such as an increase in involuntary movements) were comparable to those caused by conventional surgery—but the patients were spared the usual surgical trauma.

ON THE HORIZON

Focused ultrasound is still at an early stage of development. We're likely to see a rapid expansion of uses beyond those already approved by the FDA within the next five or six years—but a lot of uncertainty remains.

Most procedures are being done only in laboratories or as a part of clinical studies,* and the procedures (and equipment) are very expensive. Even the procedures that have FDA approval may not be covered by insurance. For more information, go to the website of the Focused Ultrasound Foundation, *FUSFoundation.org*.

HOW IT WORKS

When you were a kid, did you ever use a magnifying glass to burn a hole through a leaf using the sun's rays? The principle is the same with focused ultrasound, except that ultrasound waves (ultrafast vibrating sound waves) are used instead of sunbeams.

These are not the same low-intensity sound waves that are used in diagnostic scans. With high-intensity focused ultrasound, multiple beams of high energy pass through an acoustic lens (instead of a magnifying glass) and then converge to focus on a small area. The beams pass harmlessly through the body until they reach the desired location. There, they generate enough energy to destroy tumors, break down blood clots or create openings in the walls of blood vessels—all without affecting nearby tissues, unlike radiation, which impacts everything in its path.

There's no incision, so recovery times are quicker. And there's little risk of bleeding (the heat

*To find a clinical trial in your area, go to *Clinical Trials.gov*. In the search box, type in "high-intensity focused ultrasound."

of ultrasound closes bleeding vessels) or infection (no external germs are introduced). Patients might experience burning sensations during the procedure, but the discomfort is usually slight.

New Imaging Technique "Lights Up" Cancer Cells in Early Trial

David G. Kirsch, MD, PhD, professor, department of pharmacology and cancer biology, and department of radiation oncology, Duke University Medical Center, Durham, North Carolina.

Stephen Freedland, MD, professor, surgery, and director, Center for Integrated Research on Cancer and Lifestyle, Cedars-Sinai Medical Center, Los Angeles.

Lisa Richardson, MD, director, Division of Cancer Prevention and Control, U.S. Centers for Disease Control and Prevention, Atlanta.

Science Translational Medicine

A new imaging technique that "lights up" cancer cells may eventually help surgeons remove all of a cancer the first time, according to a preliminary study.

"When a patient has cancer, the surgeon tries to find the tumor and cut it out," explained study senior author David Kirsch, MD, PhD, a professor in the department of pharmacology and cancer biology, and the department of radiation oncology at Duke University Medical Center in Durham, North Carolina. "However, there can sometimes be microscopic residual cancer left behind that the surgeon can't see.

"So this imaging technique," he added, "is meant to help the surgeon see the cancer during the operation, to avoid the patient having to go in for a second operation."

HOW THE IMAGING WORKS

The early trial, involving both mice and a small number of human patients, used a preoperative injection of a blue liquid called LUM015 directly into the region where the cancer is located. The liquid then spreads into tumor tissue instead of healthy tissue. According to the study authors, the liquid seeks out a particular enzyme called protease that is believed to be critical to cancer growth, and is found in large quantities in malignant cells.

Once the tumor tissue is removed during surgery, a specially designed hand-held imaging probe is placed at the surgical site. Cancer cells left behind glow roughly five times brighter than healthy tissue, the researchers said. Surgeons can then remove the malignant cells on the spot, theoretically reducing the need for a follow-up operation.

IMPLICATIONS

Stephen Freedland, MD, director of the Center for Integrated Research on Cancer and Lifestyle at Cedars-Sinai Medical Center in Los Angeles, noted that one of the biggest challenges facing surgeons is determining where is the cancer.

"So better imaging is always needed. Because with a big, massive tumor it's easy to see the cancer. But when it's just a few cells or a small tumor, it's very hard to see and properly target therapy," said Dr. Freedland, who was not involved with the study.

"But if this [experimental approach] pans out, which is still a huge 'if' at this point, it holds the promise to do that," Dr. Freedland added. "I do think using these little enzymes, these protease, to tell us where the cancer is absolutely does make sense. And in theory this concept should work for the vast majority of cancers. So although it's at a very early stage, there's a lot of promise here. And hopefully they [the study researchers] are on the path to something great."

The new technology was developed through a collaboration between Duke, the Massachusetts Institute of Technology and Lumicell, a company started by the MIT researchers, involving Dr. Kirsch. Findings from the study were published online in *Science Translational Medicine*.

The researchers say theirs is the first such approach to specifically use the protease enzyme to guide imaging.

To date, the study has involved research with mice and a group of 15 patients, all of whom were diagnosed with either breast cancer or soft-tissue sarcoma.

With human patients, the research team has so far studied the fluorescent impact on tumor tissue already removed from each patient. Among mice, the team has performed real-time removal of cancerous cells based on identification by the technique.

The study authors said the technique has produced no side effects and appears safe.

A follow-up trial involving 50 breast cancer patients is already underway, and Dr. Kirsch said the hope is to make the technology available by 2017.

Lisa Richardson, MD, director of the U.S. Centers for Disease Control and Prevention's division of cancer prevention and control, said the reason people are living longer after a cancer diagnosis is "because of advances in early detection and treatment."

"[And] a complete and accurate diagnosis of cancer at the time of surgery is always the goal," she said. "Any new technique to improve cancer diagnosis is a step forward to help improve the desired outcome: eliminating cancer for an individual and improving their chances of surviving. This new technique may help surgeons be sure that cancer is completely removed during the procedure. If it pans out, the need for additional surgeries will also be decreased."

info There's more on cancer surgery at the American Cancer Society website *cancer. org* search "cancer surgery."

Transplant from Incompatible Living Donor Boosts Kidney Patients' Survival

Dorry Segeu, MD, PhD, associate professor of Surgery, Johns Hopins University School of Medicine, Baltimore.

Michael Flessner, MD, program director, division of kidney, urologic and hematologic diseases, U.S. National Institute of Diabetes and Digestive and Kidney Diseases.

Harold Helderman, MD, professor, medicine, Vanderbilt University Medical Center, Nashville, Tennessee.

New England Journal of Medicine

In what experts call a possible "paradigm shift," a new study shows kidney disease patients may live far longer if they receive a transplant from an incompatible living donor rather than wait for a good match.

The findings could offer another choice for kidney patients who might otherwise die waiting for a compatible deceased donor.

Specifically, experts said the results offer hope to "highly sensitized" transplant candidates.

That refers to patients who have a large number of immune system antibodies ready to attack a donor organ. It's common among people who've had a prior kidney transplant, according to the United Network for Organ Sharing. Patients who have had multiple blood transfusions while on dialysis, or who have been pregnant several times, can also become sensitized.

Finding a compatible donor for sensitized patients is "nearly impossible," said study lead researcher Dorry Segev, MD, PhD, an associate professor of surgery at Johns Hopkins University School of Medicine, in Baltimore.

An alternative is to transplant a kidney from an incompatible donor, with the help of special "desensitization" therapies that reduce the risk of an immune system attack on the donor organ.

Johns Hopkins pioneered the approach 15 years ago, and other transplant centers have followed suit.

Only now, though, is the long-term benefit becoming clear. Using data from 22 U.S. hospitals, Dr. Segev's team found that more than three-quarters of patients who received a kidney from an incompatible living donor were still alive eight years later.

"This is potentially a paradigm shift," said Michael Flessner, MD, a program director in the division of kidney, urologic and hematologic diseases at the U.S. National Institute of Diabetes and Digestive and Kidney Diseases, which funded the study.

Dr. Flessner expects incompatible living-donor transplants will become standard practice.

Such donations are not a panacea: There is a higher risk of rejection than with transplants from compatible living donors, said Harold Helderman, MD, a professor of medicine at Vanderbilt University Medical Center, in Nashville.

And because patients receive especially powerful immune-system suppressing drugs, they can be at increased risk for infections, he noted.

"But these results show that at the end of the day, these patients have a longer lifespan," Dr. Helderman said. "So, you accept that there are risks."

STUDY DETAILS

For the study, Dr. Segev's team followed just over 1,000 sensitized patients who received a kidney from an incompatible donor at one of 22 transplant centers in the United States. They compared the patients' survival with that of two "control" groups: slightly over 5,000 patients on the transplant waiting list who eventually received a kidney; and roughly the same number of wait-list patients who had to remain on dialysis.

After eight years, more than 76% of the incompatible-donor patients were still alive. That compared with 44% of dialysis patients and 63% of those who ultimately received a deceased-donor organ.

The findings were published in the *New England Journal of Medicine*.

WHAT IS INVOLVED IN AN INCOMPATIBLE TRANSPLANT

An incompatible transplant is no easy process. To be desensitized, patients need a procedure called plasmapheresis, which clears the blood of antibodies that could attack the donor organ. Afterward, they receive immune-suppressing drugs aimed at preventing an antibody re-emergence.

Plasmapheresis has to be repeated several times before the transplant—and often afterward as well, Dr. Flessner noted.

The desensitization process also adds about $20,000 to $30,000 to the cost of getting a transplant, according to the University of Wisconsin's transplant center, one of the U.S. programs that performs the procedure.

But it's still far cheaper than dialysis in the long run, Dr. Segev said in a news release from Johns Hopkins.

Right now, just over 100,000 Americans are on the waiting list for a donor kidney, according to the National Kidney Foundation. Dr. Segev and his team estimate that 32,000 of them are sensitized.

When those patients have a willing, but incompatible, living donor, Dr. Segev said, it may be in their "best interests" to have the transplant rather than wait.

Dr. Flessner agreed. "This holds out the hope of more family members being able to give this great gift," he said. "And it really is the gift of life."

info The National Kidney Foundation has more on kidney transplantation at *kid ney.org/atoz/atozTopic_Transplantation*

New Dangers to Your Kidneys

Orlando Gutiérrez, MD, an associate professor of medicine in the division of nephrology and assistant professor of epidemiology at The University of Alabama at Birmingham School of Medicine. He is also the chair of the Medical Affairs Committee for the American Kidney Fund. KidneyFund.org

Your kidneys are two of your body's best friends. Besides filtering and cleaning your blood, they also regulate fluids, acidity and key minerals...produce hormones that control blood pressure...and manufacture a form of vitamin D that strengthens bones.

But modern life can really clobber your kidneys—high blood pressure, elevated blood sugar and obesity all can damage these vital organs and are major risk factors for chronic kidney disease (CKD).

THE BEST DEFENSE

Controlling the big risk factors mentioned above are the best ways to prevent or control CKD. But recent studies have revealed several new risk factors that might threaten your kidneys. *These include...*

PROTON PUMP INHIBITORS

Americans spend about $11 billion yearly on acid-reducing, heartburn-easing proton pump inhibitors (PPIs), such as *esomeprazole* (Nexium) and *omeprazole* (Prilosec).

New finding: Researchers at Johns Hopkins University studied more than 10,000 people with normal kidney function. After 15 years, those using PPIs were 20% to 50% more likely to develop CKD.

Possible explanation: PPIs may cause interstitial nephritis—inflammation and scarring in the kidneys.

What to do: The researchers found that people who took an H2 blocker—such as *ranitidine*

(Zantac) or *famotidine* (Pepcid)—instead of a PPI for heartburn did not have a higher risk for CKD.

Note: Many of my patients find that TUMS and lifestyle changes, such as avoiding spicy and fatty foods and eating more slowly, can greatly reduce heartburn.

HIGH ACID DIET

Just as our oceans are becoming more acidic and threatening marine life, scientists are finding that an acidic diet threatens our kidneys.

New finding: When researchers analyzed 14 years of health data for nearly 1,500 people with CKD, they found that those who ate a high-acid, junk food–laden diet that included red meat, processed foods, sweets and few fruits and vegetables were three times more likely to develop kidney failure.

What to do: Adopt a more alkaline diet. In a recent study, researchers from Columbia University Medical Center followed 900 people for nearly seven years and found that those who routinely ate a Mediterranean-type diet—rich in alkaline foods such as vegetables, fruits, beans and heart-healthy fats like olive oil—were 50% less likely to develop CKD than those who didn't eat these foods.

TOO MUCH PHOSPHORUS

The mineral phosphorus is a must—for cellular health, energy and digestion, a steady heartbeat and strong bones and teeth. But too much phosphorus damages the kidneys and the circulatory system.

New findings: In a study I conducted with fellow kidney specialists involving nearly 10,000 people, we found that an excess of phosphorus in the diet was linked to more than double the risk of dying from any cause and three times the risk of dying from heart disease. In another study, higher levels of dietary phosphorus sped up the decline from CKD to end-stage renal disease.

Red meat and dairy products are rich in phosphorus, but about 40% of the phosphorus in our daily diets is from phosphorus-containing additives used to extend shelf life and improve flavor and texture. Those additives are just about everywhere—including in many flavored waters, iced teas, nondairy creamers and bottled coffee beverages.

What to do: Whenever possible, choose a natural food over a processed food—eat fresh green beans, for example, rather than canned… and homemade bread rather than highly processed bread.

Also helpful: If you must eat a processed food, check the label for the word phosphate or phosphoric acid, which indicates the presence of phosphorus—and try to pick a product without the additive.

SITTING TOO MUCH

It's not just lack of regular exercise that contributes to chronic health problems such as heart disease— it's also excessive sitting. And sitting takes a toll on your kidneys, too.

New finding: In a study of nearly 6,000 people, every 80-minute period of sitting during the day increased the likelihood of CKD by 20%, according to research from the University of Utah School of Medicine. That was true whether or not the person exercised regularly or had diabetes, high blood pressure or obesity.

What to do: When the same team of researchers looked at people with CKD, they found that standing up and/or walking around for just two minutes an hour lowered the risk for death by 41%. Research also shows that regular exercise is good for your kidneys.

My advice: Walk at least 30 minutes, three times a week (in addition to getting up every hour you sit)…or check with your doctor for advice on the best type of exercise for you.

Should You Be Tested for Kidney Disease?

Orlando Gutiérrez, MD, an associate professor of medicine in the division of nephrology and assistant professor of epidemiology at The University of Alabama at Birmingham School of Medicine. He is also the chair of the Medical Affairs Committee for the American Kidney Fund. KidneyFund.org

More than 25 million Americans have chronic kidney disease (CKD)—but only 6% know it!

Beware: The symptoms of kidney disease (such as swollen legs, feet and/or ankles…frequent urination…fatigue…and/or dry, itchy skin) are not likely to be noticed until you reach end-stage renal disease because the body is very good at adapting to loss of kidney function until most of the function is gone.

Blood test for measuring kidney function: Estimated Glomerular Filtration Rate (eGFR). A filtration rate of less than 60 mL/min for more than three months means that you have CKD. Most insurance companies pay for the cost of the test if the patient has a risk factor for kidney disease—such as high blood pressure…type 2 diabetes…obesity…age (65 or older)…or a family history of the disease (a parent or sibling who has CKD). If you have a risk factor for CKD, get the test every year. Otherwise, there's usually no need for testing, but be sure to consult your doctor for advice.

Doctors Report Groundbreaking HIV-to-HIV Organ Transplants

David Bernstein, MD, chief, division of hepatology, Northwell Health, Manhasset, New York.
Media briefing with Dorry Segev, MD, PhD, professor, surgery and director, epidemiology research group in organ transplantation, and Christine Durand, MD, assistant professor, medicine and oncology, both Johns Hopkins University School of Medicine, Baltimore.

Trailblazing liver and kidney transplants from an HIV-positive donor to HIV-positive recipients were recently completed by surgeons at Johns Hopkins University.

"We performed the first HIV-to-HIV liver transplant in the world and the first HIV-to-HIV kidney transplant in the United States," Dorry Segev, MD, PhD, said during a midday media briefing.

BACKGROUND

Before 2013 and passage of the HIV Organ Policy Equity Act, this kind of medical advance would not have been possible, because it was illegal for HIV-positive patients to donate organs

New Test Predicts Surgical Recovery Time

In development: A presurgical blood test that measures the immune response to stress. It could help identify patients who need additional treatments to speed recovery.

Anesthesiology

in the United States. The act allows HIV-positive donors to donate organs to patients infected with the AIDS-causing virus, Dr. Segev said.

Until the law was changed, thousands of patients with HIV in need of organ transplants often risked death while waiting for a donated organ, he said.

At the same time, "we were throwing away organs from donors infected with HIV just because they were infected. These were potentially good organs," said Dr. Segev, a professor of surgery and director of the epidemiology research group in organ transplantation at the Baltimore-based medical school.

HIV-TO-HIV TRANSPLANTS

Christine Durand, MD, an assistant professor of medicine and oncology at Hopkins, said the transplant operations went well and both patients are doing "extremely well."

The patient who received the kidney has already gone home, and the liver transplant patient is expected to leave the hospital in a couple of weeks, she said.

Both the liver and kidney came from a deceased HIV-infected donor, the doctors said.

Now that HIV can be controlled with medications, there's no reason why donor organs from HIV-positive people can't be used for HIV-positive patients in need of transplants, Dr. Segev said.

According to Dr. Segev, approximately 122,000 people are on transplant waiting lists in the United States at any time. Each year, about 500 to 600 potential organ donors who are HIV-positive die, he said.

Dr. Segev said his team is now teaching transplant centers across the country "the protocols we put together and sharing our experience and safety measures."

At the moment, these protocols only cover deceased donors, but Dr. Segev said he and his colleagues have started researching the possible use of organs from living HIV-positive donors.

IMPLICATIONS

"It's a tremendous advancement that will help the HIV population," said David Bernstein, MD, chief of the division of hepatology at Northwell Health in Manhasset, New York, who was not involved in the transplants.

"This should open up transplantation to a significant segment of the population that has had a difficult time getting transplants," he said.

HIV-positive patients aren't restricted to getting organs from HIV-positive donors. They can opt to accept an organ from a non-HIV-infected donor, potentially cutting their waiting time for a transplant, Dr. Durand said.

Transplanting organs from HIV patients carries some risks, Dr. Durand said. "These patients will be exposed to a second strain of HIV from the donor and may be infected with that strain," she said.

It's important, therefore, to consider if the donor has drug-resistant HIV, she said. "All the recipients are on HIV medications already, so we have to take into account matching regimens of drugs," she said.

In addition, it's important to ensure that the immunosuppressant drugs needed to prevent rejection of the transplanted organ don't interfere with the HIV drugs, Dr. Durand said.

"We are encouraged by these first transplants and now it is our hope and our aim to extend this possibility to other patients who are waiting on the transplant list," she said.

info To learn more about organ transplants, visit the United Network for Organ Sharing at *UNDS.org*.

Scientists Say They've Created New Type of Stem Cells

Hebrew University of Jerusalem, news release

Scientists say they have created embryonic stem cells with just one copy of human DNA instead of the normal two, and they believe their achievement might help further genetic and medical research.

These stem cells are the first human cells capable of dividing and replicating with just one copy of DNA, according to the paper published in the journal *Nature*.

"This study has given us a new type of human stem cell that will have an important impact on human genetic and medical research," said study principal co-author Nissim Benvenisty, MD, PhD, director of the Azrieli Center for Stem Cells and Genetic Research at Hebrew University of Jerusalem, in Israel.

"These cells will provide researchers with a novel tool for improving our understanding of human development, and the reasons why we reproduce sexually, instead of from a single parent," Benvenisty said in a university news release.

ABOUT THE STUDY

Human cells typically inherit two sets of chromosomes, 23 from the mother and 23 from the father, the researchers explained.

Only egg and sperm cells contain a single set of 23 chromosomes, and they cannot divide to make more eggs and sperm, the scientists added.

Other efforts to generate embryonic stem cells using just human egg cells did not work, the researchers noted. But in their latest study, they triggered unfertilized human egg cells to divide. They then highlighted the DNA with a fluorescent dye, and isolated the stem cells that had only 23 chromosomes.

The researchers showed that these stem cells could differentiate into many other cell types, including nerve, heart and pancreatic cells.

IMPLICATIONS

Because these stem cells have just one copy of DNA, they may improve genetic analysis in areas such as cancer research and regenerative medicine, the researchers noted.

And they said the stem cells could also prove useful in developing cell-based therapies for diseases such as blindness, diabetes and other conditions in which genetically identical cells could offer a treatment advantage.

Finally, the researchers said the stem cells might be important in the field of reproduction science.

info The U.S. National Institutes of Health has more on stem cells at *stemcells.nih. gov/info*.

A Pill to Ward Off Cavities? Scientists Say It Could Happen

University of Florida, news release

A new discovery might one day lead to an anti-cavity pill, researchers report.

The University of Florida scientists identified a strain of bacteria in the mouth that may keep cavity-causing bacteria in check.

The investigators said it might be possible to use this beneficial bacteria to develop a supplement taken by mouth that prevents cavities.

A healthy mouth requires a relatively neutral chemical environment, the researchers explained. When the environment in the mouth becomes too acidic, it can lead to cavities and other dental problems, study lead author Robert Burne, PhD, said in a university news release.

"At that point, bacteria on the teeth make acid, and acid dissolves the teeth. It's straightforward chemistry," said Dr. Burne, chair of the department of oral biology at the University of Florida College of Dentistry. "We got interested in what activities keep the pH elevated."

The seemingly beneficial bacteria the researchers discovered is a strain of streptococcus called A12, according to the study published recently in the journal *Applied and Environmental Microbiology*.

The researchers also mapped out the entire genetic code of A12, and said they hope to use it as a tool to screen people to see who is at higher risk of developing cavities.

According to study co-author Marcelle Nascimento, DDs, PhD, "If we get to the point where we can confirm that people who have more of this healthy type of bacteria in the mouth are at lower risk of cavities, compared to those who don't carry the beneficial bacteria and may be at high risk, this could be one of the factors that you measure for cavities risk." Dr. Nascimento is an associate professor in the College of Dentistry's department of restorative dental sciences.

The research team recently received a five-year, $3 million grant from the U.S. National Institute of Dental and Craniofacial Research to study A12 and related bacteria in the mouth.

info The U.S. Office of Disease Prevention and Health Promotion explains how to take care of your teeth and gums at *health finder.gov*. Search "teeth and gums."

Amputee "Feels" With Bionic Fingertip

École Polytechnique Fédérale de Lausanne, news release

A bionic fingertip enabled an amputee to feel different textures, researchers report.

The fingertip was linked to electrodes surgically implanted into nerves in Dennis Aabo Sorensen's upper arm. Sorenson was able to feel smoothness and roughness with the fingertip, the researchers said.

A machine controlled the movement of the fingertip over pieces of plastic with different rough or smooth patterns. As the fingertip moved over the plastic surfaces, sensors generated electrical signals that were sent to the nerves in Sorensen's upper arm.

He could tell the difference between smooth and rough textures 96% of the time, the researchers said.

Paralyzed Patients Could Regain Movement

Paralyzed patients may regain leg movement without surgery someday. A new technique called transcutaneous stimulation, which uses an external device to deliver an electrical current to the spine, helped five paralyzed men make steplike movements.

Study led by researchers at University of California-Los Angeles, published in *Journal of Neurotrauma*.

The successful test of the bionic fingertip could help speed efforts to develop artificial limbs that provide sensory feedback, according to Silvestro Micera, PhD, from École Polytechnique Fédérale de Lausanne (EPFL) in Switzerland and colleagues.

"The stimulation felt almost like what I would feel with my hand," Sorensen said in an EPFL news release. "I felt the texture sensations at the tip of the index finger of my phantom hand."

In addition to benefiting amputees, the technology could also be used to create artificial touch in robots used in surgery, rescue and manufacturing, the scientists said.

Their research was published in the journal *eLife*.

info The Amputee Coalition has more about limb loss at *amputee-coalition.org/limb-loss-resource-centre*

Advanced 3D Printer Shows Potential for New Tissues, Organs

Anthony Atala, MD, director, Wake Forest Institute for Regenerative Medicine, Winston-Salem, North Carolina.
Glenn Green, MD, associate professor, pediatric otolaryngology, University of Michigan C.S. Mott Children's Hospital, Ann Arbor, Michigan.
Nature Biotechnology, online

A new type of 3D printer may be capable of making muscle, bone and other types of tissue that are good enough for implanting in humans, scientists report.

So-called 3D "bioprinters" are machines that can print out cells in layered patterns, with the goal of creating human body tissue or even complex organs. But until now, a major stumbling block has been the scale of the printed structures.

"If you try to make something that's larger, it turns gooey and falls apart," explained Glenn Green, MD, an associate professor of pediatric otolaryngology at the University of Michigan.

Another limitation, Dr. Green said, has been the lack of blood vessels in bioprinted tissue: Larger structures are not possible without blood vessels to supply nutrients and oxygen.

The new technology, described in the online edition of *Nature Biotechnology*, seems to surmount those challenges.

Ultimately, the hope is to have 3D printers that can churn out any kind of human tissue—to replace tissue damaged by trauma, disease or birth defects, said Anthony Atala, MD, the senior researcher on the new study.

But that's the goal for the future, and many hurdles remain before the technique might be used in humans.

HOW BIOPRINTERS WORK

For now, Dr. Atala said, his team has shown that it's feasible to create ear, bone and muscle tissue that are "human-scale."

The researchers developed the new printing system over 10 years. It creates a biodegradable, plastic-like material that gives the printed tissue its shape, along with cells suspended in a water-based "ink." The tissue also has a system of "micro-channels" that allows nutrients and oxygen from the body to diffuse into the structure until a system of blood vessels can form.

Dr. Atala's team found that when it implanted bioprinted bone, muscle and cartilage into rodents, the structures matured into functional tissue, complete with a network of blood vessels.

The researchers also printed a human jawbone fragment that was the right size and shape to be used in facial reconstruction surgery.

Dr. Atala said his team plans to implant bioprinted cartilage, bone and muscle tissue into patients in the future, with funding from the Armed Forces Institute of Regenerative Medicine. The institute, which partly financed the current study, focuses on using regenerative medicine to treat battlefield injuries.

EXPERT COMMENT

According to Dr. Green, there's "no technical barrier" to implanting such printed tissues into humans—but there are some critical questions.

"We don't know what happens with these tissues long-term," Dr. Green said. Plus, he added, the experiments described in this study used materials that are not approved for use in humans. The jawbone fragment, for instance, was created with stem cells from human amniotic fluid.

As 3D bioprinting moves forward, Dr. Green said it will probably focus first on simpler structures that don't move or bear weight—including the ears, nose or bones in the skull—before trying to tackle more complicated tissue, or organs such as the heart, kidneys and pancreas.

info The U.S. National Institutes of Health has more on regenerative medicine at *nibib.nih.gov/science-education/science-topics/ tissue-engineering-and-regenerative-medicine*.

CHAPTER 16

Medication Smarts

Surprising Drug Side Effects

We all know that drugs can have side effects, but we don't always make the connection between the drug and the adverse reaction. That's because some drug side effects are surprisingly hard to recognize. That can be dangerous. A recent Harvard study found that adverse drug reactions accounted for more than 4 million annual visits to ERs and outpatient clinics. *Troubling symptoms that could actually be caused by a drug you're taking...* *

SYMPTOM: A dry, hacking cough that gets worse when you lie down at night— and that you don't think is caused by a cold, allergies or smoking.

Possible cause: An angiotensin converting enzyme (ACE) inhibitor, such as *lisinopril* (Zestril, Prinivil), *captopril* (Capoten) or *enalapril* (Vasotec). Patients are usually told that this class of blood pressure–lowering drugs can sometimes cause dizziness. But doctors don't always mention that a nagging cough will plague up to 20% of patients.

More clues: An ACE-related cough usually develops several months after starting the drug (although it may begin immediately)...is more common in women and the elderly...and usually will go away after a few days of stopping the drug (but this can sometimes take up to four weeks).

My advice: You might be able to switch to a different ACE inhibitor, but the "class effect" means that similar drugs often have similar side effects. You will probably need to discontinue the drug and switch to an angiotensin receptor blocker (ARB), such as *losartan* (Cozaar) or *valsartan*

*Never stop taking a prescribed drug or change your dose without consulting your doctor.

Robert Steven Gold, RPh, a hospital pharmacist and affiliate instructor of clinical pharmacy at Purdue University in West Lafayette, Indiana. He is the author of *Are Your Meds Making You Sick?*—a book that examines several adverse drug reactions.

(Diovan). These drugs work in much the same way as ACE inhibitors but don't cause coughing.

SYMPTOM: Irregular heartbeat (arrhythmia) that often occurs when you stand up after sitting or lying down—and feels as though your heart is pounding or racing as if you just exercised heavily.

Possible cause: A broad-spectrum antibiotic, such as *levofloxacin* (Levaquin) or *ciprofloxacin* (Cipro). Drugs in this class, known as quinolone antibiotics, can trigger *torsades de pointes*, a dangerous type of arrhythmia. Macrolide antibiotics, such as *azithromycin* (Zithromax), can also have this effect.

The risk for arrhythmias is particularly high in patients who take a quinolone antibiotic plus a thiazide diuretic, such as *hydrochlorothiazide* (Microzide), typically used for high blood pressure. Some diuretics can lower levels of potassium and change the heart's normal rhythm, which can magnify the arrhythmia caused by the antibiotic.

Lengthy episodes (10 seconds or more) of torsades de pointes can cause seizures, a loss of consciousness or even death.

My advice: Get to an ER immediately if you develop a rapid heartbeat. Tell the doctor that you're taking a quinolone or macrolide antibiotic. He/she will probably prescribe a different drug (assuming that you still need the antibiotic). In most cases, the heart will "reset" itself fairly quickly after treatment. This type of arrhythmia won't come back once the drug is discontinued.

SYMPTOM: Sudden psychosis, a change in mental status that affects you emotionally and physically, causing severe confusion, nervousness, slurred speech and/or poor coordination.

Possible cause: *Phenytoin* (Dilantin), commonly used to treat epileptic seizures and, in some cases, an irregular heartbeat. It's a tricky drug to use because there's a fine line between a therapeutic dose and a toxic dose. Most people who develop psychosis have been given a dose that's too high.

My advice: Don't neglect the laboratory tests recommended by your doctor. Patients who take phenytoin require regular tests—every three months or monthly if the drug dose changes or

adverse drug effects are suspected—to measure drug levels in the blood. Routine tests also measure albumin, a protein that binds to the drug. Phenytoin is more likely to cause problems in patients with low albumin levels (less than 3.4 g/dL).

Patients who experience a change in mental status will recover quickly once the drug is discontinued for a few days, then restarted at a lower dose. If toxic levels of phenytoin occur regularly despite decreasing the dosage, a different medication should be considered.

SYMPTOM: Sudden hearing loss. You might notice that you're having trouble hearing high frequencies (high music notes, women's voices, etc.) or that everything sounds a little "muddy."

Possible cause: *Furosemide* (Lasix), a diuretic that's often used to treat high blood pressure and swelling in the feet and/or legs. At high doses, it can cause a loss of potassium, which can impair the hair cells in the inner ear and the nerves that transmit sounds to the brain.

Most cases of ototoxicity (damage to the inner ear) occur in patients who take the drug intravenously. But it can also occur with standard oral doses, particularly when furosemide is paired with other drugs (such as the painkillers Celebrex and Advil) that also have hearing loss as a side effect.

My advice: If you're taking furosemide and notice any degree of hearing loss—or you suddenly develop tinnitus (ringing sounds in the ears)—see your doctor right away. Hearing loss is a rare side effect, but the damage can be permanent if the drug isn't stopped quickly enough. Careful monitoring is crucial, especially when using a high dose.

SYMPTOM: Intense abdominal pain that isn't accompanied by fever or other signs of illness.

Possible cause: Codeine or other narcotic painkillers. Many people know that these drugs can cause constipation, which occurs in up to 90% of those who take them. What they don't realize is that constipation that lasts for more than one or two weeks can lead to fecal impaction, an intestinal blockage that completely stops the passage of stools, causing intense pain.

My advice: Ask your doctor to prescribe the lowest possible dose. It won't completely prevent constipation, but it will reduce the risk for impaction. Be sure to drink a glass of water every few hours and get regular exercise. Fluids and exercise moisten stools and increase the frequency of bowel movements.

Also helpful: Take a daily dose of a stool-softening medication, such as *docusate* (Colace)…or use stimulant laxatives such as *bisacodyl* (Dulcolax) when you haven't had a bowel movement for several days.

Another option: Ask your doctor if you can use nonopiate forms of pain control, such as lidocaine patches.

---

1 in 6 Seniors Takes Dangerous Combos of Meds and Supplements —Don't Be a Victim!

Dima Qato, PharmD, MPH, PhD, assistant professor, pharmacy systems, University of Illinois, Chicago.

Judy Jou, MA, School of Public Health, University of Minnesota, Minneapolis.

Michael Steinman, MD, professor, medicine, University of California, San Francisco.

JAMA Internal Medicine, online

Millions of older Americans are taking prescription drugs in combinations that are extremely dangerous. Something as seemingly innocuous as taking a blood pressure medication with a statin…or taking a heart drug with an over-the-counter heartburn drug—even a nutritional supplement—could do irreversible harm.

What's even more disturbing: The number of people taking these combos has nearly doubled in less than a decade, finds a new study. It's now one in six—more than five million people.

Read on to learn the most dangerous drug combinations—and how to protect yourself or a loved one.

WHEN DRUGS COLLIDE

Between 2005 and 2006, University of Illinois researchers went into the homes, literally, of more than 2,000 adults between ages 62 and 85 (average age 71). They looked through their medicine cabinets to see what prescription medications, over-the-counter medications and dietary supplements they were taking. Five years later, they repeated the home drug inventory with a similarly representative group. The study was published in 2016.

Here's what they found: We're taking more drugs—and more supplements. The number of people taking more than five prescription medications—a threshold that makes adverse drug-drug reactions much more likely—went up from 31% to 36%. Use of supplements—especially omega-3 fish oil, vitamin D and coenzyme Q10—went up, too. Fish oil supplements alone went from 4.7% to 18.6%. These drugs and supplements may each play an important role in a patient's treatment plan, but they open the door to adverse interactions.

To explore that, the researchers zeroed in on 15 specific combinations of prescription drugs with other drugs (both prescription and OTC) as well as with supplements. They were looking at combos that could cause serious, possibly life-threatening, adverse effects such as kidney failure, uncontrolled bleeding and heart attacks.

In 2005, the percentage taking such dangerous combinations was 8.4%. By 2011, it was 15.1%, a near doubling. The percentage taking two or more of these extremely dangerous combos nearly tripled—from 1.6% to 4.2%.

THE MOST DANGEROUS COMBINATIONS

Most common dangerous drug-drug combo: Amlodipine (a calcium channel blocker for blood pressure) and simvastatin (a statin for cholesterol). When taken together, the result can be kidney failure, myopathy (severe muscle weakness) or rhabdomyolysis (a dangerous breakdown of muscle tissue). Over the course of the study, the percentage with this scary combo went up from 1% to 4%. Simvastatin or other statin medications taken with either niacin (to lower cholesterol) or warfarin (to prevent blood clots) also increases the same risks. While it's possible to take both drugs together safely, it requires careful management of doses by a doctor, while keeping a close watch on possible side effects.

Another common dangerous combo: Many people were taking blood-thinning medications, such as *clopidogrel* (Plavix) or *warfarin* (Coumadin), and also taking other supplements or OTC drugs that can greatly increase the risk for uncontrolled bleeding or clotting.

Major culprits: *Omeprazole* (Prilosec), a proton pump inhibitor for GERD…or aspirin… or *naproxen* (Aleve), an NSAID, for pain…or omega-3 fish oil…or garlic. Each of these can also "thin" the blood so the combination with Plavix can be dangerous.

Most common drugs and supplements involved in dangerous combos: Statins, blood thinners, NSAID painkillers and omega-3 fish oils. One contributor to the problem, according to the researchers—new guidelines that have led to more statins being prescribed to prevent heart attacks. More doctors are also prescribing fish oil supplements to patients, but many people also take these on their own— without realizing their interaction with other drugs they may be taking.

Frightening example: Plavix taken with Prilosec or an NSAID (aspirin, Advil, Aleve) is associated with increased risk for a heart attack or stroke—and death from cardiovascular causes. Despite this risk, nearly one million older adults now are regularly using Plavix in interacting combinations. In the five years of the study, Plavix use increased by 58% and aspirin use by 33%.

MORE ABOUT SUPPLEMENTS… NOT SO SAFE?

The most common supplements used were multivitamins or mineral supplements and calcium, the study authors noted.

It's not enough to know the number of medications and supplements patients are taking, because it doesn't tell which are helping and which are hurting, said Michael Steinman, MD, author of a journal editorial in *JAMA Internal Medicine*. Dr. Steinman is a professor of medicine at the University of California, San Francisco.

"We need to identify what the problems are and devise ways to help people avoid these problems," he said.

For example, St. John's wort, which is often taken for depression, can affect how other drugs work. These drugs include immunosuppressants, some HIV/AIDS drugs, birth control pills, the blood thinner warfarin, the heart drug digoxin and some tranquilizers (such as Xanax), according to the U.S. National Center for Complementary and Integrative Health.

Another study in the same journal found that doctors are often remiss in asking their patients about their use of complementary and alternative medicines.

On the flip side, many patients are often afraid to tell their doctor about the supplements they are taking, the researchers said.

For the study, Judy Jou, from the School of Public Health at the University of Minnesota in Minneapolis, analyzed survey data for nearly 7,500 adults. Of these, just over 42% did not tell their doctor about the supplements they were taking or alternative treatments they were trying.

"Not telling primary care providers about using complementary and alternative medicines can be dangerous, especially if the type being used creates adverse interactions with any medical treatments that a patient might be undergoing concurrently," Jou said.

Examples of this include the use of herbs and supplements that interact negatively with prescription drugs or movement-based therapies,

Just Fill Part to Start

Fill only part of a prescription for a new drug, advises Charles B. Inlander. "Split filling" a prescription lets you find out if the drug has undesirable side effects before you pay for a full prescription. Ask your doctor to write the prescription so that you can fill only part of it at first, then fill the rest later…or talk to your pharmacist about dispensing only some of what is prescribed. Most insurance plans allow split fills—but check with your insurer.

Charles B. Inlander is a consumer advocate and health-care consultant, Fogelsville, Pennsylvania.

such as yoga, that counteract prescribed physical therapy, she explained.

The study participants who were least likely to report alternative therapies were those who did yoga, tai chi or qi gong, and those who practiced meditation or mindfulness. Adults who used herbs or supplements and who had acupuncture were more likely to disclose, the researchers found.

When patients didn't tell their doctor about these practices, it was most often because their doctor didn't ask or patients felt the doctor didn't need to know, Jou said.

"Encouraging discussion of complementary and alternative medicine use can help prevent medical complications that may arise from simultaneous use of conventional and complementary and alternative medicines and treatments, as well as improving communication and trust between patients and providers," she said.

Don't be a victim: Let your health-care provider know every drug—prescription or OTC—and every supplement that you're taking. One key ally is your pharmacist, who is trained at spotting potential drug-drug or drug-supplement interactions.

Outsmart High Drug Costs

Rebecca Shannonhouse, editor, *Bottom Line Health*.

Just when you thought that drug-company greed couldn't get any worse, entrepreneur Martin Shkreli smirked and grinned as he pled the Fifth when being grilled by lawmakers at a recent congressional hearing. Shkreli, as you may recall, became the human face of mind-bending drug prices when his previous company raised the price of a lifesaving toxoplasmosis medication from $13.50 to $750 per pill!

No one has to be reminded that even if you have insurance, your share of drug costs—in the form of high co-payments or deductibles—can add up to thousands of dollars a year.

Simple price-matching secret: Use the Internet before you order your prescription. The latest resource is a new online company called Blink Health, which offers steep discounts—with the added convenience of ordering and paying for your drugs online...all you do is pick them up at your local pharmacy. (Check first to make sure your drugstore participates.)

Other cost-saving sites: GoodRx.com and NeedyMeds.org.

Another little-known fact: Pharmacies in the same town—and even in the same zip code—can charge wildly different prices. In one town, for example, a month's supply of the generic statin drug *atorvastatin* (Lipitor) cost $61 at Kroger and $196 at Kmart. At Blink Health, the same drug is priced less than $10. That's a huge savings.

PS: Shkreli is now facing criminal charges unrelated to drug pricing. Some call it justice. I call it karma!

Don't Buy Drugs at Drugstores

Secret-shopper and online surveys and analyses by *Consumer Reports*, ConsumerWorld.org and MarketWatch.com.

Drugs cost more at drugstores. Costco usually is the least expensive place to buy prescription medicines. Walmart and Kmart also have low prices. CVS was the most expensive drugstore chain for the drugs being studied, followed by Rite Aid. Over-the-counter medicines also cost less at big-box retailers than at drugstores.

Other items that cost more at drugstores: Food (example: Ben & Jerry's ice cream averaged $5.52 at drugstores but only $4.42 at grocery stores—a 25% difference), but special promotions can be good deals...certain makeup products...cleaning products, such as laundry and dishwashing detergent...office supplies, which generally cost less at big-box stores...gift wrap and greeting cards, which are less expensive at dollar stores...and photo prints, which are usually cheaper at Snapfish and Shutterfly.

OTC Painkillers That Can Be Deadly

Lynn R. Webster, MD, vice president of scientific affairs with PRA Health Sciences, a research organization, Salt Lake City, and past president of the American Academy of Pain Medicine. He is author of *The Painful Truth: What Chronic Pain Is Really Like and Why It Matters to Each of Us.* ThePainfulTruthBook.com

The Food and Drug Administration recently strengthened an existing label warning that non-aspirin nonsteroidal anti-inflammatory drugs (NSAIDs) increase the risk for heart attack and stroke. Popular over-the-counter medications including *ibuprofen* (Advil and Motrin) and *naproxen* (Aleve) are among the products affected. Taking these regularly for as little as a few weeks can put people's lives at risk…as could exceeding recommended dosages.

What to do: If you take an NSAID, keep your dose as low as possible and your duration of use as short as possible. People who have a history of heart disease, kidney disease or stroke should be especially careful to limit NSAID use.

Hidden danger: When you take a cold medication or sore throat medication, check the ingredients on the label for NSAIDs. If you see these, avoid extended use and do not take these medications if you also are taking a painkiller that contains any NSAID—the combined dose could put you in danger.

If you must take a painkiller for more than a week or so or if you have a history of stroke, heart problems or kidney issues, speak with your doctor about options other than NSAIDs. Acetaminophen could be a safer choice in certain circumstances, for example. Also, acupuncture and mindfulness meditation can help.

HIV Drug Offers Protection

High-risk people who took the drug Truvada were 86% less likely to contract HIV than those who took a placebo.

University of Montreal.

Heartburn Drugs Are Linked to Kidney Disease

James W. Lohr, MD, is a nephrologist and professor at Jacobs School of Medicine and Biomedical Sciences, University at Buffalo, The State University of New York.

Proton pump inhibitors (PPIs), such as Prilosec, Nexium and Prevacid, are recommended for only 14 days of use but sometimes are used on an ongoing basis for chronic conditions. Patients who need heartburn drugs for extended periods should talk to their doctors about alternative medicines such as H2-blockers, a group that includes Tagamet and Zantac.

The Overdose Danger

Jack E. Fincham, PhD, RPh, a professor of pharmacy administration at Presbyterian College School of Pharmacy in Clinton, South Carolina. He is also a former panel member of the FDA Nonprescription Drugs Advisory Committee and currently serves on grant review panels for the Canadian Institutes of Health Research Drug Safety and Effectiveness Network.

When you get a new prescription, the first thing your doctor does (after choosing the drug) is decide on the dose.

What most people don't think about: Your doctor's dosing decision is crucial—getting even slightly more of a medication than you need can greatly increase your risk for side effects. Correct dosing, however, can lessen (or even eliminate) side effects.

Each year in the US, drug side effects are estimated to cause more than one million hospitalizations and more than 100,000 deaths. Yet many doctors reflexively prescribe "average" doses without checking recommendations for optimal dosing based on such factors as age, sex and body weight.

For example, a 100-pound woman might be given the same dose as a 200-pound man…and a 75-year-old may be given the same dose as a healthy college student. It's not hard to guess who is more likely to have preventable side effects. While many people know that taking a blood thinner in a dose that's too high can have devastating consequences, recent research is focusing on other drugs that can also have dangerous side effects.

Important new finding: With blood pressure drugs and diabetes medication, in particular, excessive doses can increase risk for dizzy spells, confusion, falls and even death—especially among adults age 70 and older, according to recent research in *JAMA Internal Medicine*.

DOSING DANGERS

Common drugs to watch out for…*

• **Blood pressure drugs.** About 25% of patients who take one or more of these medications stop using them within six months because of side effects, and up to half quit taking them within a year. The majority of people who take blood pressure drugs will initially suffer from dizziness, unsteadiness, falls or other side effects. Alert your physician if you experience any of these side effects. Even though the discomfort typically wanes over time, it can often be prevented altogether by starting with a lower dose of medication.

Beta-blockers, such as *metoprolol* (Lopressor) and *propranolol* (Inderal), are particularly dose-sensitive. So are alpha-blockers, such as *prazosin* (Minipress). Women who take these drugs tend to have a greater drop in blood pressure/heart rate than men, so they typically need a lower dose. The same may be true of patients who have both high blood pressure and lung disease, who often suffer shortness of breath when they take excessive doses. People who take multiple blood pressure medications are also more likely to have side effects.

My advice: Tell your doctor that you would like to start with one drug. Emphasize that you'd like to take the lowest possible dose—and that you're willing to be retested (or check your own blood pressure at home with an automated blood pressure monitor) to make sure that the treatment is working.

• **Diabetes medications.** The risks for diabetes complications—such as nerve damage, blindness, stroke and heart attack—are so great

*Never change a medication dose without consulting your doctor.

that doctors tend to treat it aggressively. But oral diabetes drugs given in high doses can easily cause blood sugar to fall too low.

Example: Patients who take *glyburide* (Micronase) or *repaglinide* (Prandin) often develop hypoglycemia, excessively low blood sugar that can cause dizziness, confusion and other symptoms. Even if the initial dose was correct, physiological changes as you age and/or changes in your lifestyle could make that starting dose too potent. For example, suppose that you start exercising more and eating a healthier diet. You'll probably need a lower drug dose than you did before, but your doctor might not think (or know) to change the prescription.

My advice: Tell your doctor right away about any lifestyle changes that could affect your blood sugar levels, such as exercise frequency (or intensity), changes in meal timing, etc. Keep careful tabs on your blood sugar with home tests. If your blood sugar is consistently testing at the lower end of the recommended range (or below it), call your doctor and ask whether you should switch to a lower drug dose.

• **Painkillers.** Aspirin, *ibuprofen* (Motrin) and other nonsteroidal anti-inflammatory drugs (NSAIDs) are widely available and effective. But they're also dangerous at high doses. One study found that more than 70% of people who take these drugs daily on a regular basis suffer at least some damage to the small intestine. Like the blood thinner *warfarin* (Coumadin), they're a common cause of excessive bleeding.

My advice: Take the lowest possible dose… use painkillers as rarely as possible…and always take them with food. People assume that over-the-counter drugs are safe, but none of these medications are meant to be used long term (more than four weeks).

If you can, switch to one of the many brands of acetaminophen (such as Tylenol). It has about the same pain-relieving effects, but even with its increased risk for liver damage, acetaminophen (taken at the recommended dosage) is less likely than an NSAID to cause side effects.

• **Sedatives.** Valium and related drugs, known as benzodiazepines, are commonly prescribed sedatives in the US, but the standard doses can be much too high for women as well as older adults.

Medications such as *diazepam* (Valium), *triazolam* (Halcion) and *zolpidem* (Ambien) accumulate in fatty tissue. Since women have a higher percentage of body fat than men, the drug effects can linger, causing next-day drowsiness or a decline in alertness and concentration. In older adults, the drugs are metabolized (broken down) more slowly, causing unacceptably high levels to accumulate in the body.

My advice: Women who are given a prescription for one of these drugs should always ask if the dose is sex-specific. They can ask something like, "Do I need a lower dose because I'm a woman?"

Also, in my opinion, people age 65 or older should avoid these drugs altogether unless they have to take them for a serious problem, such as a seizure disorder. If your doctor says that you need a sedative, ask if you can use a shorter-acting drug such as *lorazepam* (Ativan)…if you can take it for a short period of time (less than a month)…or if you can get by with a lower dose.

Important: These drugs should never be combined with alcohol. The combination increases the sedative effects.

info To read more about a drug you're taking, go to *Drugs.com*.

These Four Common Drugs Can Sabotage Your Health…Here's What to Do

Spencer Nadolsky, DO, a board-certified obesity and family physician practicing in Olney, Maryland, focuses on lifestyle as medicine to treat his patients. He writes the "Lifestyle Medicine" column on *MedPage Today* with his brother Karl Nadolsky, MD, and is author of *The Fat Loss Prescription: 9 Step Plan for Losing Weight and Keeping It Off.*

Your medications may be interfering with what has been shown, time and again, to be the best medicine for most of what ails you…

Lifestyle medicine.

The problem: Common medications that you may be taking for allergies, high blood pressure, diabetes, depression and other conditions can cause you to gain or lose too much weight—or to be too tired to exercise.

And a whole lot of bad comes from that.

Read on to see whether you're taking any of these medications…and how to fix the situation if you are.

MEDS THAT FIGHT A HEALTHY LIFESTYLE

•Mood meds.

Problem: Certain antidepressants commonly prescribed for depression, anxiety and other mood disorders can affect weight. For example, *paroxetine* (Paxil) and *mirtazapine* (Remeron) often cause weight gain, while *bupropion* (Wellbutrin) can cause weight loss. (For some conditions, such as cancer, losing weight can be a problem.)

Solution: If an antidepressant you are taking is having a bad effect on your weight—by making you gain or lose when you don't want to—you might be able to switch to a different antidepressant that has the opposite effect on weight, says Spencer Nadolsky, DO, a board-certified obesity and family physician in Olney, Maryland, who co-writes a monthly "Lifestyle Medicine" column for *MedPage Today*. And most antidepressants don't affect weight at all, so switching to one of those is another option. "Or, if it's mild depression, you can consider cognitive behavioral therapy—talking to a psychologist—which is shown to work very well, too," Dr. Nadolsky says.

•Allergy pills.

Problem: Antihistamines can stimulate overeating. "There are histamine receptors in the brain that are on the appetite pathway, so if you're blocking the histamine, it may increase your appetite," Dr. Nadolsky explains. You might keep gaining weight over time, or you might just have a harder time losing weight over time—either way, it's not good.

Solution: If your allergy symptoms are primarily nasal, try switching from an antihistamine pill to an antihistamine nasal spray, which doesn't have the same effect on appetite. If you find that you can't get through the allergy season without a pill—for example, because you also have itchy eyes—then the best defense is awareness. Make sure that you counter the appetite impact of your antihistamine by keeping closer tabs on portion sizes and snacking—and try adding more exercise to your routine.

•Diabetes drugs.

Problem: Insulin reduces blood sugar levels but also causes weight gain. That's an issue if you need to inject insulin, but it's also a concern if you take oral drugs called sulfonylureas—they reduce blood sugar by making your pancreas push out more insulin. Again, weight gain can result. For many patients, "The underlying issue is that the weight problem is the cause of their insulin resistance and type 2 diabetes in the first place, so while they're getting their sugars down, they're worsening the underlying cause—which is the weight, especially around their waist."

Solution: Optimize your diabetes medications to support weight loss. To do so, talk with your doctor about the possibility of getting off sulfonylureas. "Those drugs have fallen out of favor, but I still see them prescribed a lot," Dr. Nadolsky says. The alternatives are metformin, SGLT2 inhibitors and GLP1 agonists. In some cases, these drugs, along with lifestyle strategies, can even help diabetics go off insulin. Says Dr. Nadolsky, "I've gotten a lot of people off insulin by using these medicines—and lifestyle, of course."

•Blood pressure pills.

Problem: Beta-blockers such as *atenolol* (Tenormin) slow your heart rate, which can make you feel tired…a huge obstacle to getting exercise. They also cause weight gain. "They block adrenaline, the hormone that causes your fat stores to come out so you can use them as energy," Dr. Nadolsky says. Beta-blockers also slightly reduce your metabolic rate, so you'll naturally burn fewer calories over the course of the day.

Solution: Get off beta-blockers if you can. Some people—such as those who have had heart attacks in the past or who have arrhythmias or heart failure—need beta-blockers to control their blood pressure. For most others, however, these drugs shouldn't be the first line

of treatment, says Dr. Nadolsky. Ask your doctor whether it's safe for you to switch to a different type, such as an ACE inhibitor, a calcium channel blocker or water pills (diuretics).

KEEPING YOUR EYE ON THE BALL: LIFELONG HEALTH

If this article helps you spot a specific prescription you take that's a problem, and you work with your doctor to swap it for another, that's a good start. But a more fundamental insight is that lifestyle medicine—which uses nutrition, exercise, adequate sleep and stress management to improve your health—can and should be your primary approach to staying healthy and managing chronic conditions. Medications have their place, but don't let them get you off a healthy path.

"With lifestyle medicine, the side effects are generally good, like looking better and feeling better," says Dr. Nadolsky.

We'll take those side effects any day of the week!

The Aspirin Question

Randall S. Stafford, MD, PhD, a professor of medicine at the Stanford Prevention Research Center and the director of the Program on Prevention Outcomes and Practices, both at the Stanford School of Medicine in Palo Alto, California. Dr. Stafford is a member of the Council on Aspirin for Health and Prevention and a leading developer of the content for The Aspirin Project, its educational program (AspirinProject.org).

I t seems harmless enough…popping an aspirin from that familiar little bottle tucked away in your medicine cabinet.

In fact, millions of Americans take an aspirin daily as a blood thinner to help prevent the artery-clogging blood clots that cause most heart attacks and strokes. But for many of these people, aspirin is doing more harm than good.

Recent finding: In a study of 68,800 adults taking daily aspirin therapy for heart attack and/ or stroke prevention, nearly 12% were doing so unnecessarily based on their limited chances of actually suffering from one of these conditions over the next decade. In doing so, these individuals were found to be increasing their risk for potentially dangerous side effects, such as internal bleeding, for no good reason.

A tragic toll: Among the more than 16,000 deaths each year linked to bleeding associated with use of nonsteroidal anti-inflammatory drugs (NSAIDs), about one-third of these deaths occur in those who take low-dose (81-mg) aspirin.

IS ASPIRIN RIGHT FOR YOU?

You may assume from these frightening statistics that aspirin is never worth the risk, but that would be a mistake. Whether you're trying to prevent a heart attack, stroke or cancer, to make the best decision about using aspirin, you and your doctor need to weigh your potential benefits against your potential harms and then make a choice based on your preferences. *When aspirin use may help…*

HEART ATTACK OR STROKE

If you've already had coronary bypass surgery, a heart attack or ischemic stroke (caused by a blood clot), taking aspirin and/or another blood-thinning drug, such as *clopidogrel* (Plavix) or *warfarin* (Coumadin), is wise. That's because study after study shows that aspirin significantly reduces the risk for a second heart attack or stroke. (A person whose risk for bleeding is extremely high may be an exception.)

If your goal is to prevent a first heart attack or stroke, the decision is a bit more complicated. Guidelines from the American Heart Association (AHA) and the US Preventive Services Task Force recommend aspirin for primary prevention in people at high risk for cardiovascular disease. In 2014, the FDA weighed in, releasing a statement that warned against widespread use in people of average risk.

My advice: I advise some—but not all—of my male patients who are over age 45 to take aspirin for primary prevention. For women, I advise aspirin for most who are age 65 and older. There are exceptions, especially for those who are at high risk for bleeding. Meanwhile, men and women younger than these ages sometimes have enough risk factors for heart attack and stroke that they will benefit from aspirin.

Scientific evidence: An analysis of multiple studies published in *The Journal of the American Medical Association*, involving nearly 100,000 people, showed that daily aspirin can decrease heart attacks in men age 45 and older by 32%. In women, research has found that the greatest benefit—for reduction in ischemic stroke and heart attack—occurs for those age 65 and older.

What's my criteria for recommending aspirin? If the patient's chance of having a heart attack or stroke in the next 10 years is higher than 5% to 10%.

To determine your heart attack and stroke risk: Use the cardiovascular disease (CVD) "risk calculator" created by the American College of Cardiology and the AHA. To download the calculator onto your computer or an app onto your smartphone, go to *My.AmericanHeart. org* (click on "Guidelines & Statements," then on "Prevention Guidelines").

If your risk is above 5% to 10%, talk to your doctor about whether you should be taking aspirin.

Important: Once you have your result from the risk calculator, you must balance your potential benefit from taking aspirin to prevent a heart attack or stroke against possible harm. Have you had gastrointestinal (GI) bleeding in the past? Are you regularly taking another anti-inflammatory medicine such as *ibuprofen* (Motrin), which also increases your risk for GI bleeding?

Are you age 80 or over? Aspirin might help you, but there's no solid evidence to guide your decision. Nonetheless, older adults have the most to gain from aspirin, but need to be particularly careful to avoid bleeding problems.

PREVENTING CANCER

In weighing your decision to take aspirin for heart attack and stroke, you also may want to take into account recent research showing that aspirin may help prevent cancer—and perhaps even extend the lives of people who have had a malignancy.

Landmark findings: When researchers at the University of Oxford analyzed dozens of studies on aspirin, they found that regular use of the medicine may help prevent cancer—with a 38% reduction in the risk for colon cancer and similar reductions in breast, esophageal and stomach cancers.

Check Up on Your Penicillin Allergy

Penicillin may actually be safe for most people who think they are allergic to it. In a small study, 15 patients who had been told by doctors that they were allergic to penicillin all tested negative for the allergy and could be treated safely when penicillin was given intravenously. Patients who are truly allergic must be treated with antibiotics that can be higher risk and more costly. To find out for sure whether you are allergic, be tested by an allergist.

David Khan, MD, program director, allergy and immunology fellowship program, University of Texas Southwestern Medical Center, Dallas, and author of a study presented at the recent annual meeting of the American College of Allergy, Asthma, and Immunology.

Note: There is some debate about whether low-dose aspirin is always enough, and it appears to take years of aspirin use to see a reduction in risk.

According to a study published in 2014 in *Anticancer Research*, regular aspirin users who had colon cancer were 60% less likely to have a recurrence or to die from the disease than colon cancer patients who weren't taking aspirin. Researchers theorize that cancer cells may spread throughout the body behind a protective shield of platelets—and aspirin may disrupt that process.

What this means for you: If you're a man over age 45 or a woman over age 65…and considering taking aspirin for primary prevention of a heart attack or stroke…and your risk for cardiovascular disease is "borderline" (around a 5% chance of having a heart attack or stroke in the next 10 years, according to the calculator)—your desire to prevent cancer (particularly colon cancer) may tip the scales in favor of regular use of low-dose aspirin.

With this level of evidence, however, no one should take daily, low-dose aspirin solely for the purpose of preventing cancer.

Medications That Hurt Your Eyes

Jeffrey R. Anshel, OD, optometrist and founder of Corporate Vision Consulting, which addresses visual demands in the workplace. He has written six books on computer vision concerns and nutritional influences on vision, the latest being *The Ocular Nutrition Handbook*.

Are your eyes dry or sensitive to light? Do you have blurred vision or "floaters"? These and other eye problems could be side effects of common medications.

Few people make the connection between changes in their eyes and medications they take—yet the truth is that many prescription and over-the-counter drugs cause ocular side effects. *Here are common symptoms and the drugs that could be causing them…*

Important: Contact your physician (eye doctor or primary care) if you have any of these symptoms. Most are not dangerous, and minor eye problems may be a reasonable trade-off for a potentially lifesaving drug. Always bring with you to the doctor a complete list of the medications you take—prescription and over-the-counter—and the doses. Stopping the medications can reverse the symptoms in many cases.

•**Abnormalities in pupil size.** Discrepancies in how your pupils react to light (called anisocoria) can be caused by a variety of medications, including Catapres (for hypertension), Donnatal (irritable bowel syndrome/ulcers), Humulin (diabetes) and Tavist (allergies).

If your pupils aren't always the same size—especially if only one pupil is abnormally enlarged—it's important to go to the emergency room immediately. The brain controls pupil size, so a disturbance there can cause pupils to be different sizes.

•**Cataracts.** If you live long enough, you eventually will develop cataracts (lenses that have clouded over, making it more difficult to see). Certain drugs may speed the process, including Coumadin (for heart disease), Plaquenil (malaria, rheumatoid arthritis and lupus) and most steroids.

•**Difficulty focusing.** The medical term for this condition is "accommodative insufficiency."

It grows more common with age and also is a side effect of some medications. These include Adipex (for obesity), Enduron (hypertension), Norpramin (depression) and Xanax (anxiety).

•**Double or blurred vision.** There are many potential causes for seeing double or for vision that suddenly blurs. Medications that can cause this include Adipex (for obesity), Celebrex (inflammation), Lamictal (seizures), Mevacor (elevated cholesterol), Tylenol (pain relief) and Zantac (ulcers).

If your blurred or double vision is sudden, severe and unrelenting, go to the emergency room immediately. This visual impairment is not only unsafe (for instance, when you are driving), but it could be a sign of a serious medical problem such as a stroke or brain lesion.

•**Dry eyes.** Many factors (including computer use, wearing contact lenses and allergies) can reduce tear production and cause dry eyes—and so can certain medications, such as Actifed (for allergies), Catapres (hypertension), Detrol (bladder control) and Paxil (depression).

Until you see your doctor, self-treatment options for dry eyes include blinking as often as possible…use of artificial tear solutions (available in drugstores and chain stores)…avoiding irritants, including eye makeup and air pollution… and wearing sunglasses. Or try an oral gamma-linolenic acid (GLA) product such as BioTears.

•**Eye irritation.** Redness in the whites of your eyes or irritations on your eyelids can be caused by medications such as Aricept (taken to improve cognitive loss), Cardizem (heart disease), Enduron (heart disease) and Voltaren (rheumatoid arthritis, osteoporosis).

•**Floaters and other visual disturbances.** Flashes of light or color, floaters and other visual disturbances can occur for a host of reasons, including as a side effect of a drug. Medications linked to visual disturbances include Benadryl (for allergies), Cardizem (heart disease), Elavil (depression) and Xanax (anxiety).

The causes of visual disturbances can range from inconsequential to potentially serious, so they should be checked out by your eye doctor as quickly as possible. This is especially true if you suddenly see flashes of light or if numerous new floaters appear—that could be a sign of a retinal detachment.

•**Light sensitivity.** Though there are other possible causes, light sensitivity may be a side effect of drugs (including recreational drugs such as cocaine and amphetamines). Drugs linked with light sensitivity include Diabinese (for diabetes), Dilantin (epilepsy), Lipitor (high cholesterol/heart disease), Pepcid (gastric ulcers) and Viagra (erectile dysfunction). If light sensitivity is severe and your pupils are enlarged—especially if only one pupil is enlarged—go to the ER. It could be a sign of stroke or a brain tumor.

•**Yellowed eyes.** Several conditions can cause the white parts of the eye to turn yellow, including illness, sun exposure and drugs such as Diabinese (for diabetes), Elavil (depression) and Librium (anxiety). Yellowing may be a sign of cirrhosis or hepatitis. It is important to see your doctor quickly to have this checked out.

To Sleep Better, Make Your Own Placebo

Article titled "The Placebo Effect: History, Biology, and Ethics," by Patrick Lemoine, MD, professor of psychiatry and director of clinical studies, University of Claude Bernard of Lyon, France, published in *Medscape*.
Ted. J. Kaptchuk, director, Program in Placebo Studies, Beth Israel Deaconess Medical Center, Boston.

Wouldn't it be great if you could just take a "sugar pill" to get to sleep?

Maybe you can. Recent research has shown that placebos—sugar or other non-active material given to patients in place of actual drugs—make good sleep medicine. About half of the effectiveness of prescription sleep medications comes from the placebo effect, research shows. The "real" drugs, meanwhile, may leave us groggy, memory-impaired and more accident-prone—and can lead to a drug dependency. They are widely overprescribed, especially amongst the elderly.

But if you know you're just taking a sugar pill, is it really a placebo? Don't you need to believe you're really taking a sleeping pill for the placebo effect to work?

One French doctor has devised a clever method that lets his patients use the power of the placebo to wean themselves from reliance on prescription or over-the-counter sleeping pills. *Here's how you can do it yourself...*

THE POWER OF PLACEBOS

First, a little background. The term placebo (Latin for "I shall please") has been used to refer to medicine for more than two centuries (Thomas Jefferson wrote about them), but most physicians believed these inert pills exerted no real physiological action—they simply allowed patients to fool themselves into feeling better.

Now we know better. The belief that you are taking medicine can unleash powerful, positive physical changes in your body. "A host of studies have shown that treatment with placebos elicits an array of physiological responses," says Harvard Medical School professor Ted J. Kaptchuk, who directs the Program in Placebo Studies at Beth Israel Deaconess Medical Center in Boston. "These include stimulating neurotransmitters such as the body's own opioids, cannabinoids, dopamine and serotonin, all of which can alleviate pain, depression, anxiety and fatigue. We have an entire pharmacy of substances within us—and placebos help trigger their action."

YOUR RECIPE FOR ZZZS?

Patrick Lemoine, MD, a professor of psychiatry at the University of Claude Bernard of Lyon in France, finds that many of his patients have trouble letting go entirely even if they have cut back. For them he uses homemade placebos to wean his patients off prescription pills. "It's a bit like when a child learns to swim and refuses to let go of a floating device the instructor has gradually deflated," he writes.

His weaning technique entails transferring prescription sleep medication into empty capsules and doing the same with sugar, then mixing the drug capsules and sugar capsules together so that on any given night, you won't know whether you're taking a real or fake pill.

Below is a plan based on his recommendations for patients who are used to taking a sleeping pill every night.

Make sure to first ask your pharmacist whether your prescription sleeping tablets can be safely crushed and ingested in capsules...

•**First, gather your materials.** Buy a bag of at least 150 empty capsules—choose the opaque sort over the clear—at your drugstore or online. Next, you'll need sugar, or, if you'd rather not take in even a tiny amount of sugar, you can substitute cornstarch. Finally, you'll need something with which to crush your sleeping pills—a mortar-and-pestle or, if you prefer, a capsule-filling kit (easily found online).

•**Next, count out 30 empty capsules.** Insert one finely crushed sleeping pill into each of 25 of the capsules. Now put about the same amount granulated sugar or whatever placebo material you have chosen into each of the remaining five capsules.

•**Put all of the capsules in a jar or empty pill bottle,** and shake gently to mix them around.

•**For the next month, take one capsule from this bottle each night.** On any given night, you won't know whether you've taken the sleeping drug or a placebo. But you will know that on any given night, there's a very good chance that you are taking the sleeping drug, because 25 out of the 30 capsules contain the drug.

•**The second month,** fill 20 capsules with the sleep aid and 10 with the placebo.

•**The third month,** make it even-steven—15 drug-filled caps, 15 placebo-filled caps. For the fourth month, it's 10 drugs/20 placebos. Fifth month, five drugs/25 placebos. For the last month, one drug/29 placebos.

By the end of the process, if all goes well, you'll be sleeping like a baby with almost no help from drugs. You may want to wean yourself from sleep drugs in just a few months rather than the full six, and that's fine. What's described above is not a scientifically proven method, but just one doctor's approach that works for some of his patients, so feel free to adapt the approach as you see fit.

For example, there's no reason to start taking a pill every night if you're in the habit of taking sleeping pills only when you feel that you need them. In that case, mix up a batch of sleeping pills plus some number of placebos beforehand, and take one pill when you feel that you need a little help. And if you have trouble giving up the idea that you might be taking a sleeping pill, you could go back to the 5/25 or even the 1/29 formula. You'll still be taking a lot fewer sleeping pills. (*Note*: If you're traveling, especially if you're flying, leave these pills at home. You won't be able to show that they are prescription medicines if you are asked.)

Another approach: Try a half dose of your standard sleeping pills, either cut in half (check with your pharmacist to see if yours can be cut in half safely) or mixed in with placebos as above. You can also use the placebo effect to make other types of prescriptions work better.

Finally, it's also possible that taking a placebo might work for you even if you know it's a placebo. "We've done several studies using 'open label' or 'honest' placebos (where the person taking them knew they were ingesting an inactive substance) with very good results," says Professor Kaptchuk.

In the end, learning to harness the power of placebos to get better sleep is really about activating your own abilities—and there are many paths you can take.

The Truth About Blood Thinners

Stephen Kimmel, MD, MSCE, professor of medicine and epidemiology at University of Pennsylvania School of Medicine in Philadelphia. Dr. Kimmel is the editor of two textbooks about pharmacoepidemiology and the author of nearly 200 medical journal articles.

For people at risk of developing dangerous blood clots—a main cause of stroke and other serious conditions—*warfarin* (Coumadin) has long been the granddaddy of anticoagulant medication. This pill is taken by about 3 million Americans.

Now: The FDA has approved four newer oral anticoagulants. (Other anticoagulants such as *enoxaparin* and *heparin* are available only as injections.) While the newer oral anticoagulants may offer certain benefits over warfarin, they are not the best choice for everyone.

Why this matters: Using the wrong anticoagulant drug (or dose) can have dire con-sequences, such as life-threatening bleeding in the brain or gastrointestinal tract.

WHY AN ANTICOAGULANT?

Anticoagulants are used by people who are at increased risk for ischemic (caused by a blood clot) stroke and transient ischemic attacks, or "ministrokes"…or deep vein thrombosis (a blood clot in a deep vein), which can lead to a deadly pulmonary embolism (a blood clot in the lung). Anticoagulants also help prevent clots from forming in people who have an abnormal heartbeat (atrial fibrillation)…or have received a heart-valve replacement.

THE WARFARIN STANDARD

Warfarin has been used in the US for decades and is very effective at protecting high-risk people from blood clots. It's the only anticoagulant approved for use in people with mechanical heart valves.

Here's the catch: The amount of warfarin in the body must be regularly measured via a blood test called the International Normalized Ratio (INR). This allows doctors to monitor and customize the dosage for each individual patient, but it also means that you'll need frequent blood tests—weekly or monthly—to make sure that the drug is working properly. This testing is crucial, but not all patients do it as often as they should.

In addition, when you take warfarin, you must closely monitor your diet. Foods that contain vitamin K, such as leafy greens, broccoli and spinach, help your body make normal clotting proteins, which means they will work against the drug's action. For this reason, you should be consistent in the amounts of vitamin K–rich foods that you eat. Otherwise, the drug's effectiveness will be affected.

Also, warfarin interacts with more than 700 prescription and over-the-counter drugs as well as many supplements, including ginkgo biloba, St. John's wort, coenzyme Q10 and others. You need to keep your doctor informed about everything you take. The newer drugs have far fewer interactions.

BETTER THAN WARFARIN?

Four alternatives to warfarin are now available in the US—*dabigatran* (Pradaxa), *rivaroxaban* (Xarelto), *apixaban* (Eliquis) and *edoxaban* (Savaysa). Clinical trials show a lower risk for hemorrhagic (bleeding) stroke with the newer drugs compared with warfarin. There is also a reduction in overall strokes with some of the newer drugs.

Other differences include…

•**No regular blood work.** There is no good way to monitor levels of these new drugs in the body, but they have proved effective without monitoring levels, so you won't have to endure weekly or monthly blood tests, as needed when using warfarin. However, the complete safety profile of new drugs is also unknown, and doctors cannot customize dosing for each individual.

•**There are no foods that work against the newer drugs,** as there are with warfarin. The newer drugs are as effective as warfarin no matter what you eat.

•**No antidote.** If a patient's blood becomes too thin and bleeding becomes uncontrollable, there is nothing to reverse it when using one of the newer anticoagulants. Warfarin does have an antidote.

Editor's note: More than 100 lawsuits have been filed on behalf of patients who were injured or died due to a major bleeding event after taking Xarelto. The manufacturer of Pradaxa agreed to pay $650 million last year to settle about 4,000 similar claims.

•**A link to kidney function.** The newer drugs can be affected by your kidney function, so your doctor will need to consider this when choosing a medication and its dose.

HOW TO CHOOSE?

If you're taking warfarin and doing well, you don't need to think about trying one of the newer drugs—unless there are strong, compelling reasons to do so (such as an inability to get necessary blood work). Remember, newer drugs don't have as long a track record as older ones. That's why it's important to thoroughly discuss your medication options with your doctor.

What to consider…

•**If you have difficulty remembering to take pills throughout the day,** once-a-day Xarelto or Savaysa may be best for you.

•**If you play sports or have a hobby that may cause a bleeding accident,** warfarin might be best, since it is the only anticoagulant with an antidote that allows doctors to stop uncontrolled bleeding.

•**If you have a history of stomach problems or gastrointestinal bleeding,** you may want to avoid Pradaxa and Xarelto—both medications have the highest risk for these complications.

•**If cost is an issue, you may want to consider warfarin.** The newer anticoagulants are marketed only in brand-name versions that are much more expensive (even with insurance coverage) than warfarin, which is available in generic form. With warfarin, you also have the cost of the necessary routine blood work, but this expense may be covered by your insurance.

Caution: Do not stop using an anticoagulant without consulting your physician—this drug helps control your increased risk for stroke and other blood clot complications. Because of the bleeding risk associated with anticoagulants, people who use these drugs should wear a medical identification bracelet.

Antianxiety Medication Can Slow Recovery

Study led by researchers at Timone Hospital, Marseille, France, of 1,062 patients admitted to French hospitals, published in *JAMA*.

Antianxiety medication can slow recovery from surgery. Patients sometimes take antianxiety drugs to calm themselves before surgery. But people who took *lorazepam* (Ativan) before a surgical procedure requiring general anesthesia needed ventilation tubes longer, had poorer-quality postsurgical sleep, had more postsurgery amnesia and took longer to recover cognitive abilities than people who took a placebo or nothing.

New Antidote for a Sometimes Fatal Blood Thinner

US Food and Drug Administration, Medscape and other media sources.

Dabigatran (Pradaxa), one of a new generation of blood thinners, has led to hundreds of fatal bleeding incidents, according to the manufacturer.

That's because there hasn't been an antidote. By contrast, if you're taking the blood thinner *warfarin* (Coumadin) and you get a cut, your doctor can give you an antidote so that your blood can clot normally and your wound can heal. When it's safe to do so, you can go back on warfarin.

Now the FDA has approved the first-ever antidote for Pradaxa—*idarucizumab* (Praxbind), an intravenous drug. The most common side effects include headache, low potassium, constipation, confusion, fever and pneumonia. Antidotes for other newer blood thinners such as *rivaroxaban* (Xarelto) are in development but not yet available.

The new blood thinners are more convenient than warfarin...no special dietary restrictions and no regular blood checks as you need with warfarin...but for many people, warfarin is still the best choice.

CHAPTER 17

Men's Health

Latest Thinking on the PSA Debate

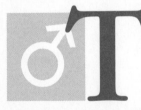

The prostate-specific antigen (PSA) test is the most controversial health issue facing men today. Many consider it crucial for early detection and treatment of prostate cancer, noting that in the years after it was approved, the number of prostate cancer deaths dropped by 40%.

The catch-22: Even though some experts believe that PSA testing has played a key role in reducing the number of deaths from prostate cancer, it can't differentiate harmless cancers (the majority) from aggressive ones. Studies have shown that men whose levels test high are only marginally less likely to die from prostate cancer, on average, than those who were never tested... and they're more likely to have biopsies, surgeries and other risky treatments that will make no difference in their long-term health.

That's why a 2012 task force advised against widespread screening. Within a year, PSA testing had dropped by 28%—but there was a corresponding decline in the diagnoses of potentially risky cancers.

To sort through the issues, we spoke with H. Ballentine Carter, MD, an internationally recognized expert in the diagnosis and treatment of prostate cancer.

Isn't early cancer detection always a good thing?

Not for prostate cancer. Most tumors discovered by routine PSA tests are indolent—slow-growing cancers that pose no risk to a man's long-term health. The tests do find some dangerous cancers, but not many. Over a 10-year period, only one life will be saved for every 1,000 men who are screened.

H. Ballentine Carter, MD, a professor of urology and oncology and the director of adult urology at Johns Hopkins University School of Medicine in Baltimore. He has published more than 200 papers and 32 textbook chapters on male urologic health. Dr. Carter is also coauthor of *The Whole Life Prostate Book.*

It's tempting to argue that saving the lives of a few men (particularly if you're one of them) outweighs the inconvenience for the thousands who aren't helped. But the test isn't merely a bother for those who test positive. Many of these men will be subjected to biopsies and other treatments, including surgery—and possible complications such as incontinence and impotence—for cancers that never would have been a threat.

Do you agree with the guidelines for curtailed testing?

It's worth pointing out that no government agency has ever recommended mass PSA screening. It's an important test for select men, but it's not for everyone—and it needs to be used more judiciously.

Consider an 80-year-old man who is expected to live for another five or 10 years. Does he need to have a PSA test? Probably not, because most prostate cancers are slow-growing. He's unlikely to die from prostate cancer, even if cancer cells are already present.

But a man in his 50s should consider having the test every two years. If his PSA is low—for example, between 0 ng/ml and 2.5 ng/ml—he can rest easy. If his level is high—10 ng/ml or above—he can work with his doctor to decide if he needs a biopsy or other tests/treatments.

Won't reduced screening cause more cancer deaths?

In the year after the 2012 task force recommended against routine PSA testing, the number of prostate cancer diagnoses dropped. Much of the reduction involved low-risk cancers, but there was also a reduction in the diagnoses of higher-risk cancers, according to a study published in *The Journal of Urology*. This is potentially worrisome, although it's unclear whether the "missed" diagnoses will eventually lead to more cancer deaths. The goal for now is smarter testing, not more testing.

What do you mean by "smarter"?

The PSA test can't distinguish meaningless tumors from lethal cancers. Yet some doctors urge men to undergo biopsies based on a single high reading. That's a mistake.

If a man's PSA is, say, 10 ng/ml, that's concerning. But what if the high reading is transitory and caused by something other than cancer? What if the lab made an error?

Even when a high PSA is caused by cancer, a single high reading might not mean it's a lethal cancer. I worry more about PSA velocity—the amount that PSA increases over time and how quickly it rises. A continuously rising PSA—especially more than one point per year—can point to an aggressive cancer.

What if my PSA tests high?

Don't panic. All sorts of things besides cancer can cause a high PSA reading—infection, inflammation and even ejaculation within the past 48 hours can cause a temporary increase. Your doctor should recommend a repeat test within a few weeks or months, possibly followed by annual or semiannual testing. Do not agree to a biopsy unless your doctor is convinced that cancer is a strong possibility.

Also helpful: A new test approved by the FDA in 2012, the prostate health index (PHI), looks at different types of prostate cancer-specific biomarkers—total PSA, free PSA and pro-PSA. The score from the combined factors is more reliable than PSA alone. Research has shown that this type of testing—along with even newer tests, such as the 4Kscore, that look for other cancer "markers"—can reduce unnecessary biopsies by about 30%.

What's the "sweet spot" between too much testing and not enough?

When the task force guidelines were issued, PSA tests were overused. Also, only about 10% of men who were tested and diagnosed with prostate cancer were managed with active surveillance. This approach doesn't rush men into treatment—they undergo monitoring that may include digital rectal exams and biopsies. The goal is to determine more precisely which men will truly benefit from treatment.

Active surveillance is now used in up to 40% of patients. This is good and might encourage more testing because men will be reassured that they'll be treated only for cancers that pose a real threat.

What advice do you have for men who want to be tested?

A healthy man, without a family history of prostate cancer (in his father, brother or son), should consider having a PSA test between the ages of 50 and 55 and then every two years but only after a conversation with his doctor about potential risks and benefits. Men with a family history of prostate cancer and African-American men—both of whom are at increased risk—should ask their doctors about earlier testing.

A man needs to ask himself if he can deal with the stress if his PSA is high, suggesting that he might have cancer. Can he live with the idea that he might have a "harmless" cancer? Onnecessary surgery or other treatments? That's exactly what we're trying to avoid.

Better Prostate Cancer Test

James McKiernan, MD, chair of urology, Columbia University College of Physicians and Surgeons, New York City.

An experimental urine test for genetic changes indicating prostate cancer identified 92% of men with elevated prostate-specific antigen (PSA) levels who had high-grade, deadly cancers, in a recent study of more than 700 men over age 50. The commonly used current PSA blood test cannot distinguish between high- and low-grade cancers, resulting in many unnecessary, painful and risky biopsies. The new test is at least a year or two away.

Low Vitamin D Levels May Signal More Aggressive Prostate Cancer

Adam Murphy, MD, assistant professor, urology, Northwestern University, Chicago.
Anthony D'Amico, MD, PhD, chief of radiation oncology, Brigham and Women's Hospital, Boston.
Journal of Clinical Oncology, online.

Prostate cancer may be more aggressive in men who are deficient in vitamin D, new research suggests.

A study of nearly 200 men having their prostate removed found those with low vitamin D levels were more likely to have rapidly growing tumors than those with normal levels of the "sunshine" vitamin.

"If men with vitamin D deficiency are more likely to have [more advanced disease] at the time of prostate surgery, then perhaps men should be tested for this when they are diagnosed with prostate cancer and subsequently supplemented with vitamin D if they are deficient," said researcher Adam Murphy, MD. He is an assistant professor of urology at Northwestern University in Chicago.

However, another expert isn't ready to go that far.

This study can't prove that vitamin D deficiency causes aggressive prostate cancer, only that the two are associated, said Anthony D'Amico, MD, PhD, chief of radiation oncology at Brigham and Women's Hospital in Boston.

But Dr. D'Amico thinks the results are important enough to spur further study into the possible connection between vitamin D and prostate cancer. "It's a hypothesis that's worth testing," he said.

For now, though, Dr. D'Amico doesn't think enough evidence exists to recommend vitamin D supplements to prevent prostate cancer or make it less aggressive.

Dr. Murphy said he has been exploring the link between prostate cancer and vitamin D for some time. He said racial distinctions were noted in this study, too, with black men having more aggressive tumors and lower vitamin D levels than white men.

These findings suggest that one reason black men have higher odds of developing—and dying of—prostate cancer is because of their "higher propensity for having vitamin D deficiency from the sun-blocking effects of melanin and perhaps dietary intake differences," Dr. Murphy said. The study could not prove this, however.

VITAMIN D SOURCES

The human body gets vitamin D from certain foods. These include fortified products (such as milk, orange juice and cereal), and certain fish (such as salmon), according to the U.S. National Institutes of Health. The body also makes the vitamin when the skin is exposed to sunlight.

Dark-skinned people have more melanin, which prevents burning.

RECOMMENDATIONS

Dr. Murphy said men with dark skin, low vitamin D intake or low sun exposure should be tested for vitamin D deficiency when diagnosed with prostate cancer or elevated PSA (prostate specific antigen), which is associated with the cancer. He believes supplementation is warranted for those with low vitamin D levels.

The study included 190 men having prostate surgery. The researchers found that nearly 46% of the men had aggressive cancer, and these men had vitamin D levels about 16% lower than men with slower-growing tumors.

After accounting for age, PSA levels and abnormal rectal exams, Dr. Murphy and his colleagues found that vitamin D levels below 30 nanograms per milliliter (ng/mL) of blood were linked to higher odds of aggressive prostate cancer.

The report was published online recently in the *Journal of Clinical Oncology*.

info For more about prostate cancer, visit the American Cancer Society website, *cancer. org*.

Why Men with Cancer Should Consider Sperm Banking

Pasquale Patrizio, MD, MBE, HCLD, professor of obstetrics, gynecology and reproductive sciences, director of the Yale In Vitro Fertilization and Preservation Program at the Yale School of Medicine in New Haven.

Cancer is no reason for a man to give up plans to father a baby. If you've been given a diagnosis of cancer and there's even a slight possibility that you will want to father a child in the future, have a discussion with your doctor about sperm banking. Technological advances now make it a feasible option for nearly any man who wants to pursue it.

Here's why you should discuss this before cancer treatment starts—chemotherapy, radiation and some surgeries can result in infertility by making you azoospermic (no measurable

---

Natural ED Alternative

Move over Viagra! Men who consumed the most flavonoid-rich foods (such as blueberries, apples, citrus fruits and red wine) had a 10% reduced risk for erectile dysfunction (ED) compared with those who ate the least, a recent 30-year study has found.

Possible reason: Flavonoids enhance blood vessel function and reduce inflammation, both of which improve blood flow to the penis.

Bonus: Men who were also physically active (brisk walking for two to five hours per week) cut their risk for ED by up to 21%.

Eric Rimm, ScD, professor of epidemiology and nutrition, Harvard T.H. Chan School of Public Health, Boston.

---

sperm count), by causing ejaculatory dysfunction or by removing reproductive organs. There's also some evidence that cancer itself can negatively affect sperm production, although not all studies show this.

What's stopping more men from doing this? Simple ignorance plays a part—one-third of men awaiting cancer therapy don't even know sperm banking is an option. But there are many misconceptions as well. To clear them up, we spoke with Pasquale Patrizio, MD, director of the Fertilization and Preservation Center at the Yale School of Medicine.

SIX MYTHS ABOUT SPERM BANKING

MYTH 1: It's too expensive.

Truth: It's probably far cheaper than you think. Collecting and initially freezing (technically called "cryopreserving") sperm costs only a few hundred dollars, and storage fees are about $50 per month. Some insurers will cover a portion of the cost of freezing if it's for a cancer patient.

MYTH 2: My sperm count is already too low, so banking sperm won't help.

Truth: Even if you haven't started treatment yet, your illness might have already taken a toll on your sperm count. This would be revealed during a semen analysis before cryopreservation. But the science has come a long way, and these days more sperm survive the freezing process. That's true even if there are only a few "units" of sperm—a unit is the contents of one ejaculate.

"With the technology that's now available in the laboratory, that can be sufficient to have a pregnancy," says Dr. Patrizio. As long as you have some sperm, you're a candidate for sperm banking, he says, "so freeze no matter what."

MYTH 3: I don't have time. I need to start cancer treatment ASAP.

Truth: Sperm banking is not time-consuming, and your treatment can wait a few hours or a day. A desire to get your cancer treatment started ASAP may be one reason why your primary care doctor or oncologist doesn't bring up sperm banking to you. (One study found that only 10% of oncologists offered sperm banking to all eligible men.) You have every right to start the conversation yourself if you're at all interested in fathering a child in the future. Even if you're too weak from your illness to ejaculate, surgical sperm retrieval is a possibility.

MYTH 4: It's too late—I already started cancer treatment.

Truth: Although it's highly recommended and ideal that men freeze their sperm before they start treatment, it's not absolutely a contraindication to freeze after cancer treatment has started. Have a conversation with a fertility specialist, who can educate you (and your partner if you already have one) about the risks of using sperm that have been exposed to chemotherapy or radiation, which include possible genetic abnormalities and an increased risk for miscarriage. But here again, technology is on your side—if you decide to use this sperm down the line, pre-implantation genetic screening can identify many chromosomal abnormalities in embryos before they are used to create a pregnancy.

MYTH 5: It's really too late. I never banked sperm, went through all my treatments, and now I don't have any sperm…but we still want to have a baby.

Truth: Don't despair! Many men begin sperm production again after a period of months or longer. After around a year, if you're still azoospermic, a specialist can perform a biopsy to see if any sperm can be extracted from your testicles. "In about 25% to 30% of cases, there is some very minute amount of sperm that can be detected in the testicle but is not enough to spill over into the ejaculate," Dr. Patrizio says. This sperm can be inserted into a partner's or donor's egg. Dr. Patrizio says he waits 18 months before diagnosing an azoospermic patient infertile.

MYTH 6: I'm too old.

Truth: Men can father children throughout their life spans. The real concern related to aging has nothing to do with cancer, actually. There's growing evidence that men of "advanced paternal age"—over age 50—"may have a slightly higher risk of fathering children with chromosomal disorders or diseases due to gene mutations, such as autism, Down syndrome or dwarfism," says Dr. Patrizio. That risk is worth discussing with a fertility specialist if you're considering fathering more children. But it has nothing to do with sperm banking.

More Prostate Help from Vitamin D

Bruce Warren Hollis, PhD, is a professor of pediatrics, biochemistry and molecular biology at Medical University of South Carolina, Charleston, and coinvestigator of a study of 37 men scheduled for elective prostatectomies, presented at the 249th National Meeting & Exposition of the American Chemical Society.

Vitamin D may eliminate the need for prostate cancer surgery. A man who is diagnosed with low-grade prostate cancer can consider taking 4,000 IU of vitamin D a day during a one-year waiting period. It slows the progression of low-grade prostate cancer and even may reverse it—eliminating any reason to remove the prostate.

How it appears to work: Vitamin D fights inflammation within the prostate gland.

ED Could Mean Low D

Erin D. Michos, MD, MHS, FACC, is associate director of preventive cardiology at the Ciccarone Center for the Prevention of Heart Disease, Baltimore, and leader of a study presented at a recent American Heart Association meeting.

Erectile dysfunction linked to vitamin D deficiency. Men with vitamin D deficiency are

32% more likely to have ED than men who are not deficient. Men with ED symptoms should have cardiovascular risk factors measured—such as blood pressure and lipid and glucose levels—because up to 80% of ED is thought to have vascular causes. But vitamin D measurement also is useful—the vitamin has a role in regulating blood pressure, glucose and inflammation.

VA Hospital Care Improving, Study Suggests

Harlan Krumholz, MD, professor, medicine, Yale University School of Medicine, New Haven, Connecticut.

Ashish Jha, MD, MPH, professor, health policy and medicine, Harvard T.H. Chan School of Public Health, Harvard Medical School, Boston.

Journal of the American Medical Association.

Veterans Affairs hospitals seem to do just as well as other US hospitals when it comes to treating older men with heart disease or pneumonia, a new study suggests.

The findings, published online in the *Journal of the American Medical Association*, were called "reassuring" in light of recent negative news about the nation's VA health care system.

Researchers found that between 2010 and 2013, men treated for a heart attack, heart failure or pneumonia at a VA hospital were slightly less likely to die in the next month, compared to similar men treated at a non-VA center.

They were, on the other hand, somewhat more likely to be readmitted to the hospital in that same time frame.

Still, the differences between the VA and non-VA groups were so small—usually less than one percentage point—that the outcomes really are comparable, said senior researcher Harlan Krumholz, MD, a professor of medicine at Yale University School of Medicine in New Haven, Connecticut.

"There've been many news stories in recent years suggesting that veterans aren't being well-served by the VA health system," Dr. Krumholz noted.

This study, he said, offers some reassurance.

Much of the negative press has focused on sick veterans who've been forced to wait months

for treatment—for everything from hepatitis to post-traumatic stress. In 2014, President Barack Obama ordered a system overhaul to address the issue, but it's not yet clear what the impact will be. By 2015, the number of vets on waiting lists had only grown, the VA reported.

Amid the controversy, Dr. Krumholz said, an "ongoing question" has been whether veterans ultimately fare worse than other Americans with the same health conditions.

Past studies have suggested that, at least when it comes to short-term death rates after hospitalization, VA patients do better. But those studies are at least a decade old, according to Dr. Krumholz and his colleagues.

STUDY DETAILS

The current study looked at records for men treated at 104 VA hospitals for one of three conditions: heart attack, heart failure or pneumonia. They were compared with men treated for the same conditions at 1,500 non-VA hospitals. All of the men were age 65 or older, and received care between 2010 and 2013.

Overall, the study found that VA patients had slightly lower rates of death in the month after being hospitalized. Among men treated for heart failure, for instance, 11.4% of vets died, versus 11.9% of men at non-VA hospitals.

VA patients were somewhat more likely to be readmitted within a month. Among heart failure patients, 24.7% were readmitted, compared with 23.5% of non-veterans, the study found.

EXPERT COMMENT

"I think the findings offer some reassurance that on at least one critical outcome measure—mortality—VA hospitals seem to be doing as well, if not better, than non-VA hospitals," said Ashish Jha, MD, a professor of health policy and medicine at Harvard T.H. Chan School of Public Health in Boston.

Dr. Jha, who wrote an editorial published with the study, said the slightly higher readmission rate is unlikely to reflect poorer care during the first hospital stay. That's in part because factors like income and education have a more "profound" effect on readmission rates than on death risk, Dr. Jha explained.

"We know that VA patients are poorer and more often minorities," compared to non-VA patients, Dr. Jha said.

Dr. Krumholz agreed that readmissions can depend on a range of factors, including hospitals' practices.

But while he saw the findings as positive, on the whole, he said there are still questions to be answered. For one, this study focused on older men with only three medical conditions.

Future studies, Dr. Krumholz said, need to look at other health problems, younger vets and women. Plus, he added, there are issues other than death rates and readmissions—including how well people recover after being hospitalized.

VA HOSPITAL SYSTEM STILL NEEDS IMPROVEMENT

It's already clear that the VA needs to do better, according to Dr. Jha. He pointed to a couple potential ways: The system could, for instance, focus on improving a small number of performance measures that "actually matter" to veterans.

"The VA actually measures a lot of different things, some of which are important and many of which are not," Dr. Jha said. "I think important measures for performance accountability include patients' experience, hospital-acquired infection rates and, of course, mortality rates."

He said the VA could also create incentives for hospitals that would improve patients' care, but are hard to "game." Employees at some VA hospitals were caught falsifying waiting list data to hide veterans' treatment delays, according to published reports.

"I think the key part is to ensure that incentives are tied to measures that matter to patients and clinicians," Dr. Jha said. "When you have large incentives tied to a bad measure—such as the 30-day waiting time—it's easier for some hospitals to just game it than to try to improve. That's what we saw happen."

The White House has more on veterans' health care reform at *whitehouse.gov/issues/ veterans/health-care*.

Better Prostate Cancer Recovery

Neha Vapiwala, MD, associate professor of radiation oncology, University of Pennsylvania Perelman School of Medicine, Philadelphia.

Radiation therapy for prostate cancer often results in side effects such as fatigue, erectile dysfunction and urinary incontinence.

New study: Men who did 75 minutes of yoga twice weekly during their six- to nine-week regimen of radiation reported stable or fewer side effects than those who did not do yoga.

Why: Yoga may help to strengthen pelvic-floor muscles and increase blood flow to the area.

Better Prostate Cancer Treatment

Christopher Sweeney, MBBS, associate professor of medicine, Harvard Medical School, Boston.

Men with hormone-sensitive stage IV cancer that had spread beyond the prostate to bones, lymph nodes or other organs lived an average of 14 months longer (58 months versus

Wait-and-Watch Warning

A review of more than 3,600 prostate cancer patients undergoing "watchful waiting" found that less than 5% were monitored appropriately, which means receiving routine prostate-specific antigen (PSA) tests, physical exams and at least one additional prostate biopsy within a two-year period. Inadequate monitoring puts these men at risk of having their cancer progress without them knowing it.

Karim Chamie, MD, MSHS, assistant professor of urology, David Geffen School of Medicine, University of California, Los Angeles.

44 months) when they received both chemotherapy and androgen-deprivation therapy (ADT) than those receiving the standard treatment of ADT alone.

Explanation: Adding chemo at the start of ADT, for those who could tolerate it, kept tumors dormant longer with relatively minor side effects (such as fatigue, low white blood cell count and infection).

Prostate Cancer–Alzheimer's Link

Kevin T. Nead, MD, is a resident physician, radiation oncology, Perelman School of Medicine, University of Pennsylvania, Philadelphia, and leader of an analysis published in *Journal of Clinical Oncology.*

Prostate cancer treatment is linked to Alzheimer's.

Recent finding: Androgen deprivation therapy (ADT) extends the lives of some men with prostate cancer—but those receiving ADT (a hormone therapy) were 88% more likely to be diagnosed with Alzheimer's disease than men not receiving ADT over a median follow-up period of 2.7 years.

Low Fertility Linked to Cancer

Analysis of more than 20,000 patients by researchers at University of Utah, Salt Lake City, published in *Fertility and Sterility.*

Lower fertility is associated with testicular-cancer risk. Men who sought infertility treatment were three times more likely to develop testicular cancer than men who were known to be fertile. The risk was 10 times higher in men with an abnormally low sperm count.

ED Drugs Don't Make You Good in Bed

Study of more than 2,600 men, ages 51 to 87, by researchers at The University of Manchester and NatCen Social Research, London, both in the UK, published in *International Journal of Impotence Research.*

Erectile-dysfunction drugs don't ensure good sex. Many older men with erectile dysfunction (ED) who used Viagra, Cialis, Levitra and similar medicines still expressed concern about their level of desire, frequency of sexual activity, erectile function and other aspects of their sex lives. Doctors need to give patients realistic expectations...and treat any psychological or relationship issues.

The Man's Sex Cure for Kidney Stones

Study titled "Can Sexual Intercourse Be an Alternative Therapy for Distal Ureteral Stones? A Prospective, Randomized, Controlled Study" by researchers in the department of urology, Clinic of Ankara Training and Research Hospital, and in the department of biostatistics and medical informatics, Akdeniz University Faculty of Medicine, both in Turkey, published in *Urology.*

You're a man. You develop a kidney stone. Ouch. It's not too large, so it's the kind that sometimes passes on its own. *Your doctor gives you three choices...*

•**Just wait and hope that it passes.**

•**Take a prescription medication such as *tamsulosin* (Flomax),** which relaxes muscles in the bladder, so stones can pass more easily.

•**Have sex three or four times a week.**

And the winner is...sex! In a study published in the journal *Urology,* 75 men with moderate-sized kidney stones were put into one of the three groups above. The results...

•**26 of the 31 men in the "have sex" group passed a kidney stone.** That's about 84%. It took an average of 10 days.

•**10 of the 21 patients in the Flomax group—about 48%—passed a stone.** It took an average of 17 days.

•**Only eight of the 23 patients in the control group—about 35%—passed a stone.** It took an average of 18 days.

Of course, the men didn't actually get to choose which group to be in—they were randomly assigned to a group, to make it a more reliable study.

PRESCRIPTION: SEX?

Before you call your friend who just got diagnosed with a kidney stone and give him the good news, be aware that this unique treatment is appropriate for only certain kinds of kidney stones. Stones that are larger than seven millimeters (mm) in diameter (a little more than one-quarter inch) are less likely to pass on their own, and those over 10 mm almost never do. These larger stones are generally treated with extracorporeal shock wave lithotripsy, in which shock waves from outside the body are targeted to the stone (or stones) to break it up so it can pass.

In this study, the average stone size was about 5 mm. These men also had stones on the lower end of the ureter—the tube that runs from the kidneys to the bladder. Kidney stones stuck in the middle of the ureter do pass on their own, but slightly less often, on average, than those lower down.

So these were the right guys for this experiment. How did it work? One urologist commenting on the study speculated that nitric acid, which is released to create an erection, relaxes the ureter, so stones may pass more easily. Male orgasm itself may also relax the muscles of the ureter.

The study prescribed sex with a partner, so there's no data on whether masturbation may also help pass kidney stones, although it's reasonable to assume that it may. And don't worry about passing a stone during sex—since kidney stones come from the bladder, it's not going to happen!

So...if you have a kidney stone—or have a friend who has one—and it's not too big...and you're not in unbearable pain...and you have a willing partner, go ahead and check in with your doctor about the kidney stone "sex cure." And if you don't have a partner who can help with your multiple weekly "treatments," there's probably no harm in, well, taking things into your own hands. Frequent ejaculation is already known to help protect the prostate from cancer, and for both men and women, having sex more than once a month is linked with both marital and personal happiness.

When you start to sweet talk your partner, explain that it's doctor's orders.

ED Might Also Mean Diabetes

Sean C. Skeldon, MD, is a family-medicine resident at University of Toronto, Ontario, Canada, and corresponding author of a study published in *Annals of Family Medicine*.

Among men ages 40 to 59 with ED, the probability of having undiagnosed type 2 diabetes was one in 10—compared with one in 50 for men who did not have ED. In men with diabetes, ED is likely due to damage to the blood vessels and nerves involved in erectile function. Screening for diabetes should be part of ED management—simply using a pill to achieve an erection will not treat the underlying condition.

Many Men Have Body Image Issues, Too

David Frederick, PhD, assistant professor, psychology, Chapman University, Orange, California.

Rick Gardner, PhD, professor emeritus, psychology, University of Colorado, Denver.

Aaron Blashill, PhD, assistant professor, psychology, San Diego State University.

Psychology of Men and Masculinity, online.

Women aren't the only ones at risk of worrying about their looks: A new study finds many men also fret about their physique, especially gay men.

Surveys on male body image found that 20% to 40% of men were unhappy with some aspect of their looks, including physical appearance, weight, and muscle size and tone.

Those feelings spilled into their health and sex lives, as well.

Many straight and gay men, for example, reported exercising (55% and 57%, respectively) and dieting (29% and 37%, respectively) to lose weight in the past year.

Twenty percent of straight men and 39% of gay men reported trying to hide one aspect of their bodies during sex, usually their bellies.

David Frederick, PhD, assistant professor of psychology at Chapman University in Orange, California, and the study's lead author, said men's body image is an issue that gets overlooked.

"We know so many women are dissatisfied, so it kind of gets lost that there's also a lot of men who are dissatisfied," he said.

The study was published online by the journal *Psychology of Men & Masculinity*.

Gender differences in "body dissatisfaction" are shrinking, likely because of media influence, said Rick Gardner, PhD, professor emeritus of psychology at the University of Colorado, Denver.

"Men are increasingly bombarded by messages related to weight and fitness," Dr. Gardner said. "And you rarely see a very overweight man in a TV ad or in a TV program or movie, unless they are playing the role of a buffoon or a bad guy," he observed.

Previous body image studies have shown gay men are at higher risk than straight men for developing body dissatisfaction. But those studies were based on small, biased samples that recruited participants from gay-affiliated political and support organizations, Dr. Frederick explained.

STUDY DETAILS

To overcome potential bias, Dr. Frederick and co-author Jamal Essayli, of the University of Hawaii at Manoa, drew data from more than 116,000 men across five national online surveys posted to general news websites.

Study participants' average ages ranged from 35 to 50.

Not only were gay men more dissatisfied with their appearance, but they were more vulnerable to social pressures regarding their appearance, the study found. *For example...*

• **77% of gay men felt they were judged,** or objectified, versus 61% of straight men.

• **58% of gay men routinely thought about how they looked,** compared with 39% of straight men.

• **58% of gay men,** but only 29% of straight men, felt pressure from the media to look attractive.

• **Gay men were also more likely than straight men to report interest in cosmetic surgery (51% versus 23%).**

Gay men "tend to mirror levels of body dissatisfaction found among heterosexual women," said Aaron Blashill, PhD, assistant professor of psychology at San Diego State University. That's likely due to both groups being attracted to men, he said.

"Men, regardless of their sexual orientation, place greater emphasis on physical appearance [of prospective mates], compared to women," Dr. Blashill continued. As a result, he said, gay men "may be more likely to both objectify their partners and themselves."

Being "overweight"—as defined by body mass index—did not register as a negative, but being "obese" did, the study found. Overweight men (63% straight, 48% gay) were satisfied with their weight.

Male Sexual Enhancement Supplements Often Ineffective, Possibly Harmful

Wake Forest Baptist Medical Center, news release.

There's no proof that over-the-counter sexual enhancement supplements for men work, and some are potentially dangerous, a new study reports.

Many men seeking medical help for sexual health issues report using dietary supplements. But with little regulation of dosage or ingredients, the health effects of these products are unknown, the researchers said in background notes.

Don't Pluck Those Nose Hairs!

Trim nose hairs, but do not pluck them. The hairs filter impurities in the air when you breathe, so pulling them out is not a good idea—and can lead to ingrown hairs and skin infections.

Neal Schultz, MD, dermatologist in private practice, New York City, and host of DermTV.com.

And many of these products contain traces of an ingredient used in drugs like Viagra that can be dangerous to men with certain health problems, the researchers added.

The researchers identified top-selling male sexual-help supplements and analyzed the ingredients, including those in products marketed to enhance erections, desire and sexual performance.

"While certain natural supplements we reviewed show promise for improving mild sexual dysfunction, they lack robust human evidence," study senior author Ryan Terlecki, MD, an associate professor of urology at Wake Forest Baptist Medical Center in Winston, Salem, North Carolina, said in a center news release.

"In addition, because of concerns that some products are impure or weak, we do not routinely recommend these products to our patients," he added.

Some of the most commonly used products include horny goat weed, ginseng, DHEA, ginkgo biloba, fenugreek and maca, the researchers found.

For many of the products, there's no scientific evidence to support claims they can improve libido, erectile dysfunction or sexual performance, the researchers said.

They also found that some of the supposedly "natural" products have traces of phosphodiesterase-5-inhibitors (PDE5Is), the medication found in prescription drugs—such as Viagra—used to treat impotence.

One study reviewed by the researchers found that 81% of tested samples of over-the-counter male sexual enhancement products bought in the United States and Asia contained PDE5Is.

"PDE5Is cannot yet be legally sold over the counter in this country," Dr. Terlecki said. "Men who use these medications without a physician's supervision run the risk of taking them inappropriately. Patients with advanced heart disease, for example, or who take nitrates, such as nitroglycerin, should not use PDE5Is as it may cause an unsafe drop in blood pressure. Likewise, men with severe liver impairment or end-stage kidney disease requiring dialysis should avoid these products."

Also, men who take medications such as *tamsulosin* (Flomax), *terazosin* or *doxazosin* to treat an enlarged prostate are at risk for dizziness and falls if they take PDE5Is at the same time, the researchers said.

The study was published recently in the *Journal of Sexual Medicine.*

Men, Avoid Impotence Drugs Before Surgery

American Association of Nurse Anesthetists, news release.

Men should not take erectile dysfunction drugs such as Viagra and Cialis just before surgery, experts say.

The drugs contain nitric oxide, which opens blood vessels and relaxes muscles. This can cause a patient's blood pressure to become dangerously low when combined with anesthesia and other drugs used during surgery, according to the American Association of Nurse Anesthetists (AANA).

The group advises men not to take Viagra or Cialis the day before surgery because the drugs take more than 24 hours to clear the body.

It's also important for men to inform the person administering their anesthesia about their use of erectile dysfunction drugs.

"Patients should never feel embarrassed about telling their anesthesia professional that they use these products," Juan Quintana, CRNA, DNP, AANA president, said in a new release from the association.

"Anesthesia professionals need to know this information to prepare the anesthesia plan, and to keep patients safe. As with all sensitive information, we honor the patient-provider trust," Quintana added.

It's also important for patients to share information about any other prescription drugs or complementary and alternative medicines they are using, such as ginseng, ginger or other dietary supplements.

Impotence Not an Inevitable Part of Aging

Texas A&M University, news release.

While the risk of impotence—erectile dysfunction—increases with age, men should know it's not an inevitable part of growing older, experts say.

About 30 million American men have erectile dysfunction. Worldwide, the number is expected to reach 320 million by 2025, researchers have estimated.

The problem affects 22% of men older than 60, and 30% of men older than 70. But the condition is most likely due to an underlying physical or mental health condition rather than older age, according to doctors from Texas A&M University in College Station.

Heart disease and other serious medical conditions—such as diabetes, kidney disease, multiple sclerosis and Parkinson's disease—can cause erectile dysfunction, the experts explained.

Certain medications, including antidepressants, antihistamines and blood pressure drugs, can also cause erectile dysfunction. These medications can affect nerves, blood circulation or hormones. If you suspect that's the case, talk to your doctor, the experts said.

Another potential cause of erectile dysfunction is emotional distress caused by relationship problems, depression, anxiety, low self-esteem, guilt and fear of sexual failure.

Unhealthy lifestyle habits—such as being overweight, smoking and excess drinking, and drug abuse—can also lead to erectile dysfunction. Eating foods high in flavonoids, such as blueberries, may reduce the risk of impotence, the experts noted in a university news release.

In addition, injuries to the lower body may also cause erectile dysfunction. So while exercise is healthy, men should be cautious about any activity that may put their lower body at risk for injury. However, despite concerns that cycling may contribute to erectile dysfunction, the experts said recent research has found this isn't true.

Regular Exercise May Boost Prostate Cancer Survival

Ying Wang, PhD, senior epidemiologist, Epidemiology Research Program, America Cancer Society, Atlanta.

Elizabeth Kavaler, MD, urology specialist, Lenox Hill Hospital, New York City.

Manish Vira, MD, vice chair, urologic research, Northwell Health's The Arthur Smith Institute for Urology, New Hyde Park, New York.

American Association for Cancer Research, news release.

Sticking to a moderate or intense exercise regimen may improve a man's odds of surviving prostate cancer, a new study suggests.

The American Cancer Society study included more than 10,000 men, aged 50 to 93, who were diagnosed between 1992 and 2011 with localized prostate cancer—meaning it had not spread beyond the gland. The men provided researchers with information about their physical activity before and after their diagnosis.

Men with the highest levels of exercise before their diagnosis were 30% less likely to die of their prostate cancer than those who exercised the least, according to a team led by Ying Wang, PhD, senior epidemiologist at the cancer society's epidemiology research program.

More exercise seemed to confer an even bigger benefit: Men with the highest levels of exercise after diagnosis were 34% less likely to die of prostate cancer than those who did the least exercise, the study found.

While the study couldn't prove cause-and-effect, "our results support evidence that prostate cancer survivors should adhere to physical activity guidelines, and suggest that physicians should consider promoting a physically active lifestyle to their prostate cancer patients," Dr. Wang said in an AACR news release.

Meat Intake Affects Fertility

Meat intake may influence men's fertility. The sperm of men who ate a lot of processed meats, such as bacon and sausage, were less likely to successfully fertilize a woman's egg than the sperm of men who ate more poultry.

Study of 141 men involved in fertility treatment led by researchers at Harvard T.H. Chan School of Public Health, Boston, published in *Fertility & Sterility*.

The researchers also examined the effects of walking as the only form of exercise. They found that walking for four to six hours a week before diagnosis was also associated with a one-third lower risk of death from prostate cancer. But timing was key, since walking after a diagnosis was not associated with a statistically significant lower risk of death, the study authors said.

"The American Cancer Society recommends adults engage in a minimum of 150 minutes of moderate or 75 minutes of vigorous physical activity per week," Dr. Wang said, and "these results indicate that following these guidelines might be associated with better prognosis."

Two experts in prostate cancer care said the findings shouldn't come as a big surprise.

"Physical activity helps all aspects of health," said Elizabeth Kavaler, MD, a urology specialist at Lenox Hill Hospital in New York City. "This study reinforces that a healthy lifestyle, including exercise, is one of the few aspects of post-cancer outcome that a patient can control."

Manish Vira, MD, of Northwell Health's Smith Institute for Urology, in New Hyde Park, New York, agreed.

The study "adds to the growing body of evidence that regular exercise is associated with better prostate cancer outcomes," he said. "Multiple studies have shown improvements in other cancers as well, including breast, colon and lung cancer."

"Regular exercise improves patients' cardiovascular health, quality of life, and likely, their overall ability to fight disease," Dr. Vira added.

Dr. Wang stressed that further research is needed to see if the findings might differ by patient age at diagnosis, weight or smoking.

Aspirin May Decrease Death from Prostate Cancer, Study Finds

Christopher Allard, MD, urologic oncology fellow, Harvard Medical School, Boston.

Sumanta Pal, MD, ASCO expert, and oncologist, City of Hope, Duarte, Calif.

Howard Scher, MD, chief, Genitourinary Oncology Service, Memorial Sloan Kettering Cancer Center, New York City.

Presentation, American Society of Clinical Oncology meeting, San Francisco.

Men who take aspirin regularly may have a lower risk of dying from prostate cancer, a new study suggests.

"We found that regular aspirin intake after prostate cancer diagnosis decreased the risk of prostate cancer death by almost 40%," said lead researcher Christopher Allard, MD, a urologic oncology fellow at Harvard Medical School in Boston.

However, he added, "It is premature to recommend aspirin for prevention of lethal prostate cancer, but men with prostate cancer who may already benefit from aspirin's cardiovascular effects could have one more reason to consider regular aspirin use."

Since this was an observational study, no one can draw a direct cause-and-effect link between aspirin use and risk of death from prostate cancer, said Sumanta Pal, MD, an ASCO expert and an oncologist at City of Hope in Duarte, California.

"These studies are certainly thought-provoking, but are best followed by formal clinical trials where we compare use of aspirin to either no treatment or perhaps a placebo," Dr. Pal said.

HOW ASPIRIN WORKS AGAINST CANCER

Still, Dr. Allard speculated that aspirin's ability to suppress platelets in the blood—which is why aspirin can cause bleeding as a side effect—might help explain how aspirin could prevent the lethal progression of prostate cancer.

"Platelets probably shield circulating cancer cells from immune recognition," he said. "By depleting those platelets, you're allowing the immune system to recognize the cancer."

Dr. Allard added that aspirin likely helps prevent the cancer from spreading to other areas of the body, such as the bone.

STUDY DETAILS

In the study, men without a diagnosis of prostate cancer who took more than three aspirin tablets a week had a 24% lower risk of getting a lethal prostate cancer. However, aspirin didn't affect the overall likelihood of being diagnosed with prostate cancer or even high-grade prostate cancer, Dr. Allard said.

Among men with prostate cancer, regular aspirin use after diagnosis was associated with a 39% lower risk of dying from prostate cancer. Use of aspirin before diagnosis didn't have a measurable benefit, the researchers said.

The study included information from more than 22,000 men in the Physicians' Health Study. The study began in 1982 to test the benefits and risks of aspirin and beta carotene in the prevention of heart disease and cancer.

Nearly 3,200 men were diagnosed with prostate cancer over the almost three-decade study. Just over 400 men developed lethal prostate cancer. Lethal prostate cancer was defined as either death from prostate cancer or the spread of prostate cancer to other organs.

Dr. Allard said men thinking about taking aspirin regularly for any reason should consult their doctor to discuss individual risks and benefits.

NEW BLOOD TESTS

Another study from the same meeting suggests that an experimental new blood test can be used as a "liquid biopsy." This test can then help determine the best medicines for prostate cancer patients.

Solid tumors shed cancer cells into the bloodstream. This test uses a computer to analyze the appearance of those cells, said lead researcher Howard Scher, MD, chief of the Genitourinary Oncology Service at Memorial Sloan Kettering Cancer Center in New York City.

Patients with circulating cancer cells that varied widely in appearance didn't respond well to hormone therapy, and survived for shorter lengths of time on average, the researchers said.

"It's remarkable that a blood test could help us profile cancers in real time, gleaning insights

that directly affect patient care decisions," Dr. Pal said. "Eventually, we may be able to spare some men with prostate cancer the significant side effects of hormone therapy."

Testosterone Therapy— Who Needs It? (And Who Doesn't)

Study titled "Effects of Testosterone Treatment in Older Men" by researchers at Perelman School of Medicine, University of Pennsylvania, Philadelphia, Harvard Medical School, Boston, et al., published in *The New England Journal of Medicine*.

Editorial titled *"Establishing a Framework—Does Testosterone Supplementation Help Older Men?"* by Eric S. Orwoll, MD, department of medicine, Oregon Health and Science University, Portland, published in *The New England Journal of Medicine*.

Eric S. Orwoll, MD, professor of medicine and attending physician, bone and mineral section, division of endocrinology, diabetes and clinical nutrition, Oregon Health and Science University, Portland.

Put 25 men in their 60s in a room, and odds are one is taking testosterone. Between 2011 and 2013, the number of American men prescribed the male hormone nearly doubled, from 1.3 to 2.3 million men.

Yet we still know so little about this huge human experiment. It's true that levels decline with age, which might contribute to low sex drive, muscle weakness, fatigue and depressed mood. But does taking testosterone really help? Is it safe? Or is it an ineffective, perhaps even dangerous fad created by a massive advertising campaign—to "treat" normal aging in men?

The best way to find out—careful medical studies. Now there is one. It doesn't answer all the questions, but it does identify the benefits—

Bro Out to Lose Weight

Men who want to lose weight should eat with other men.

New study: Men who shared a meal with one or more women ate 93% more pizza than when they ate with other men.

Cornell University

modest though they are—for a specific group of men.

Are you, or is someone you know, one of them?

THE TESTOSTERONE TRIALS

The new study homes in on men 65 and older with clinically low blood testosterone levels (less than 275 nanograms per deciliter) and symptoms, such as low libido/sexual function, difficulty walking or inability to walk at a normal pace (faster than 2.7 miles per hour for six minutes) or low vitality such as fatigue. It's the first large double-blind, placebo-controlled study—the gold standard—to study testosterone-replacement therapy in older men.

Even before the study got going, there was a significant finding. Most of the men who volunteered for the study didn't actually have low testosterone. When their blood was tested, only 1.5% actually qualified for inclusion. This is in line with other studies that find that many men being treated for "low T" don't have it—many don't even get tested. In this study, men who qualified got either topical testosterone gel—enough to raise their levels to the average for a man in his 20s or 30s—or a placebo gel. *Results...*

•**Sexual function improved—modestly.** On a scale of 0 to 12, scores for sexual activity went from 1.4 to 1.6 for the testosterone group, with no improvement for the placebo group. On a scale of 0 to 33, sexual desire improved from 11.9 to 14.15 for the testosterone group, while the placebo group showed no improvement. And increased erectile function went up only 3.1 points on a scale of 0 to 30—from 8.0 to 11.1—among those who got the testosterone.

•**Mood improved and depressive symptoms went down—slightly.**

•**There was no improvement in vitality or the ability to walk more easily or more briskly.**

UNANSWERED QUESTIONS

One big question that the study didn't answer—is testosterone therapy safe? It's still a muddy issue. There is concern that testosterone therapy may increase the long-term risk for prostate cancer, for example. Some studies have also shown that using testosterone might increase the risk for cardiovascular disease, while others have found no risk or even a protective effect. To be prudent, the study excluded men with significant symptoms of prostate enlargement and those at high risk for either prostate cancer or heart disease. In this short-term study of testosterone (one year of therapy), there were no serious adverse effects. But we'll need more research to fully answer the safety questions.

Also, this study does not shed any light on whether middle-aged men, who are the biggest consumers of testosterone, would benefit...or whether men with slightly higher levels than the study cut-off might improve, too. But it does find that there is a small group of older men for whom this may be an appropriate treatment. Just don't expect the world.

"On average, the effects are generally small, and it's not clear that they are clinically important," says Eric Orwoll, MD, in the department of medicine at Oregon Health and Science University in Portland, who wrote an accompanying editorial to the study. "It may be that the benefits of testosterone are more important in some men than others. Right now, however, there's no way to predict just who will benefit the most—or the least."

SHOULD YOU TRY TESTOSTERONE?

As a practicing physician, Dr. Orwoll would consider prescribing testosterone to men who fit the criteria of the study, have relevant symptoms and who want to give it a try. He usually prescribes a trial period of, say, three to six months to see if there is benefit.

So if you do feel your sex drive has diminished, talk to your doctor about getting tested for testosterone to see if it is low and to rule out other causes of your symptoms such as depression, stress, heart conditions and sleep apnea. Your doctor should also rule out any reasons not to take testosterone, such as high risk for heart disease or prostate cancer.

Whatever you choose, it's also important to realize that there are many ways to boost your testosterone level without drugs—such as by losing weight.

CHAPTER 18

Natural Cures

Natural Cures Tailored to Your Sleep Problem

Let's say you have trouble sleeping. You want to avoid prescription and even over-the-counter sleep drugs, which can be habit-forming and have bad side effects. You're leaning toward a safer, natural alternative...possibly melatonin.

You're wondering, What's the best sleep supplement?

But that's the wrong question.

Here's the right one—What's the best supplement to help me with my specific sleep problem?

To get answers, we spoke with Laurie Steelsmith, ND, LAc, a licensed naturopathic physician and acupuncturist in private practice in Honolulu. "There are lots of herbs and supplements to choose from that can help with sleep problems," she said. "In my experience, some work better for certain situations than others. In fact, melatonin, the most popular sleep supple-

ment, is usually not the best choice." (We explain why below.)

She also prescribes lifestyle changes that may help with each specific situation. For most of her patients, these lifestyle changes—and, if needed, specific herbs and supplements tailored to their particular situations—can help restore good sleep.

One caveat: "If you have a chronic medical condition or take any kind of medication, check with your doctor before taking supplements."

Here's what Dr. Steelsmith advises patients in her own practice....

IF YOU HAVE TROUBLE FALLING ASLEEP

"This is usually due to a busy mind, anxious thoughts and high levels of the stress hormone cortisol in the evening, when it should be low," said Dr. Steelsmith.

Before taking supplements, do this for a week: Try a calming bath to unwind at night, or relaxation therapy such as meditation or lis-

---

Laurie Steelsmith, ND, LAc, a licensed naturopathic physician and acupuncturist in private practice in Honolulu and author of *Natural Choices for Women.* DrSteelsmith.com

tening to a guided imagery recording. Lower the lights, quiet the house, turn off all electronics. "If you're still experiencing insomnia after a week, try taking one of the following supplements to help you drop more easily into sleep…and make sure you continue with the lifestyle changes."

•**Phosphatidylserine.** This supplement, usually derived from cabbage or soy, decreases cortisol at night. "Phosphatidylserine can help optimize your reaction to stress and support the proper release of cortisol," Dr. Steelsmith explained. She prescribes a product called Seriphos—she has been doing so for 23 years with good results—that contains 90 mg of phosphatidylserine. "Start with one pill an hour or two before bedtime taken with a small high-protein snack (such as a cracker with almond butter) for better absorption and to prevent stomach upset. If you tolerate it well and you need more support, take two pills. You can take up to two pills before bed and two in the middle of the night if you're waking up." Side effects are rare—occasionally, you might feel a little sleepy the next day, and very rarely, a paradoxical feeling of being more awake at bedtime. Avoid phosphatidylserine if you have kidney problems.

•**Valerian root and GABA.** Valerian root (an herb) and GABA (gamma-aminobutyric acid, an amino acid supplement) help to calm the nervous system. "They both bind to GABA receptors in the brain and can be taken alone or together," said Dr. Steelsmith. The standard dose of valerian root is 300 mg to 500 mg of a standardized extract of 0.5% essential oils taken one hour before bedtime. The standard dose of GABA is 250 mg to 1,000 mg taken one hour before bed. "Start with GABA first to see if you get the desired effect," she said. "I usually start patients with 250 mg at night, and increase the dose to up to 1,000 mg if necessary," she said. (GABA can cause serious cardiovascular side effects and nightmares in very large doses—10,000 mg—and should be avoided entirely by pregnant and lactating women.) Valerian root is safe and effective for most people, but side effects can occur, such as headaches, insomnia, excitability and a feeling of uneasiness. "If falling asleep is still a huge effort, take both at the same time. It's safe to take valerian root (up to

500 mg at night) and GABA (250 mg to 500 mg at night) for up to three months—while working on the underlying causes of your insomnia."

IF YOU HAVE TROUBLE STAYING ASLEEP

"Nighttime wakening can be one of the most difficult-to-treat sleep conditions," said Dr. Steelsmith.

One lifestyle tip: Make sure you're eating adequate calories for dinner. "Skipping dinner causes your blood sugar level to drop, which increases cortisol in your body and can wake you up," Dr. Steelsmith explained. "Eating a solid, healthful dinner that contains all three macronutrients—protein, fat and carbohydrate—can mitigate this."

•**5-HTP.** Another common culprit is too little serotonin. "This neurotransmitter makes us feel happier, calmer and more balanced and plays an important role in sleep," Dr. Steelsmith said. To boost serotonin, she often prescribes 5-HTP. This supplement is the active form of tryptophan, an amino acid that your body needs to make serotonin. It's often used to help people who are depressed, a condition that can be characterized by low serotonin levels. But your levels can be lower than ideal even if you aren't experiencing depression—and if so "5-HTP supplements can help you stay asleep," Dr. Steelsmith said. "Start with 100 mg taken at least one hour before bed, and gradually increase to 300 mg if you need it." At these doses, side effects are rare—but don't take this supplement if you are taking a prescription antidepressant (such as an SSRI) that also increases serotonin levels.

IF MENOPAUSAL SYMPTOMS ARE WAKING YOU UP…

Women who are in the menopausal transition (perimenopause) often have sleep problems due to hormonal fluctuations.

First step: Get your hormone levels assessed to see if your estrogen is too high and progesterone too low, or if both hormones are low. If progesterone is low, chaste tree berry (see next page) can balance levels, "but sometimes bioidentical hormones can help, too," Dr. Steelsmith explained. She starts with bioidentical progesterone, and if that isn't enough, may prescribe an estrogen cream to apply to the vagina or vulva. (For more on this topic, see *Bottom Line's* video, "Bioidentical Hormones" at *bottomline inc.com/bioidentical-hormones*.)

•**Chaste tree berry.** For women in perimenopause, this herb can help to naturally increase waning progesterone levels. "Progesterone is a calming hormone and can help even out a woman's fluctuating hormonal levels through its action on the pituitary gland," Dr. Steelsmith explained. It has been shown to help support healthy ovulation, which is essential for supporting progesterone levels, even during perimenopause." She presribes the product Asensia, a chaste tree berry–containing product that also contains other ingredients, including L-arginine and green tea extract, which in combination help the chaste tree berry be better utilized by your body. "It is very safe to use," she said. "It can be used long-term, but I prescribe up to one year."

•**Especially for night sweats.** "Asensia can help in women who are waning in progesterone," said Dr. Steelsmith, "and I have also found that Seriphos works great for insomnia associated with night sweats. I know, I have them!"

•**Got to pee?** Try to get up and do your business without turning on the lights or peeking at the clock. "But if every night you're being wakened about the same time, you could try taking a drop of a homeopathic sleep remedy such as Quietude by Boiron. It contains homeopathic doses of hyoscyamus niger, nux moschata, passiflora incarnata and stramonium. The tablets can be placed under the tongue and allowed to dissolve while you drift off to sleep."

IF YOU HAVE JET LAG OR WORK THE NIGHT SHIFT

If you've crossed a few time zones or regularly work through the night, you know that it throws off your circadian rhythm, making it hard to get back into a regular sleep pattern. Expose yourself to sunlight, especially morning sunlight, when you can, which will help regulate your internal clock. *A few specific tips…*

•**For jet lag, before your trip,** wake up and go to sleep earlier several days before a trip heading east…go to sleep later for a westward trip… and when you get to your destination, make yourself get up in the morning and work out.

•**For shift work,** you'll sleep better and be more awake on the job if you stick to the same sleep and wake schedule every day, even on days you're not working.

If these approaches don't work for you, consider…

•**Melatonin.** "A lot of people think they should pop melatonin whenever they have trouble sleeping," said Dr. Steelsmith, "but it's really only best for resetting a body clock that has been thrown off by shifting time zones or shift work." A typical dose is 3 mg under the tongue to be taken within one hour of when you want to fall asleep. "For jet lag, you can use it for a few nights to settle into a new time zone…or it can be used longer by people who have night shifts. It's often used long term for men and women who change their day/night sleep cycle frequently—such as doctors and nurses." Side effects can include headache, short-term depression, daytime sleepiness, dizziness, cramps and irritability. "Some people are very sensitive to melatonin, and even a typical 3-mg dose may be too much for them—I start patients with a 1-mg dose and slowly increase to 3 mg if they tolerate it well. I would not prescribe it to children or to young women who want to get pregnant. Because melatonin levels tend to naturally drop as people get older, I am most apt to prescribe it to patients older than 50."

NOURISH YOUR CALM

"All these strategies can help you feel rested and restored," said Dr. Steelsmith, "but to truly improve sleep, I believe that you need to take stock of how your energies are being spent—and adjust your lifestyle so that you nourish a calm nervous system. This alone will do wonders for people who are having trouble sleeping."

After all, you can't expect to be mentally overstimulated all day and then have your mind turn off at night like a switch. Exercise is also key—it "discharges stress and tension, and encourages sound sleep." She recommends getting regular physical exercise but avoiding exercising in the three hours before bedtime, when it could rev you up.

Finally…as a last resort, Dr. Steelsmith occasionally prescribes prescription sleep aides. "I think there is a time and place for them. I have prescribed them to patients who had intractable insomnia." Some patients need these only occasionally, but others stay on these long term. She prefers drugs such as Benadryl, which allow a person to wake up, rather than others such as Ambien, "which could put a person into a trancelike state where he/she doesn't remember what he has done if he gets up in the middle of the night."

A Natural Way to Treat Ulcers Without Antibiotics

Mark Liponis, MD, chief medical officer, Canyon Ranch, Lenox, Massachusetts. CanyonRanchDestinations.com

Andrew Rubman, ND, medical director, Southbury Clinic for Traditional Medicines, Southbury, Connecticut. SouthburyClinic.com

---

If you have an ulcer and tests show that you are infected with the common stomach bacterium H. pylori, the standard medical treatment is two antibiotics and a proton pump inhibitor (PPI)—sometimes with bismuth, the active ingredient in Pepto-Bismol.

This treatment works quite well most of the time. But there are serious drawbacks. Antibiotics can seriously disrupt your gut biome—the balance of bacteria that is essential to health.

It's no wonder that many complementary health practitioners, including naturopaths, often prescribe different regimens, relying on botanical and other supplements to bring H. pylori under control. But do they really work? Can readily available, over-the-counter, natural supplements treat ulcers as well as standard medical treatment can?

A trio of medical professionals at Canyon Ranch, a health resort with multiple locations that specializes in integrative and preventive medicine, decided to find out. Says lead study author Mark Liponis, MD, chief medical officer of the Canyon Ranch, "We wanted to find a treatment for H. pylori that avoided antibiotics and their side effects."

H. PYLORI: WHEN AN OLD FRIEND TURNS NASTY

Before we get into the details, one point is important to make. H. pylori isn't always a bad thing to have in your gut. The persistent bacteria has co-evolved with humans over tens of thousands of years—about half the people on Earth are infected with it, and in the US, it's about 20%—with both positive and negative effects. While it can cause ulcers and has been implicated in other stomach problems such as irritable bowel syndrome (IBS), H. pylori may protect against certain cancers and also helps ward off gastroesophageal reflux disease (GERD).

The truth is, most people who harbor the bacterium do just fine—about 80% of people with it don't get ulcers, for example. So if you don't have symptoms, there's no reason to mess with your H. pylori. But if you do have ulcers, which are lesions in the stomach lining that can be painful and debilitating, getting rid of this bacterium is the way to go.

AN EFFECTIVE COMBINATION

Dr. Liponis's team searched the existing literature for herbs with known activity against the bacterium that are also available in a commercial preparation. Once they had a formula, they tested it on 39 patients who were found to be infected with H. pylori and who had digestive issues such as peptic ulcer disease, irritable bowel symptoms or endoscopy-confirmed gastritis or esophagitis (inflammation of the lining of the stomach or esophagus)—all linked to overgrowth of the bacterium. Treatment lasted two weeks.

Results: 74% were free of the bacterium after two weeks, and all of these "responders" had improvement in their symptoms. None of the participants stopped taking the treatment because of side effects, although a few experienced minor abdominal cramping or increased gas.

It's a small study, and there was no control group, so more research is needed to establish this as a new treatment. But other studies have found that the standard antibiotic/PPI regimen is effective roughly 80% of the time, so the results are comparable.

SHOULD YOU TRY IT?

If you want to try this protocol, do so under the supervision of a health-care professional. An ulcer, gastritis, esophagitis and IBS are serious conditions, so you don't want to self-treat. According to Andrew Rubman, ND, naturopathic physician and *Health Insider* contributing editor, who has long used natural botanical treatments for ulcers, it's better and more effective to work with a physician who is expert in digestive issues and who can help you learn to encourage your body's own natural healing processes to cope with ulcers and other stomach and digestive challenges.

When you do talk with your doctor, you can share these details about this study's treatment protocol. *For two weeks, patients took...*

•**Mastic gum,** which comes from a plant grown in Greece. This is a traditional stomach remedy in the Mediterranean, and it has shown anti-H. pylori activity in the lab.

Source: Jarrow Formulas.

Dose: One 500-mg capsule, taken three times a day.

•**Oil of oregano,** which also has shown anti-H. pylori effects in lab studies.

Source: Biotics Research Corporation.

Dose: Emulsified oil of oregano, one 50-mg tablet, three times a day.

•**Bismuth,** which is already part of standard medical treatment for H. pylori. The team used Pepto-Bismol as a source, since it's readily available.

Dose: Four to six tablets a day in divided doses between meals.

•**A probiotic.** Why? While these supplements are kinder on the gut than antibiotics, they can still upset the balance of bacteria.

Source: Vital 10, which contains five billion bacteria from 10 different bacterial strains.

Dose: One capsule, taken twice daily.

•**A fiber supplement,** to "feed" the probiotic.

Source: Herbulk, a supplement that includes both cellulose, a source of insoluble fiber, and psyllium, a source of soluble fiber. "Soluble fiber promotes the growth of friendly bacteria," explains Dr. Liponis.

Dose: 14 grams a day (a heaping tablespoon) mixed in a large glass of water.

Then, for the next two weeks, patients continued just with the probiotic and the fiber supplement. The researchers also made a few adjustments for individuals. Some participants were sensitive to aspirin, so they were given a different bismuth supplement because Pepto-Bismol contains salicylates, the active ingredient in aspirin. Some patients already had such high-fiber diets that they didn't need a fiber supplement. But the goal was to find a standard regimen that relied on standard over-the-counter supplements.

Surprising Problems Hypnosis Can Cure

Roberta Temes, PhD, a psychotherapist, hypnotist and former faculty member in the department of psychiatry at Downstate Medical School, SUNY Health Science Center, Brooklyn, New York. She is author of *The Complete Idiot's Guide to Hypnosis: Mesmerizing Facts About Using Hypnosis for Mind and Body Health.* DrRoberta.com

You've probably heard that hypnosis can help you lose weight or quit smoking. But it can do so much more! It can provide quick relief—typically in one session—for a number of health symptoms. And unlike many medications, it has no unpleasant side effects. *Here are common problems that it can help...*

FEAR OF PUBLIC SPEAKING

Many of us get a little nervous about speaking in front of groups. Those who are truly terrified suffer from glossophobia, a severe fear of public speaking that can cause intense anxiety, a rapid heartbeat, profuse sweating and the strong desire to run away.

Some of my clients have been promoted to management positions that require regular presentations. They're grateful to advance their careers, but the public-speaking component frightens them.

During the hypnosis session: When my client is in a hypnotic state (see the box on the next page), I might ask him to visualize walking toward the stage and actually getting there and speaking.

Example: "You are walking with ease. You feel secure. You are comfortable. You are well-prepared and know your subject matter thoroughly. As you walk onto the stage, you begin to feel extremely pleased...you are a fine speaker...and you are enjoying yourself."

Then I will ask him to visualize himself actually making the speech and visualize the audience as friendly, approving people. I may have him visualize a particular person in the audience cheering him on. Or I may suggest that he is speaking to an empty room if that is what he has indicated comforts him. Once he sees himself, while hypnotized, speaking with calmness and confidence, he can easily replicate that in real life.

DENTAL PHOBIAS

Dental visits are rarely pleasant, but they cause much less pain than in the past. Yet many people are so frightened that they put off necessary visits for years.

During the hypnosis session: I'll often use a technique called dissociation, which permits a client to mentally escape from her immediate experience and drift off to a more pleasant place.

Example: "You are absorbed in a beautiful scene in your mind. You will be at the beach, and while you are concentrating on that image of a sunny day, the mouth will have no feeling."

Notice, I say, the mouth. That immediately dissociates it from her body. It is no longer her mouth—she no longer feels it.

If the particular dentist does not know any hypnosis, then I end our hypnosis session with the suggestion, "When you sit in the dentist's chair, every word said to you during this hypnosis session will be remembered and you will immediately take your mind to your scene of nature and all the hypnotic suggestions that you have received will be in force."

ANGER MANAGEMENT

Hypnosis can help you manage the expression of your anger.

During the hypnosis session: When an anger-management client is in a deep hypnotic

What Happens During Hypnosis?

Medical hypnosis is different from entertainment hypnosis, which you may have seen in a movie or on TV. You cannot be hypnotized against your will—you cannot be made to quack like a duck or reveal your deepest secrets. Hypnosis is simply a technique that changes the ways in which your brain interprets experiences.

About 15% of the population responds exceptionally well to hypnosis. They are the folks who can use hypnosis as anesthesia during surgery. About 20% respond only a little bit to hypnosis. For most situations, that little bit is all that's needed. The rest of the population falls somewhere in between.

A hypnotist's talent lies not so much in the ability to help the client become hypnotized but in the ability to choose the most appropriate words to say to the hypnotized client. We call those words the hypnosis script.

An induction is the technique that helps the client reach that state of suggestibility—the trance state. In movies, the client follows a swinging watch or pendulum. In my office, I ask the client to stare at a fixed spot on the wall, and then I'll speak in a slow, quiet voice, using words such as comfortable, calm, safe and secure.

You may have already experienced hypnosis and not known it.

Example: You drove to a destination and then couldn't actually remember having driven there. You were so absorbed in your inner world that you were oblivious to your surroundings. You essentially put yourself in a hypnotic trance.

The best way to find a good hypnotist is through word of mouth. There are scholarly hypnosis researchers who are poor clinicians and plenty of minimally trained lay hypnotists who do a good job. Sadly, there is no government licensing for hypnotists. You also can buy hypnosis CDs at *HypnosisNetwork.com*.

Roberta Temes, PhD.

trance, I suggest that he replay a recent anger situation in his mind. I then guide him through a visualization exercise in which he handles the original scene by counting to 10 before responding, and then he responds with calmness. I encourage him to reflect and analyze, rather than personalize, the confrontation. Habits rehearsed while a client is hypnotized can translate to the waking state.

PAIN RELIEF

Research has shown that hypnosis is an effective way to reduce or even eliminate pain. A study of burn patients found that those who underwent hypnosis experienced much less pain and that their need for painkillers was reduced by half. Many hospital burn units employ hypnotists.

Hypnosis can reduce anxiety, fear, negative expectations and feelings of helplessness and victimization. When those feelings are reduced, pain is diminished. But what I consider a fascinating use of hypnosis for pain control is reframing the pain. Reframing permits the patient to experience the pain from a new perspective.

During the hypnosis session: I might tell a patient, "When your body starts to heal, you'll feel some discomfort. That's good. Your body is letting you know that it is recovering. You will enjoy receiving these messages." This suggestion reframes pain so that it means something good.

Example: Imagine that two soldiers have each been shot in the leg. One feels terrible pain because he is focusing only on the injury. The other reframes the shooting and introduces a new aspect—perhaps this injury will cause him to be discharged and go home. With that thought, the pain becomes bearable.

ERECTILE DYSFUNCTION

Many men have physical problems—diabetes, vascular disease, etc.—that make it difficult to achieve or maintain an erection. But this problem also can be caused by sexual self-consciousness. A man who worries about his bedroom performance is more likely to have erection problems than one who is relaxed.

During the hypnosis session: I will encourage the man not to concentrate on himself or how his body is responding.

Example: "Think only about pleasing your partner. From this moment on, whenever you are having sex, you will be focusing on your partner. You will know that your mind can control your body, and without your conscious intervention, your brain will send the correct message to your penis."

Men who are self-conscious in bed sometimes feel the same way out of bed, so I might include a hypnotic script that fosters self-confidence. I also give a suggestion about expecting success.

Example: "In your body, your lungs function automatically. Your pancreas functions automatically. Your liver functions automatically. And so, your penis can function automatically, too. No need for you to worry about it."

I end the session with a confirmation that "you will always remember that your body is exactly the way it should be and that it is just right."

Natural Remedies to Save Your Sight

Jeffrey R. Anshel, OD, founder of the Ocular Nutrition Society and president of Corporate Vision Consulting, based in Encinitas, California, where he also has the private optometry practice E Street Eyes. He is author of *What You Must Know About Food and Supplements for Optimal Vision Care: Ocular Nutrition Handbook.* SmartMedicine ForYourEyes.com

V ision problems in the US have increased at alarming rates, including a 19% increase in cataracts and a 25% increase in macular degeneration since 2000.

Why the increase? Americans are living longer, and eyes with a lot of mileage are more likely to break down. But not getting the right nutrients plays a big role, too—and the right foods and supplements can make a big difference.

Of course, people with eye symptoms or a diagnosed eye disease should work closely with their doctors. I also recommend medical supervision for people who are taking multiple supplements.

But here are common eye problems and the foods and supplements that can fight them...

DRY EYES

The eyes naturally get drier with age, but dry-eye syndrome—a chronic problem with the quantity and quality of tears—often is due to nutritional deficiencies. Poor nutrition can permit damaging free radicals to accumulate in the glands that produce tears.

What to do: Take one-half teaspoon of cod liver oil twice a week. It's an excellent source of DHA (docosahexaenoic acid, an omega-3 fatty acid) and vitamins A and D, nutrients that improve the quality of tears and help them lubricate more effectively.

Also helpful: BioTears, an oral supplement that includes curcumin and other eye-protecting ingredients. (I am on the scientific advisory board of BioSyntrx, which makes BioTears and Eye & Body Complete, see below, but I have no financial interest in the company.) I have found improvement in about 80% of patients who take BioTears. Follow the directions on the label.

CATARACTS

Cataracts typically are caused by the age-related clumping of proteins in the crystalline lens of the eyes. More than half of Americans will have cataracts by the time they're 80.

What to do: Eat spinach, kale and other dark leafy greens every day. They contain lutein, an antioxidant that reduces the free-radical damage that increases cataract risk. (Lutein and zeaxanthin, another antioxidant, are the only carotenoids that concentrate in the lenses of the eyes.)

Important: Cook kale or other leafy greens with a little bit of oil…or eat them with a meal that contains olive oil or other fats. The carotenoids are fat-soluble, so they require a little fat for maximal absorption.

I also advise patients to take 500 milligrams (mg) of vitamin C three or four times a day (cut back if you get diarrhea). One study found that those who took vitamin C supplements for 10 years were 64% less likely to have cataracts.

The supplement Eye & Body Complete contains a mix of eye-protecting compounds, including bioflavonoids, bilberry and vitamins A and D. Follow instructions on the label.

COMPUTER VISION SYNDROME

The National Institute of Occupational Safety and Health reports that 88% of people who work at a computer for more than three hours a day complain of computer-related problems, including blurred vision, headaches, neck pain and eye dryness.

What to do: Take a supplement that contains about 6 mg of astaxanthin, a carotenoid. It reduces eyestrain by improving the stamina of eye muscles.

Also helpful: The 20/20/20 rule. After every 20 minutes on a computer, take 20 seconds and look 20 feet away.

REDUCED NIGHT VISION

True night blindness (nyctalopia) is rare in the US, but many older adults find that they struggle to see at night, which can make night driving difficult.

What to do: Take a daily supplement that includes one-half mg of copper and 25 mg of zinc. Zinc deficiencies have been associated with poor night vision—and you'll need the extra copper to "balance" the zinc. Zinc helps the body produce vitamin A, which is required by the retina to detect light.

Also helpful: The foods for AMD (below).

AGE-RELATED MACULAR DEGENERATION (AMD)

This serious disease is the leading cause of blindness in older adults. Most people with AMD first will notice that their vision has become slightly hazy. As the disease progresses, it can cause a large blurred area in the center of the field of vision.

What to do: Eat several weekly servings of spinach or other brightly colored vegetables, such as kale and yellow peppers, or egg yolks. The nutrients and antioxidants in these foods can help slow the progression of AMD. The National Eye Institute's Age-Related Eye Disease Study (AREDS) reported that patients who already had macular degeneration and had adequate intakes of beta-carotene, zinc, copper and vitamins C and E were 25% less likely to develop an advanced form of the disease.

Also helpful: The Eye & Body Complete supplement, mentioned earlier. It contains all of the ingredients used in the original AREDS study—plus many others, including generous amounts of lutein and zeaxanthin that were included in a follow-up study, known as AREDS2—and was found to have positive effects.

How to Care for Your "Other" Circulatory System

Andrew L. Rubman, ND, medical director of the Southbury Clinic for Traditional Medicines in Southbury, Connecticut.

Your body's ability to resist infections depends on a healthy lymphatic system, which drains excess fluids and captures (and kills) cancer cells, bacteria and viruses. But immunity, it turns out, may be only part of what this system does.

Intriguing new finding: For the first time, scientists have identified a "shadow" plumbing system that rapidly drains wastes from the brain. Age- or injury-related damage to the glymphatic system (named for the glial cells in the brain) could impair drainage and contribute to many neurodegenerative diseases, including Alzheimer's disease. *Key facts about the lymphatic system…*

SLUGGISH CIRCULATION

After blood delivers nutrients to the body's tissues, it "leaks" into the empty spaces between cells. The lymphatic system picks up this fluid (now stripped of red blood cells) and returns it to the circulation. Along the way, it passes through one or more of the body's hundreds of lymph nodes, which are packed with infection-fighting immune cells. The lymphatic system also includes the adenoids, tonsils, thymus and spleen. What happens when this system becomes overworked or "congested"? You might notice that some of your lymph nodes—in your neck, under the chin, in the armpits, etc.—are swollen and tender. This usually indicates that

an infection is brewing in a nearby area of the body. Your legs or arms also could feel puffy and bloated or swollen—a sign that lymphatic fluid is accumulating faster than it can be removed.

During a routine checkup, your doctor will feel for swollen lymph nodes in the neck, in front of the ears and around the armpits and groin, etc. Swelling and/or tenderness means that drainage is impaired.

Examples: Swollen lymph nodes in the groin area could mean that you have a pelvic or urinary tract infection. Swelling just in front of the ear could indicate an ear infection.

Important: If you notice swollen and/or tender lymph nodes that enlarge or persist for more than a few weeks, see your doctor—even if you have no other symptoms. It could be a sign of an immune system disorder (such as lupus) or cancer.

BETTER DRAINAGE

You're less likely to get an infection—and recover more quickly if you have one—if you follow these steps to help lymph flow efficiently…*

• **Contrast hydrotherapy.** This involves applying heat to an area, followed by immediate exposure to cold. The contrast causes tissues to alternately pump and relax, which pushes fluid through the lymphatic system.

What to do: Let's say that you notice swelling in one or both armpits. Soak a washcloth in water that's about 104°F—the temperature of a hot bath. Apply it to the area for three to five minutes, continuing to reheat the cloth when it starts feeling cool. Next, soak a cloth in ice water and apply it to the same area for a minute or two, then switch back to heat. Repeat the cycle three to five times, and do it three times a day until the swelling goes down. If there's no improvement within a few weeks, see your doctor.

• **Dry brushing.** Gently passing a brush (or a loofah) over the skin, from the extremities toward the heart (corresponding to the flow of lymphatic fluid), causes the underlying tissues to contract/relax. This pushes accumulated fluid just under the skin into deeper lymphatic ves-

*These therapies are generally safe but should be avoided by people with diabetes or other conditions that impair circulation and cause temperature insensitivities.

sels. I often recommend dry brushing that includes the face for patients with skin problems that may be caused by congested lymph, such as frequent blackheads.

What to do: Use a high-quality brush, preferably one that's made with natural bristles—it should feel stiff but still have a little "give." Slowly brush the affected area (or the whole body) with pressure that is firm but not painful. After a session, your skin should be slightly pink. If it's red or irritated, you're pressing too hard. Each session should last five to 10 minutes. Do it twice a day to keep your lymphatic system functioning efficiently.

•**Self-massage.** Some massage therapists are trained in lymphatic drainage massage. Professional treatments are a good choice for patients with lymphedema, swelling that may occur after a mastectomy or other cancer treatments. But for less serious lymphatic congestion, self-massage works just as well.

What to do: Very lightly stroke the congested area, slowly moving your fingers at least a few inches from the affected area toward your heart for a few minutes. If you are coming down with a cold, for example, gently stroke swollen lymph nodes every few hours.

•**Pokeweed salve/liquid.** I often prescribe this herbal therapy for patients with hard or tender lymph nodes due to inflammation/infection. The active ingredients are transported through the skin and act as a lymphatic solvent. Improvement usually occurs within a few days. It's typically applied two to three times daily for two weeks.

Pokeweed is available at most health-food stores, but I advise using it only under the supervision of a doctor who specializes in herbal remedies. The herb contains alkaloid compounds that can potentially cause serious side effects, including changes in heart rate and/or difficulty breathing. People with kidney disease or other chronic conditions should not use pokeweed.

•**More water.** If you're dehydrated, the kidneys are less able to filter and eliminate wastes. Buildups of cellular by-products thicken lymph and impair normal circulation. The usual advice is to drink eight glasses of water a day, but some people need more—or less. One way to ensure

proper hydration is to check your urine to see if it is pale yellow.

For a more accurate assessment: Buy a pack of urine dipsticks. They are inexpensive and sold at pharmacies with indicators to check specific gravity, a measure of urine concentration. If you're drinking enough water according to the specific gravity reading (ask your healthcare provider for your optimal reading), use the dipstick once a week. Otherwise, use it daily until your hydration status improves.

Natural Ways to Quiet Tremors

Monique Giroux, MD, a neurologist and medical director and cofounder of the Movement & Neuroperformance Center of Colorado in Englewood, CenterforMovement. org. Dr. Giroux was formerly a clinical fellow in integrative medicine at The University of Arizona and movement disorders at Emory University. She is the author of *Optimizing Health with Parkinson's Disease.*

Most people think of tremors—rhythmic trembling in your hands, voice, head or other parts of your body—as a red flag for neurological disorders such as Parkinson's disease and multiple sclerosis (MS).

That can be true. But this constant shakiness can also accompany a wide range of other conditions, including so-called essential tremor (ET), a chronic but harmless disorder that often is inherited and affects an estimated seven million Americans—a greater number than those affected by MS and Parkinson's disease. In some people, tremors also can occur as a side effect of common prescription drugs such as certain antidepressants, asthma inhalers, seizure medicines and immune-suppressing drugs. Even pain and anxiety can cause mild shaking or worsen tremors that are due to disease or medication.

If you suffer from tremors, there's no question how disruptive the problem can be to everyday life. Simple movements most of us take for granted—such as shaving, eating or simply writing a check—can turn into a shaky endurance test.

But quieting tremors is no small feat. Medications such as antiseizure drugs and mild tranquilizers are effective only about half of the time and can have troubling side effects, including drowsiness and confusion. Injections of *botulinum toxin* (Botox) can help head and voice tremors but are less effective for hand tremors because weakness can result as a side effect. An invasive procedure called deep brain stimulation (DBS) is reserved for the worst cases. This treatment, which can be quite effective, involves surgically implanting electrodes in the brain that are connected to a pacemaker placed under the skin near the collarbone. Electrical pulses are continuously delivered to block the impulses that cause tremors.

Good news: If drugs or surgery aren't for you or leave you with lingering symptoms, several natural therapies can help calm tremors by easing the stress and altering the brain chemicals and emotional responses that exacerbate the condition.

Important: Before trying natural remedies, be sure to avoid caffeine, smoking and/or excess alcohol—all of which can worsen tremors. Also, make regular exercise (especially strength training) a priority—tremors are more common when muscles become fatigued. *Natural treatments to tame any type of tremor...*

AROMATHERAPY

Breathing in the aroma of certain flowers and herbs can reduce tremors by enhancing brain levels of gamma-aminobutyric acid (GABA), a widely circulated neurotransmitter with proven stress-fighting effects. Raising GABA levels helps calm the overexcited neurons that can worsen tremors. *What to try for tremors...*

•**Lavender.** This fragrant blue-violet flower has been shown in a number of small studies to produce calming, soothing and sedative effects when its scent is inhaled. Lavender essential oil is widely available and can be inhaled in the bath (add five to eight drops to bath water for a long soak) or by dabbing a drop on your neck or temples.

SUPPLEMENTS

Certain supplements can ease tremors by enhancing muscle relaxation and/or reducing the

*Consult your doctor before trying these therapies to determine the cause of your tremors and for advice on the approaches best suited to your situation.

Your Jaw Might Be to Blame

There's a surprising source of many health problems—the jaw joint, reports Victor Zeines, DDS. The temporomandibular joint (TMJ) is a hinge connecting the jaw to the skull near the ear. According to Traditional Chinese Medicine, the joint is connected with the small intestine meridian—a line of energy based on the body's acupuncture points.

Result: TMJ problems can cause digestive disorders. They also can be responsible for trouble chewing, ringing in the ears, headaches, earaches, vertigo and neck and back pain.

Among the treatments for TMJ disorders: Jaw exercises...facial massage...stress management...and/or a nighttime mouth guard.

Victor Zeines, DDS, is a holistic dentist in New York City and author of *Healthy Mouth, Healthy Body: The Natural Dental Program for Total Wellness.* NatDent.com

---

body's overall stress levels or load of inflammatory chemicals, which can play a role in tremors caused by neurodegenerative diseases. Check with your doctor to make sure these supplements don't interact with any medication you may be taking and won't affect any chronic condition you may have...**

•**Magnesium.** This mineral helps to regulate nerve impulses and muscle contraction. Magnesium-rich foods include sesame seeds, beans, nuts, avocados and leafy greens. To ensure that you're getting enough magnesium, consider taking a supplement.

Typical dose to ease tremors: 200 mg to 400 mg daily.

•**Fish oil.** The omega-3 fatty acids in fish oil offer proven anti-inflammatory effects—systemic inflammation is implicated in neurodegenerative diseases such as MS and Parkinson's disease. Fish oil is abundant in fatty fish such as salmon, albacore tuna, mackerel and herring. Aim for two servings per week. If you don't like fish, consider trying a supplement.

**Because supplements aren't regulated by the FDA for purity, I advise looking for products that bear the "USP-verified" stamp on the label—this means they have met rigorous testing standards to ensure quality by the scientific nonprofit US Pharmacopeial Convention.

Typical dose to ease tremors: 1,000 mg to 1,500 mg daily.

•**Valerian, skullcap and passionflower.** These calming herbs have been successfully used as part of a regimen to ease tremors. The supplements can be found in combination products, including capsules, teas and tinctures. Follow instructions on the label.

BEAT TREMORS WITH YOUR MIND

If you suffer from tremors, it's common to think—Oh no...my arm (or other body part) is shaking again...this is so embarrassing! I hate this! While such thoughts are perfectly natural when tremors emerge, they are potentially destructive when trying to calm your condition.

What helps: Mindfulness can reset this negative thought pattern so that you stop viewing tremors as a problem, which only leads to distress that often worsens the condition.

Mindfulness is more than just relaxation. Often done in conjunction with deep-breathing exercises, mindfulness helps you simply observe your thoughts, feelings and sensations and let them pass without judging them, labeling them or trying to control them. By reducing the distress you feel about the tremors, you are no longer fueling the condition.

You can learn mindfulness from CDs or books.

My recommendations: Consult your local hospital to see if it offers mindfulness-based stress-reduction classes. Also consider trying other mind-body therapies that may help, such as hypnosis, biofeedback and breath work.

Natural Cures for Anger

Jamison Starbuck, ND, is a naturopathic physician in family practice and a guest lecturer at the University of Montana, both in Missoula. She is past president of the American Association of Naturopathic Physicians and a contributing editor to *The Alternative Advisor: The Complete Guide to Natural Therapies and Alternative Treatments.*

When it comes to human emotions, explosive and out-of-control anger is one of the toughest. It's not only hard on relationships at home, work and/or school,

it's also hard on the health of the angry person. Heart rate, blood pressure and the digestive system can all be affected. To curb anger, conventional doctors use both psychotherapy and prescription medications (such as antidepressants and tranquilizers). These approaches can help. But among the many patients I've treated for anger problems, lifestyle changes and natural medicine offer longer-lasting results. It's important to recognize that it's normal and healthy to feel and appropriately express anger, but when it becomes excessive, problems can develop.

If you or someone you love is struggling with anger, here's my advice...*

•**Watch your diet.** A good first step is to reduce known dietary nuisances such as caffeine, alcohol and high-sugar foods—all of which affect the brain and can interfere with your ability to cope with anger.

•**Review your hormone health.** Women can experience significantly worse anger when they are premenstrual or going through menopause. In men, anger often kicks up during middle age when their testosterone levels are waning. For both males and females, anger is common during puberty—another time when hormone levels are changing. If you suspect that your anger may be tied to your hormone health, ask your doctor about testing your testosterone, estrogen and progesterone levels. Both men and women have all three of these hormones, and for optimal emotional health, all three should be correctly balanced.

•**Check for allergens.** All kinds of allergies can wreak havoc with one's emotional stability. Whether you're allergic to inhalants (such as pollen, pet dander or dust) or to foods (such as dairy, wheat or eggs), these allergens can cause big problems. Sometimes, the only symptom of an allergy is emotional distress, irritability and/or volatile anger.

If you have frequent anger: Keep a diary of explosive events and the foods you ate and possible allergens in your environment during the 12-hour period prior to your angry feelings. Look for patterns. If you suspect a link, speak to your doctor about allergy testing. For food aller-

*If you have a chronic medical condition or take medication, talk to your doctor before trying any supplements.

gy testing, I recommend IgG blood testing…for inhaled allergens, IgE scratch testing.

●**Get more B vitamins.** Anger is often linked to fatigue and low blood sugar. Vitamins B-5 (pantothenic acid) and B-6 (pyridoxine), in particular, can help with both conditions. To ensure that your B vitamin levels are balanced, look for a B-complex supplement that includes B-5 and B-6.

●**Try botanical medicines.** Gentler than pharmaceuticals, herbal remedies can calm emotions without dulling the brain.

My favorite anger-fighting herbs: Passionflower and skullcap. Pick a product (tincture, capsule or tea) containing either one or both of these herbs. Individual sensitivities vary, so start with a low dose. Take it for several days to see whether your anger is improving. If it's not, slowly increase the dose, but do not exceed the manufacturer's recommended dose. Use during high-stress periods or any time that anger is a problem.

The 8 Best Homemade Cleaners

Mandy O'Brien, Wisconsin-based biologist and coauthor of *Homemade Cleaners: Quick-and-Easy, Toxic-Free Recipes.* She also runs the website LivingPeacefullyWithChildren.com.

There's no way to know all the chemicals you are bringing into your home when you use commercial cleaning products. Thanks to loopholes in ingredient-disclosure laws, cleaning-product makers are not required to supply a complete list. But independent testing shows that many cleaners contain harsh or even toxic chemicals that have been linked to cancer, asthma, and skin and lung irritation. That includes some cleaners labeled with reassuring words such as "green," "nontoxic" and "biodegradable."

Example: The product Simple Green Concentrated All-Purpose Cleaner says "nontoxic" and "biodegradable" on its label, but testing by the Environmental Working Group, an organization

of independent scientists, found that it contains a solvent known to damage red blood cells.

If you make your own cleaning products, you can better control what comes into your home. *The following eight do-it-yourself cleaners are safe, effective, inexpensive and easy to make…*

TWO-STEP DISINFECTANT THAT KILLS GERMS BETTER THAN CHLORINE BLEACH

1. Combine white distilled vinegar and water in a spray bottle in a 1:1 ratio. Spray this on surfaces as you would bleach.

2. Thoroughly wipe away the vinegar with a cloth or sponge.

3. In a separate bottle, add hydrogen peroxide and spray on the surface. Wipe off.

A researcher at Virginia Polytechnic Institute found that this system kills germs better than chlorine-based bleach. It's safer, too. Chlorine-based bleach (and commercial cleaners that contain it) can cause skin irritation and respiratory problems including asthma attacks, among other health concerns. Hydrogen peroxide is a type of bleach but is safer.

Important: Do not skip the wipe-down step. When vinegar and hydrogen peroxide combine, they produce peracetic acid, which has respiratory health risks similar to those of chlorine bleach.

SWEET-SMELLING SINK SCRUB

1. Mix one cup of baking soda…one tablespoon of ground cinnamon…and five drops of sweet orange essential oil in an airtight container. (Essential oils are available online and in pharmacies, health-food stores and at big-box retailers such as Target and Walmart. Prices vary but start at about $3 per ounce.)

2. Sprinkle a small amount of this mixture on a wet sink, and scrub with a cloth.

3. Rinse.

Baking soda is a wonderful mild abrasive—it removes grease, grime and soap scum without scratching surfaces.

SAFE LIQUID HAND SOAP

1. Combine three tablespoons of liquid castile soap with one cup of water. (Liquid castile soap can be purchased online and in pharmacies, health-food stores and at big-box retailers such as Target and Walmart, typically for 50 cents to $1 an ounce.)

2. Add up to 10 drops of your favorite essential oil. (This step is optional. Essential oil makes the soap slightly more antibacterial, but mainly it adds scent.)

3. Stir until the soap dissolves.

4. Pour the mixture into a liquid soap dispenser.

Traditional detergent soaps contain harsh chemicals derived from petroleum. Castile soaps are instead made from plant oils and are extremely safe to use in our homes and on our skin.

Helpful: Unlike some all-natural hand soaps, this one foams. Foaming does not improve soap's cleaning power, but it could save you money—when soap does not foam, people tend to use more than necessary.

FLOOR CLEANER WITH THAT FAMILIAR LEMONY SCENT

1. Fill a bucket with hot water.

2. Mix in two tablespoons (or two large squirts) of liquid castile soap and 20 drops of lemon essential oil.

3. Allow your mop to soak in this mixture until it's saturated, then mop as normal.

This simple mixture cleans hard-surface floors including wood, tile and linoleum without harsh chemicals. It leaves behind a lemon smell that those of us raised in the era of Lemon Pledge associate with cleanliness.

Tip: If you're bored with lemon-scented cleaners, feel free to substitute another essential oil, such as lime, orange or grapefruit.

GLASS CLEANER THAT WON'T STREAK

1. Combine one-half cup of white distilled vinegar with three-quarters cup of water in a spray bottle, and shake until mixed.

2. Spray on windows and mirrors.

3. Dry with a lint-free cloth or crumpled newspaper. (Newspaper is slightly more abrasive than paper towels, so it does a better job of removing dirt and debris...and newspaper does not leave behind bits of lint.)

Commercial glass cleaners often contain detergents that can leave streaks of residue. This simple vinegar-based detergent-free cleaner will not streak. (You might see streaks the first time or two you use it—that's the lingering residue from a previously used commercial cleaner.)

Tip: If you dislike the smell of vinegar, soak lemon peels, lime peels and/or orange peels in one-half cup of vinegar for at least one week. Strain out the peels, then use the now citrus-scented vinegar in place of the standard vinegar in the recipe above.

EFFECTIVE ALL-NATURAL DISH SOAP

This soap is meant for washing dishes by hand...

1. Add one-quarter cup of tightly packed, grated bar soap (castile soap is available in bar form) to one-and-a-quarter cups of boiling water, and stir until dissolved.

2. Add one tablespoon of washing soda (washing soda can cause skin irritation, so be careful handling it) and one-quarter cup of liquid castile soap, stir again, then remove the mixture from the heat. (Washing soda can be found in the laundry aisle of many supermarkets.)

3. Allow the mixture to cool, then add 20 to 30 drops of the essential oil of your choice.

4. Store in a glass jar or a soap dispenser.

EFFECTIVE NATURAL DISHWASHER SOAP

To make a natural dishwasher soap, combine one cup of borax...one cup of washing soda...one-half cup of kosher salt...and one-half cup of citric acid. Store in an airtight container. Use one tablespoon per dishwasher load.

SAFE AIR FRESHENER

1. Mix one cup of baking soda with 20 to 30 drops of your favorite essential oil. (Citrus oils, such as grapefruit, lemon, lime or orange, are good options.)

2. Sprinkle the mixture on surfaces that require deodorization, such as carpets or upholstery. Leave on for 20 minutes or more, then vacuum up. Or place an open container of the mixture near the source of the odor.

Some commercial air fresheners actually spread neurotoxins throughout the home. Rather than remove or cover the odor, many work by deadening your sense of smell.

Create Your Own Healing Space

Esther M. Sternberg, MD, director, The University of Arizona Institute on Place and Wellbeing...research director, Arizona Center for Integrative Medicine...and professor of medicine, The University of Arizona, all in Tucson. She is the author of *Healing Spaces: The Science of Place and Well-Being.*

To create your own healing space, start by locating a specific area in your home or in the office where you can have quiet when you wish.

Then spend a few days noticing the things you see and do that make you feel comfortable and relaxed, as well as the objects that have strong positive meaning for you. To add these elements to your living space, create an area on your bookshelf or on your walls. A healing space could also be a favorite chair, a single picture or even the wallpaper on your smartphone. *Also helpful...*

•**Let nature in.** It's no coincidence that most people enjoy outdoorsy scents (such as pine and newly cut grass) and find sounds like surf and windswept trees relaxing. If your room lacks a window facing a pleasant scene, put up a landscape painting you find relaxing, and add some houseplants or cut flowers to the area. You could also add a scented cushion (for example, pillows filled with dried lavender buds give off a pleasing fragrance). Essential oils used in a spray bottle and scented candles can provide scents from nature as well.

Note: Some people are allergic to certain scents or plants. Check with your doctor before using.

•**Add soothing sounds.** Put a CD or MP3 player in your space to provide soothing music. You can find many types of relaxing music, including nature sounds, for free on the web (try *CalmSound.com* and *SoundOasis.com*).

Also: Gary Malkin, an award-winning film scorer, composes beautiful relaxing music (go to *www.musaic.biz/gary.html* and click on "The Vault").

HOW TO USE HEALING LIGHT

Exposure to sunlight has been linked to mood. For example, studies in Canada in winter have shown that depressed patients placed on the sunny side of hospital wards were discharged earlier than those on the darker side of wards. When creating your own healing space, pay close attention to light.

What to do: Use lamps that will give you the light levels you respond best to, and when possible, choose a space with ample windows for natural light. If there is little natural light in the room, try a full-spectrum light box. The devices are available online and range from $100 to $500. They may be covered by insurance if you've been diagnosed with seasonal affective disorder (SAD) or depression. People with diabetes, eye disease or bipolar disorder should check with their doctor before using a light box.

Beat Body Odors Naturally

Jamison Starbuck, ND, is a naturopathic physician in family practice and a guest lecturer at the University of Montana, both in Missoula. She is past president of the American Association of Naturopathic Physicians and a contributing editor to *The Alternative Advisor: The Complete Guide to Natural Therapies and Alternative Treatments.*

Body odor can develop for several reasons—poor hygiene, poor diet, inadequate hydration, disease and the use of certain medications, such as antibiotics. Fungi and bacteria can live on the skin and in body parts, too, causing musty, funky odors. Infections of all sorts—such as strep throat or an ear or a vaginal infection—will cause a putrid odor around the affected body part. Liver disease can result in a dusty, mousy body odor. Deodorant can help temporarily but isn't a cure.

If you don't like how you smell...

•**Consider what you eat.** A diet high in animal fat and protein—such as cheese, milk, meat and eggs—will create more body odor than a diet high in fruits and vegetables. This odor comes mainly from the by-products of fat and protein digestion.

What helps: Reduce your animal food intake by half, and double your fruit and vegetable intake. Do this for 10 days. If your diet was the culprit, you'll start smelling better!

•**Avoid garlic and onions.** These foods release sulfur-smelling compounds through the lungs and skin.

If you can't make yourself give them up, try this: Rather than having garlic or onions raw, cook them. This helps reduce the sulfuric compounds that lead to body odor. The spice cumin can also make you smell bad. If it does, avoid it.

•**Drink water as your primary beverage.** Coffee creates the infamous "coffee breath," and sugary beverages (and sweets in general) increase your risk for fungus, the organism primarily responsible for jock itch, vaginitis and stinky feet.

What helps: Drink half your body weight in ounces of water daily.

•**Try tea.** Certain herbal teas gently support liver health, reducing body odor caused by medication or high-fat foods. My favorite is a combination of the liver-healthy herbs dandelion root, burdock root, yellow dock root and milk thistle.* You may be able to find all of these herbs in a premixed tea, or you can buy small amounts of each and combine them in equal parts yourself.

What to do: Use two teaspoons of dried herb mix per 10 ounces of water. Simmer or steep for five minutes, and drink 24 ounces a day. It may take 10 or more days to notice significant changes in body odor with this tea.

•**Do a vinegar spritz.** While it won't cure the problem—smells are most often generated from the inside out—vinegar can kill fungi and bacteria on the skin, thus reducing odor caused by these organisms. Use a 50/50 white vinegar/water solution, and spray it over your feet, armpits and genitalia. Towel off after a minute or two (the vinegar smell will quickly dissipate).

Important: If your body odor persists and/or is noticed by others—and does not improve with these suggestions—see your doctor. Very strong body odor can be a sign of serious disease such as infection, cancer or organ failure.

*Avoid these herbs if you have a ragweed allergy. Check first with your doctor if you have a chronic condition or take medication, since these herbs could interact.

Pain News

The Best Foods for Chronic Pain

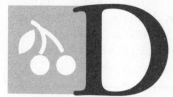**D**o you have chronic pain that has lasted 12 weeks or more? If so, you're probably popping pain-killers. But drugs should be your last resort.

Reason: You can knock out some discomfort with drugs, but side effects are common—and the pain is unlikely to go away altogether.

What's better? Most people don't realize that dietary changes—eating certain foods and avoiding others—can have a big effect on chronic pain, such as joint pain, back and neck pain, headaches and abdominal pain. I've seen for myself with patients who have a variety of chronic pain conditions (as well as my own back pain) just how effective dietary changes can be.

Where to start…

•**More cherries and berries.** All fruits contain healthy amounts of antioxidants, which are important for reducing inflammation and pain. Inflammation is associated with tissue swelling, pressure on nerves and decreased circulation, which contribute to pain. Cherries (along with blueberries, cranberries and blackberries) are particularly helpful because they're rich in antho-cyanins, chemicals that relieve pain even more effectively than aspirin. Cherries do have a fairly short season, but frozen cherries and 100% cherry juice offer some of the same benefits, though nothing takes the place of fresh organic produce.

In a study, researchers at University of California-Davis found that men and women who ate a little more than a half pound of cherries a day had a 25% reduction in C-reactive protein (CRP), a clinical marker for inflammation.

Bonus: The vitamin C in cherries and other berries has additional benefits. It's used by the body to build and repair joint cartilage, impor-

Mel Pohl, MD, a physician who specializes in treating addiction and chronic pain. He is the medical director of the Las Vegas Recovery Center and author, with Katherine Ketcham, of *The Pain Antidote: The Proven Program to Help You Stop Suffering from Chronic Pain, Avoid Addiction to Painkillers—and Reclaim Your Life.*

tant for people with joint pain caused by osteo-arthritis. Like anthocyanins, vitamin C also is a potent antioxidant that can reduce CRP.

•**Give up sugar.** By now, many of the hazards of sugar, including weight gain and cardiovascular damage, are well-known—but most people don't know that consuming sugar increases pain.

What's the link with chronic pain? A high-sugar diet causes the body to produce advanced glycation end products (AGEs), which trigger massive amounts of inflammation.

And it isn't only sugar per se that does the damage. The American College of Clinical Nutrition has reported that foods with a high glycemic index—these include white bread, white rice and other "simple" carbohydrates that are quickly converted to glucose during digestion—increase inflammation even in healthy young adults. For those with arthritis or other ongoing painful conditions, even a slight increase in inflammation can greatly increase discomfort.

My advice: Try to eliminate added sugar and processed carbohydrates from your diet. Give up candy, soda, baked goods and highly refined grains. If you really enjoy a bit of sugar in your morning coffee, go for it. Treat yourself to the occasional sweet dessert. But in my experience, people with chronic pain usually do better when they give up sugar altogether.

•**Cooler cooking.** You might struggle with pain control if grilling is one of your favorite rituals. Meats and other foods exposed to prolonged, high-heat cooking—on the grill, in the broiler, pan-frying and deep-fat frying—generate high levels of AGEs. Increased pain is just one of the risks—some research has linked AGEs to heart disease, diabetes and possibly even Alzheimer's disease.

You'll do better with cooler cooking methods, such as simmering and sautéing and moderate-heat (around 350°F) roasting. Slow-cookers are another good choice. I don't advise patients with chronic pain to give up grilling, broiling or pan-frying altogether. Just remind yourself to use these methods less often—say, once a week. Let your pain be your guide. If it's getting worse, make bigger changes.

•**Less alcohol.** Actually, no alcohol is the best choice for people with chronic pain. Alcohol irritates intestinal tissue and allows bacteria to pass into the blood more readily. The presence of bacteria will increase inflammation even if you don't develop obvious symptoms of infection.

Listen to your body. Some people can have an occasional beer or a glass of wine without noticing any change in their pain levels. If you're one of them, go ahead and imbibe on occasion.

•**Switch to olive oil.** The heart-healthy benefits aren't the only reasons to use extra-virgin olive oil in place of polyunsaturated vegetable oils (such as canola). Olive oil contains a substance called oleocanthal, which interferes with the inflammatory COX-1 and COX-2 enzymes. People who consume olive oil have lower levels of prostaglandins, the same pain-causing neurotransmitters that are blocked by aspirin.

Use olive oil just as you would other cooking oils—by drizzling some on pasta or salads, for example, or using it when you sauté vegetables or fish.

•**Eat seafood twice a week.** The omega-3 fatty acids in cold-water fish (such as salmon, sardines and trout) are among the most potent anti-inflammatory agents. Studies have shown that people who suffer from morning stiffness and joint tenderness do better when they consume more omega-3s. You can get by with fish-oil supplements, but they're unnecessary if you eat fatty fish at least twice a week.

Don't Take Tylenol for This

Tylenol doesn't relieve two common types of pain, warns study author Gustavo Machado. Acetaminophen, found in Tylenol, is ineffective for low-back pain—it worked no better than a placebo—and provides only minimal, short-term benefit for knee/hip osteoarthritis.

What may help more: Oral or topical non-steroidal anti-inflammatory drugs (NSAIDs), such as ibuprofen and naproxen...weight loss...and exercise.

Gustavo Machado, PhD candidate, The George Institute for Global Health, University of Sydney, Australia, and lead author of an analysis published in *BMJ*.

•**Drink plenty of water**—between eight and 10 glasses a day. It helps the kidneys and liver filter toxins (such as pesticide residues) from the body. Even though the liver breaks down about 95% of the toxins you ingest, the by-products can linger in the blood and other tissues. Water dilutes the concentration and reduces the inflammatory effects.

Also helpful: Green tea. It provides extra water along with catechins, antioxidants that reduce inflammation and pain.

Let Mussels Help You Build Muscle

Timothy D. Mickleborough, PhD, professor of exercise physiology and biochemistry, department of kinesiology, School of Public Health, Indiana University, Bloomington. His study appeared in the *Journal of the International Society of Sports Nutrition.*

If stiff and achy muscles after fitness workouts make exercise a literal pain, don't be discouraged. The secret to postworkout recovery may lie in the sea…not the pharmacy. No, we're not talking about soaking in sea salts (though that can help, too!) but about a novel way to repair muscle. *It turns out that the New Zealand green-lipped mussel (Perna canaliculus) might be a great workout buddy…*

INFLAMMATION PREVENTION

Plenty of folks—athletes included—reach for nonsteroidal anti-inflammatory drugs (NSAIDs) to relieve muscle soreness after exercise. But they provide only temporary relief, and regular use of certain NSAIDs can hurt your heart and stomach. Likewise, ice packs and liniments can help the symptoms, but they also provide temporary relief.

A marine oil supplement blend derived from New Zealand green-lipped mussels does provide pain relief and has nutraceutical benefits. Brands include Lyprinol, sold overseas, and Omega XL, sold in America. Studies in animals and humans have shown that, like fish oil and other omega-3 supplements, this marine oil can reduce muscle pain caused by inflammation, including arthritis pain. In fact, a recent study showed that the marine oil supplement reduced postexercise muscle pain in men not accustomed to exercise.

The study, conducted by researchers from the department of kinesiology at the Indiana School of Public Health at Indiana University, took 32 men who didn't exercise regularly and randomly assigned them to take either 1,200 mg per day of the marine oil supplement or placebo (an olive oil capsule). The men had not done any strength-training exercises for the 60 days prior to the study and had never before used a nutraceutical, such as an omega-3 supplement. They were instructed to not exercise except when instructed as part of the study. They began taking their supplement/placebo 26 days before performing muscle-damaging exercise (running downhill on a treadmill for 20 minutes) and continued the supplement/placebo regimen until four days after this exercise session.

Signs of muscle damage, inflammation, oxidative stress and fatigue were measured via blood tests, and pain, soreness and physical range-of-motion tests were taken before and at several points after the exercise session to see how the marine oil compared with placebo.

The results: The men who received the marine oil had less muscle soreness and pain, less loss of muscle strength and range of motion and less muscle fatigue than those taking placebo. Some of these effects became more noticeable with time after exercise. For example, you may have noticed that muscle soreness after newly beginning an exercise routine doesn't set in immediately—it hits a day or two later and persists for another day or two before easing up. In this study, the average level of muscle soreness, rated on a scale of 0 to 10 (with 0 being no soreness) was about the same two days after exercise—4.6 in the marine oil group and 4.8 in the placebo group. But by day 4, the average pain rating dropped to 1.8 in the marine oil group but only to 3.0 in the placebo group. And while range of motion increased over the four days post-exercise in the marine-oil group, it decreased in the placebo group. Blood work also showed that the marine oil supplement helped prevent inflammation in muscles cells.

MORE OMEGA-3 CHOICES

The marine oil, fish oil and other supplements that contain anti-inflammatory compounds—namely long-chain omega-3 polyunsaturated fatty acids (LC-PUFAs), eicosapentaenoic acid (EPA) and docosahexaenoic acid (DHA)—are known to counteract muscle inflammation, in part by inhibiting an enzyme called cyclooxygenase, which is exactly what NSAIDs such as ibuprofen, aspirin, naproxen and celecoxib do.

What's the difference between a good fish oil supplement and the marine oil? The study, which was sponsored by the manufacturer of Lyprinol and Omega XL, implied that the marine oil was superior to fish oil based on animal studies, but head-to-head human studies have not been done. The researchers based their claims on a laboratory study that showed that the fatty acids unique to the New Zealand green-lipped mussel strongly inhibit cyclooxygenase and do so more than fish oil. At best, you have more choices of PUFA-based nutraceuticals that can, among their many benefits, fight muscle pain and enhance exercise.

As with fish oil, side effects are minimal… some people may experience diarrhea, nausea and gas. Of course, if you have shellfish allergies, this supplement is not for you.

Yoga Eases Arthritis Pain

Susan J. Bartlett, PhD, associate professor of medicine, McGill University, Montreal.

Yoga eases arthritis symptoms, we hear from Susan J. Bartlett, PhD.

New eight-week study: Adults with knee osteoarthritis or rheumatoid arthritis who took hour-long yoga classes twice a week, plus did one practice session per week at home, reported a 20% improvement in pain, energy levels, mood and physical function (such as walking speed), compared with those who didn't do yoga.

Opioid Warning for Arthritis Patients

Rheumatoid arthritis (RA) patients who took opioid-based pain relievers (especially high-dose long-acting drugs such as OxyContin) had a nearly 40% increased rate of serious infections, including pneumonia and meningitis, than those who didn't take opioids. Certain opioids can affect the immune system, making users more susceptible to infection.

Andrew Wiese, MPH, researcher, Vanderbilt University, Nashville.

Don't Ignore Joint Pain If You Have This Skin Condition

Oliver FitzGerald, MD, professor of rheumatology, St. Vincent's University Hospital, Dublin.

Don't ignore joint pain if you have psoriasis, we hear from Oliver FitzGerald, MD. Having psoriasis is the single greatest risk factor for developing psoriatic arthritis (PsA), an autoimmune form of arthritis.

New research: A delayed diagnosis of even six months—from symptom onset to the first doctor's visit—can significantly increase risk for deformed joints and disability, according to a review of nearly 300 PsA patients.

Best Natural Remedies for Migraines

The late Jay S. Cohen, MD, widely recognized expert on prescription drugs and natural alternatives. He authored *15 Natural Remedies for Migraine Headaches*.

Migraine headaches can be awful—and many people find that the side effects of the prescription medications given to prevent or treat them can be just as bad. For instance, listed among the numerous possible adverse effects for *propranolol*, a commonly prescribed migraine medication, are vertigo, facial swelling, receding gums, cardiac arrhythmia—and, believe it or not, headache.

However, compelling research has shown that certain natural remedies help prevent, soothe and reduce the frequency of migraine headaches—without the side effects of drugs.

Important: Check with your doctor to make sure that none of these natural treatments will interact with any other medications that you take or conditions that you have. Then work through the following list to see what helps you. You also can combine remedies, such as riboflavin, magnesium and CoQ10, but always check with your doctor.

RIBOFLAVIN

Also called vitamin B-2, riboflavin occurs naturally in certain foods. It helps convert food into energy…it's an antioxidant that fights free-radical damage…and it helps activate other forms of vitamin B.

How riboflavin helps migraines: It's thought that some migraines occur because oxygen is not being properly metabolized in the mitochondria (the so-called "power plants" of cells), so riboflavin's energy-boosting function may help prevent this type of migraine.

The research: The first published study evaluating riboflavin for migraine therapy reported that taking 5 milligrams (mg) three times daily over several months diminished migraine frequency—some subjects said that taking hourly doses halted acute migraines. Studies done in 1994 and 1998 found that taking 400 mg/day of riboflavin helped reduce frequency and severity of migraines, with the best results seen in the third month of therapy. A 2004 study of migraine patients who had not responded to other therapies yielded a 50% reduction in migraine frequency for patients who took riboflavin daily.

How to take riboflavin: The suggested dose is 400 mg daily. It's safe to take riboflavin indefinitely. Some people notice improvement quickly, but others see benefits only after three or four months of taking riboflavin daily. A small percentage of people find that riboflavin makes their faces flush and/or report digestive upset—if that happens to you, you might try dividing your dose in half (200 mg, morning and night) or just take 200 mg/day.

COENZYME Q10

Also called *ubiquinone*, CoQ10 is a substance that occurs naturally in the body that helps with mitochondrial function and energy production. It's also an antioxidant that may help stem inflammation.

How CoQ10 helps migraines: CoQ10 works similarly to riboflavin, supporting cellular energy production. Its antioxidant power is so strong that it's often recommended for people with certain types of heart disease and muscular and nervous system problems.

The research: Several small studies found that taking CoQ10 reduced migraine frequency. In a 2002 study of 32 adults taking 150 mg/day, 61% said that the days they experienced migraines were down by 50% or more. A 2005 study found that 48% of participants experienced a 50% or greater decrease in frequency, and a 2007 study of children and adolescents had similar results.

How to take CoQ10: Start with a dose of 150 mg/day and, if needed, work your way up to taking three daily doses of 100 mg (morning, noon and night). One percent of people report some stomach upset with CoQ10—if you're in that group, stop taking CoQ10.

MAGNESIUM

The vast majority of Americans are deficient in magnesium, which is a problem because it is essential to the healthy function of muscles and the nervous system. I believe magnesium is very helpful for people with a deficiency—not so much for those whose magnesium levels already are healthy.

How magnesium helps migraines: Magnesium plays a role in many cellular processes and also is responsible for smooth-muscle activity in the nerves and arteries—both factors in migraines. Also, magnesium deficiency has been shown to cause spasms of the cerebral arteries, associated with migraine.

The research: A 1995 study reported that intravenous delivery of 1,000 mg of magnesium was effective at halting migraines. Studies examining the use of oral magnesium (600 mg/day) to prevent migraines were done in 1996 and 2008 and found that it reduced both the frequency and severity of the headaches.

How to take magnesium: A good dose to begin with is 100 mg twice daily. Gradually work your way up to 400 mg/day.

5-HTP

5-Hydroxytryptophan (5-HTP) is a building block used by the body to produce serotonin, a neurotransmitter that aids cellular communication and also is associated with mood. Available in many foods, 5-HTP is produced from the amino acid tryptophan.

How 5-HTP helps migraines: 5-HTP gets converted by the body to serotonin (found in the nervous system and the gut), which is involved in the conduction of pain signals and the dilation/constriction of blood vessels—both relevant to migraine pain.

The research: A 1973 study compared the efficacy of 5-HTP therapy (200 mg/day) and a prescription medication in 20 patients and found identical results—both treatments achieved a 55% reduction in frequency, and the 5-HTP patients who continued taking the supplement reported continual improvement. Subsequent studies found 5-HTP effective at soothing the pain of migraines already in progress.

How to take 5-HTP: Begin with a small dose (50 mg to 100 mg), and if need be, work

Vitamin D and Migraines

Many of us take vitamin D, but one-third of American adults still don't get enough. That's bad news because it affects blood pressure and immune function. Also, low levels are linked to a range of chronic diseases including diabetes, osteoporosis, fibromyalgia and numerous types of cancer.

How vitamin D helps migraines: Though research shows the benefits of vitamin D for migraines, the actual mechanisms by which vitamin D helps prevent or treat migraines aren't well-understood. Since we do know that deficiencies affect all organ systems, it makes sense that raising levels of vitamin D would be beneficial.

The research: Studies done in 2009 and 2010 found correlations between vitamin D deficiency and chronic tension and migraine headaches—and noted improvement with vitamin D therapy.

How to take vitamin D: It's a good idea to get your vitamin D levels tested and discuss the proper dosage with your doctor based on the results. Mainstream doctors typically recommend between 200 international units (IU) and 800 IU a day. Some alternative practitioners go far higher, to 5,000 IU/day, or even more.

—Jay S. Cohen, MD.

your way up to the maximum daily dosage (300 mg to 400 mg), taken at bedtime. Side effects are mild and may include gastrointestinal problems and weird dreams.

MELATONIN

This sleep-promoting hormone has numerous positive effects, including suppression of the substances that promote pain. It also fosters anti-inflammatory activity, regulation of serotonin and nerve and blood vessel interaction.

How melatonin helps migraines: A theory about one possible cause of migraine relates to an imbalance in the relationship between the hypothalamus and the pineal gland that affects adequate melatonin production.

The research: A 2004 study followed 34 adult patients who were given a nightly melatonin dose of 3 mg for three months—25% stopped getting migraines altogether and 80% reported a 50% or greater reduction in frequency. A 2008 study examining children and adolescents taking 3 mg of melatonin at bedtime found a 50% or greater reduction in frequency for 71% of participants.

How to take melatonin: Start with a dose of 0.5 mg or 1 mg and go up to 2, 3 or 5 mg, depending on your reaction. Take melatonin in the evening, preventively, or as treatment for an acute migraine. Melatonin yields superior results and has far fewer side effects when compared with common migraine drugs.

Headband That Prevents Headaches

Gary Kaye, founder and chief content officer of Tech50+, an Internet site that covers consumer electronics–related topics. Based in Oxford, Connecticut, he has reported on technology for more than 30 years at NBC News, ABC News, CNN, Fox Business Network and other organizations. Tech50Plus.com

B ioTrak Health Halo senses subtle head and neck muscle tension that can presage the onset of migraines and tension headaches. The headband sends a gentle vibration to alert its wearer to the potential problem. Then an app guides the wearer through relaxation techniques designed to ward off the headache. Bio-Trak says Halo users eventually learn to sense an oncoming headache themselves, reducing the need to wear the headband. Halo has not yet been subjected to independent studies, but research suggests that biofeedback and relaxation techniques can control certain headaches. Halo should be available sometime in 2017 for around $200. *HaloCalm.com*

A Simple Fix for Neck Pain

Shani Soloff, manual orthopedic physical therapist and founder of the Stamford, Connecticut–based ergonomics firm The Posture People.
Rebecca Shannonhouse, editor, *Bottom Line Health*.

I f you've got neck pain, you know all too well the misery it causes.

In your search for relief, don't forget to consider this: How much time do you spend on the phone? Even if it's just a few calls a day, using a handheld landline or cell phone causes you to hold your body in ways that nature never intended.

When you're talking, you naturally tip your head toward the phone—and get even more contorted when your hands are busy and you raise a shoulder to prop the phone in place. It's no wonder that these movements were widely cited in a landmark study that found more than

45% of office workers had frequent episodes of neck pain!

You may think that you've solved the problem if you've switched to a speakerphone. But chances are you haven't. A speakerphone may not be a good alternative, because many people tend to move their necks forward—and lean toward the speakerphone.

Fortunately, the solution is often as simple as investing in a good headset. Shani Soloff, a manual orthopedic physical therapist and founder of the Stamford, Connecticut–based ergonomics firm The Posture People, advises everyone who uses a phone to do this. It will help you maintain proper posture—with your body straight and your shoulders square—while talking on the phone.

It doesn't really matter what style you choose, as long as it's comfortable and easy to use. You can start by checking online at such sites as *Headsets.com, BestBuy.com* or *Staples.com*. Headsets come in corded and wireless versions…prices range from about $15 to $350. Your neck will thank you!

When Shoulder Pain Won't Go Away

Beth E. Shubin Stein, MD, an associate attending orthopedic surgeon and a member of the Sports Medicine and Shoulder Service at the Hospital for Special Surgery in New York City.

A s many as half of all Americans suffer from shoulder pain each year. For a significant number of these people, the problem lingers on…for weeks, months or even longer.

There is hope: Whether the pain stems from an injury, overuse or some unknown cause, chronic shoulder pain can be dramatically improved—and usually eliminated. The treatments may also help those whose shoulder pain is caused by arthritis. *Here are the latest approaches for the most common shoulder problems…*

ROTATOR CUFF PROBLEMS

Most people are quick to chalk up shoulder pain to tendinitis, a nagging form of inflammation. But that's usually a mistake.

New thinking: The shoulder pain thought of as tendinitis is typically a result of tendinosis, a related condition that occurs when the tendons (ropelike cords connecting muscle to bone) begin to deteriorate. Tendinosis can usually be diagnosed with a physical exam and an X-ray and/or MRI.

Red flag for the patient: The pain may be barely perceptible while the arm is at rest—but if you extend the arm outward, in front of the body or overhead, the pain can range from dull to excruciating.

Rotator cuff tendinosis develops when tendons in the rotator cuff (a group of tendons and muscles that attach the upper arm to the shoulder joint) break down over time. This can occur due to age…repetitive use…or weakness of the rotator cuff muscles.

What works best: During the first week or two, to "quiet" the inflammation around the tendon, apply ice (for 15 to 20 minutes several times daily)…and take a nonsteroidal anti-inflammatory drug (NSAID), such as *ibuprofen* (Motrin).

If pain continues, your doctor should also refer you to a physical or occupational therapist, who can recommend exercises (such as those on the next page) to strengthen the rotator cuff and shoulder blade (scapula) muscles. If pain worsens or lasts longer than a week or two, a cortisone injection into the bursa surrounding the rotator cuff tendons can help.

Good news: Within six weeks, this nonsurgical regimen alleviates the pain 90% of the time.

Beware: Chronic use of cortisone can damage tendons, so surgery (see below) should be considered if two or three injections (given no more than every three months) have not relieved the pain.

If you don't get relief after six weeks or the pain returns after cortisone therapy wears off, you may want to consider surgery. Arthroscopy (inserting a tiny camera via small incisions) allows the surgeon to assess the shoulder joint and correct the damage that has led to rotator cuff tendinosis. When performed by an experienced surgeon, the procedure has a high success rate. Complications are rare but may involve infection or stiffness.

To find an experienced surgeon, consult The American Orthopaedic Society for Sports Medicine, *SportsMed.org*.

Two approaches that are less invasive than surgery…

•**Platelet-rich plasma (PRP) injection involves the use of platelets from a patient's blood.** The platelets are separated from the blood with a centrifuge and reinfused into the affected tendons. The platelets are rich in growth factors that aid healing, and the technique is considered safe, since the patient's own cells are used.

A small study published in 2013 in *Global Advances in Health and Medicine* found that a single PRP injection significantly improved pain and function at a 12-week follow-up. More research is needed, however, for definitive evidence of its effectiveness. Some patients opt to have a series of PRP injections. Insurance rarely covers the cost—typically about $1,500 per injection.

•**Stem cell treatment.** With this therapy, which is currently experimental, certain bone marrow cells are reinjected into the shoulder area, where they can help replace degenerated tendon tissue. Though promising, this therapy is not yet widely available. Several clinical trials are now ongoing. To find one, go to *ClinicalTrials.gov*.

FROZEN SHOULDER

Frozen shoulder (or adhesive capsulitis), which usually occurs for unknown reasons, develops when the capsule surrounding the shoulder joint gets inflamed and then stiffens. A dull ache in the shoulder can come and go, slowly worsening to a ferocious pain that may awaken you during sleep or hurt even when your arm is at your side.

In the past, doctors recommended physical therapy to "thaw out" the joint and restore range of motion. But the physical therapy typically aggravated the condition—and it often did not improve for more than a year.

New thinking: With a two-part approach—a cortisone injection given early on into the joint and gentle exercises—sufferers can get pain relief and restore their range of motion within a matter of weeks to months.

Surgery is rarely needed if frozen shoulder is promptly diagnosed and treated at this stage. Cortisone injections are usually not helpful when frozen shoulder has progressed to severe stiffness, but physical therapy may help restore mobility.

After receiving a cortisone injection, the following exercises should be performed on the recovering shoulder three times a day. *Gently hold each for five seconds and do 10 reps of each exercise...*

- **Overhead stretch.**

What to do: Lie on your back with your arms at your sides. Lift your arm straight up in the air and over your head. Grab your elbow with your other arm and gently press toward your head.

- **Cross-body reach.**

What to do: Stand and lift your arm to the side until it's a bit below shoulder height, then bring it to the front and across your body. As it passes the front of your body, grab the elbow with your other arm and exert gentle pressure to stretch the shoulder.

- **Towel stretch.**

What to do: Drape a towel over the unaffected shoulder, and grab it with your hand behind your back. Gently pull the towel upward with your other hand to stretch the affected shoulder and upper arm.

Here's How to Finally Relieve Your Back Pain

Jack Stern, MD, PhD, a surgeon who specializes in spine neurosurgery and is on the clinical faculty at Weill Cornell Medical College in New York City. He has a private practice in White Plains, New York, and is the author of *Ending Back Pain: 5 Powerful Steps to Diagnose, Understand, and Treat Your Ailing Back.* SafeSpineSurgery.com

Back pain might not be as inevitable as death and taxes, but it sure comes close. About 80% of Americans will have back pain at some point in their lives.

A troubling trend: Studies show that far too many people are now having surgery in an attempt to relieve back pain.

But only about 10% of all back pain sufferers actually need surgery. Even when pain is severe, the overwhelming majority of back patients will make a full recovery within two to three months with nothing more than painkillers, exercise, physical therapy or other conservative treatments.

Most people get their first episode of back pain in their 30s. But as we age, the incidence of back pain increases. With wear and tear, the spinal discs, which act as shock absorbers and allow the spine to flex, start to dry out and weaken (a condition called disc degeneration). This can result in painful back conditions such as a herniated disc, facet joint syndrome or spinal stenosis.

More about these back problems and the best treatments for them...

HERNIATED DISC—DON'T RUSH TO HAVE SURGERY!

About 20% of adults have one or more herniated discs without symptoms, but others aren't so lucky. A herniated disc is among the main causes of low-back pain and the "shooting" pain of sciatica.

As we age, the spinal discs lose some of their water content, which makes them more prone to tearing or rupture (a herniated disc). An MRI is used for diagnosis.

My advice: Unless you're having serious neurological symptoms—foot or leg weakness, for example, or a loss of bowel or bladder control—wait at least six weeks before considering surgery.

The surgery for herniated disc, called a microdiscectomy, is frequently performed on an outpatient basis, is very safe and has a high success rate. But research has shown that about 90% of patients with a herniated disc will get better without surgery. There's a good chance that the body's natural healing mechanisms will break down the damaged portion of the disc, and the pain will clear up on its own. The catch is that it can sometimes take up to a year or more to recover.

Even though doctors often recommend steroids (oral or as an injection), many patients prefer a nondrug approach to pain relief.

A therapy that's underutilized…

•**Alexander technique.** This is an especially good treatment choice for back pain or sciatica that is caused in part by poor posture or other issues involving body mechanics. It can also help some patients with spinal stenosis (see below).

With the Alexander technique, named after its inventor Frederick Alexander, a patient's body movements are analyzed and then specific recommendations are made to relieve tension in the body and improve posture and movement.

Important finding: A study in *BMJ* involving 579 patients with chronic or recurrent low-back pain found that those who had six to 24 instructional sessions and practiced the technique had less pain than those given conventional treatments, such as massage and exercise.

FACET JOINT SYNDROME—
WAIT IT OUT?

Facet pain affects at least 15% of all people with back pain—and nearly 45% of back pain sufferers ages 50 to 60. It can be caused by trauma—twisting too hard during a round of golf or a tennis serve, for example—but it's usually due to osteoarthritis in the spine. The facet joints are the round protrusions that you can feel when you touch your spine. Arthritis in these areas can cause pain and/or stiffness, just as it does in the knees or other joints.

Clues for facet pain: The pain usually comes on quickly…can make it difficult to stand up straight or get out of a chair…and may also cause pain in the buttocks or thighs.

If you have mild/occasional facet pain: I advise you to wait it out. Many people get better on their own within four to six weeks. While you're waiting for the issue to resolve, you can take *ibuprofen* (Motrin) or other painkillers… avoid stressing the area…and try chiropractic treatments (they're safe and can realign the facet joints to reduce pressure but avoid if you have severe osteoporosis or spinal cancer).

If you have severe/lasting pain: Ask your doctor about radiofrequency nerve ablation. It's a simple surgical procedure that uses a micro-electrode to destroy the affected nerve. In one important study, the procedure was found to reduce pain by 50% to 80% in most people. Nerve ablation is unlikely to cause complications, although the nerve sometimes grows back—and could cause pain in the future. Insurance usually covers the procedure.

SPINAL STENOSIS—SURGERY IS
TYPICALLY NEEDED

With spinal stenosis, there is a narrowing of the spinal canal (the open space in the spine that holds the spinal cord), which can exert pressure on spinal nerve roots resulting in pain. Some people are born with a narrow spinal opening, but most often it's caused by age-related changes such as arthritis or the growth of bone spurs in the spinal canal. Some people with spinal stenosis have low-back pain while others have pain that radiates down the leg (it can be similar to the pain that's caused by sciatica).

Clues for spinal stenosis: Pain increases when you walk and quickly gets better with rest. With sciatica, pain is sometimes relieved by walking. Also, if there is pain relief when bending forward (this movement "opens up" spinal spaces and reduces pressure), this points to stenosis. A diagnosis can be confirmed with a CT scan or MRI of the lumbar spine.

My advice: I almost always recommend surgical decompression for patients with spinal stenosis. One large study showed that people who have surgery recover more quickly and stay pain free longer than those who have physical therapy or undergo other treatments for spinal stenosis. The procedure is usually covered by insurance.

With surgical decompression, the surgeon removes the excess bone and overgrowth of ligaments that's causing the pressure. It takes about three months for full recovery—but it's one of the most successful spinal operations, with more than 80% of patients reporting good improvement. However, surgery can't correct arthritis, so symptoms may eventually return. Risk for side effects is low but includes nerve injury and infection.

Simple Exercise to Prevent Back Pain

Do this simple exercise to strengthen your back: Stand, sit or lie on your back, and exhale all your breath while pulling your navel in and up toward your head. Hold for 10 seconds, and release. Repeat 12 times.

Todd Sinett, DC, is a chiropractor and founder/owner of Midtown Integrative Health & Wellness in New York City. He is author of *3 Weeks to a Better Back*.

Ease Back Tension in Two Minutes

Jill Miller, fitness therapist based in Los Angeles, author of *The Roll Model* and creator of the exercise program Yoga Tune Up. YogaTuneUp.com

Do you store tension in your back and sides? Chances are, you're not breathing as deeply and naturally as you could be. *Try this quick move to discharge back tension and get relief...*

How to tell if that's the problem: You experience upper or lower back pain, side stitches or bouts of difficult breathing. The reason is likely because you have poor breathing mechanics.

What to do: Lie face down on the floor with a pillow under your abdomen. As you breathe slowly and deeply, try to compress your gut into the pillow and let your body change the shape of it. This helps the deepest muscles in your core to get stronger and more pliable and balanced. Do this for one minute, then place the pillow up higher under your rib cage and repeat the breathing-and-compression exercise.

You can do this exercise any time of day, but it's best to do it 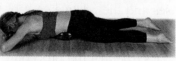 on an empty stomach—say, first thing in the morning or before dinner.

Photo courtesy of Jill Miller and Victory Belt Publishing from *The Roll Model—a Step-by-Step Guide to Erase Pain, Improve Mobility and Live Better in your Body*. YogaTuneUp.com

Nerve Block Technique Might Help Ease Chronic Back Pain

Michael Gofeld, MD, associate professor, medicine, University of Toronto, and chronic pain management specialist, St. Michael's Hospital and Women's College Hospital, Toronto.
John Mafi, MD, internist and assistant professor, David Geffen School of Medicine, University of California, Los Angeles.
Nathaniel Tindel, MD, orthopedic spine surgeon, Lenox Hill Hospital, New York City.
Presentation, American Academy of Pain Medicine annual meeting, Palm Springs, California

A procedure that uses radio waves to treat chronic low back pain provided long-lasting relief to a small group of patients, researchers report.

Called intradiscal biacuplasty (IDB), the procedure uses two water-cooled needles to blast radiofrequency energy at the nerve fibers within and around a spinal disc that's begun to degenerate but has not ruptured, explained lead researcher Michael Gofeld, MD.

"Basically you're destroying the nerve fibers, which will lead to the elimination of pain," he said. Dr. Gofeld is a chronic pain management specialist at St. Michael's Hospital and Women's College Hospital in Toronto.

A year out from treatment, half of the patients who received IDB in the study said they still were experiencing significant pain reduction, Dr. Gofeld and his colleagues reported.

The treatment is specifically to help people with discogenic back pain, Dr. Gofeld said—pain related to discs that are deteriorating but have not ruptured.

Prior studies have found that discogenic back pain accounts for 39% of cases of chronic lower back pain, he said.

The idea of using radio waves to treat back pain has been around for a quarter-century, Dr. Gofeld said. But recent breakthroughs using water-cooled needles have made the technology potentially more effective.

"If the needle gets too hot, the energy will not spread efficiently enough," Dr. Gofeld said.

The procedure takes about a half hour, followed by six weeks of physical therapy, he said.

Ideal patients have lower back pain that doesn't shoot down the legs and limited disc degeneration, with no significant tears or ruptures.

John Mafi, MD, an internist and assistant professor at UCLA's David Geffen School of Medicine, in Los Angeles, pointed out that the U.S. Food and Drug Administration approved IDB for use in 2007. But the technology has not been widely adopted in the United States, he said.

"It's not widely used," Dr. Mafi said. "Insurance doesn't seem to cover it yet, and that may be because they want to see more evidence."

For example, the U.S. Centers for Medicare and Medicaid Services (CMS) ruled in September 2008 that the government insurance plans would not cover any radiofrequency treatments for low back pain. The CMS decision memo concluded that there wasn't enough evidence to prove that the procedures would improve health outcomes.

STUDY DETAILS

Dr. Gofeld's study, which was funded by device manufacturer Kimberly-Clark Corp., focused on 22 patients who received IDB treatment alongside typical medical care for back pain.

These patients originally showed less pain at six months following treatment, and now a one-year follow-up found that their pain reduction and improved function had continued, Dr. Gofeld said.

The one-year report also included 25 members of the initial control group for the study, who at first only received typical medical care that included physical therapy and exercises.

These patients were allowed to "cross over" after six months and receive IDB. They also experienced some pain relief and improved function, the Canadian researchers reported.

However, their pain reduction was not as strong as that experienced by the original treatment group, Dr. Gofeld said.

IMPLICATIONS

"We can infer from this result that the sooner we do the procedure and get the patient into rehabilitation treatment, the better will be the result," he said.

Researchers also found no significant side effects associated with IDB.

Dr. Mafi said the small number of patients involved makes this more of a "pilot study."

"I wouldn't jump to any changes in policy based on this study," Dr. Mafi said. "This is a promising start, but now it's time to do a rigorous clinical trial from this pilot data."

Nathaniel Tindel, MD, an orthopedic spine surgeon at Lenox Hill Hospital in New York City, also sounded a cautious note, based on both the small number of participants and the fact that numerous prior radiofrequency treatments have failed to help people with low back pain.

"Whenever there are a plethora of procedures offered to treat a condition which is known to heal best when left alone, those procedures are either all very effective or equally ineffective," Dr. Tindel said. "Unfortunately, medical research has already shown us that intradiscal therapy falls into the latter category, and to date has not been shown to have long-term effect on back pain and disc disease."

info For more on thermal intradiscal procedures for back pain, visit the U.S. Centers for Medicare and Medicaid Services, *CMS.gov* and search "thermal intradiscal procedures."

Got Knee Pain?

Jordan Metzl, MD, a sports medicine physician at the Hospital for Special Surgery in New York City. He is coauthor of The Exercise Cure: A Doctor's All-Natural, No-Pill Prescription for Better Health & Longer Life. *DrJordanMetzl.com*

Why live with a bum knee when you can have less pain and more mobility with a new one? With such great promises and the relative ease of knee-replacement surgery, it's no surprise that this is now one of the most popular procedures in the US.

It's true that the procedure can be a blessing for those with severe arthritis (the main reason for surgery) that impairs their ability to live an active, pain-free life. But the decision to have surgery should not be made casually—and if you do end up getting a knee replacement, there are facts you should know before choosing between the tried-and-true approach and the newer, less invasive surgical procedure.

TO AVOID SURGERY

If you have mild-to-moderate knee pain, but you're still able to work and do normal activities, chances are you can greatly improve without surgery by following these steps…

•**Stretch and strengthen the muscles.** Studies have shown that simply strengthening the muscles that support the knees (the quadriceps in the front of the thighs and the hamstrings in the backs) can reduce damage, pain and disability.

My advice: Work those muscles three or four times a week for at least six to eight weeks before making a decision about surgery.

Examples: Leg extensions, hamstring curls and clamshells. Even if your knee is hurting, it's worth taking an over-the-counter painkiller, such as *ibuprofen* (Advil) or *acetaminophen* (Tylenol), about 30 minutes before your workout so that you can do the exercises. Curcumin supplements have also been shown to decrease inflammation and arthritis pain. A physical therapist or personal trainer can help design a workout that includes targeted stretches and strengthening exercises that are right for you.

•**Drop some excess weight.** Every pound of body weight equals several pounds of "loading force." This means if you are 10 pounds overweight, for example, your knees get an extra 40 pounds of pressure. That's enough to increase pain and limit mobility—and accelerate arthritis-related damage.

Get Your Vitamin D Levels Checked

Low vitamin D levels are linked to progression of knee osteoarthritis. Patients found to be clinically deficient in vitamin D were twice as likely to experience worsening knee osteoarthritis as people with sufficient vitamin D.

Fang Fang Zhang, PhD, MD, is an assistant professor in the Friedman School of Nutrition Science and Policy, Tufts University, Boston, and leader of a data analysis, published in *Journal of Nutrition*.

My advice: If you're overweight—even by a few pounds—it's affecting your knees. Get serious about losing those extra pounds!

•**Try hyaluronic acid.** This naturally occurring substance acts as a lubricant to the joints and may work as well as painkillers and steroids (without the side effects) for some people. It's usually injected into the affected joints once a week for three to five weeks.

My advice: There's no way to predict who will benefit from these injections. Consider them if exercise and weight loss haven't given you adequate relief. Insurance typically covers the cost.

WHAT NEXT?

If you've given the strategies described earlier your best shot and still have serious knee pain, surgery is usually the next step. *What to consider…*

•**Partial knee replacement.** This approach, also known as uni-compartmental knee replacement, is newer than total knee replacement and gets a lot of attention because it is less invasive. The advantages include an incision that is roughly half the size (about three to 3.5 inches) of that used for total knee replacement. Patients also are hospitalized for just a day or two rather than three to five days for a total knee replacement. With the partial approach, the knee may feel more "natural"—for example, it may have less "creakiness" and better range of motion—than it would after a more extensive procedure.

But a partial knee replacement isn't for everyone. To be a candidate for this procedure, the damage is generally isolated to only one part of the knee. Also, the research is not yet clear, but patients who have partial procedures may be more likely to require subsequent "revision" surgery—because of continuing arthritis, for example, or because the first procedure didn't improve pain and/or mobility. For many patients, the risks from repeat surgery could outweigh the benefits of a less traumatic initial procedure.

•**Total knee replacement.** This procedure is called a "total" replacement because the damaged surfaces of the knee bones are replaced—the tibia (shinbone)…femur (thighbone)…and sometimes the patella (kneecap). The surgery requires a large incision (usually seven to eight inches) and typically takes about two hours.

The majority of patients who opt for knee surgery require a total replacement. Surgeons have a lot of experience with the procedure—and there's strong evidence that it works. More than 90% of total knee-replacement patients report that they have a lot less pain…and about 85% of these artificial knees are still going strong after 20 years. While patients who receive total replacements have somewhat less flexibility than those who go the partial route, most are able to do light hiking, ballroom dancing and biking.

THE BOTTOM LINE

No matter which approach your surgeon suggests, make sure you're comfortable with the plan. Some patients will feel best about the decision if they get a second opinion.

Until more is known about the long-term benefits and risks of partial knee replacement, most surgeons advise their patients with severe arthritis to get it over with and have a total replacement.

Patients with osteoarthritis in all areas of the knee and those with inflammatory arthritis (such as rheumatoid arthritis), which tends to affect the entire knee, are not candidates for a partial approach and require a total knee replacement.

Consider a partial procedure only if you mainly have damage in just one part of the knee, you haven't improved after physical therapy, weight loss and the other suggestions described above, and your pain prevents you from sleeping through the night and/or performing your normal daily activities.

A Painful Stubbed Toe

Michael J. Trepal, DPM, professor of surgery, New York College of Podiatric Medicine, New York City.

Generally, when a person stubs a toe, if pain, redness and swelling subside within a few days and the toe is not crooked or the skin broken, then the injury can be treated at home.

Helpful: Keep the swelling down by staying off the foot as much as possible. Wear a wider shoe with a rigid sole until you're able to return to normal footgear.

If you stubbed your toe and symptoms persist without improvement after a few days or pain interferes with walking, you should consult a podiatrist—especially if you suffer from diabetes or peripheral neuropathy.

No More Foot and Leg Pain

Patrick O. McKeon, PhD, a certified athletic trainer and assistant professor in the department of exercise and sport sciences at Ithaca College in Ithaca, New York, where he's also a faculty member in the School of Health Sciences and Human Performance. His research focuses on ankle instability and other lower-extremity joint injuries.

Just about every workout these days includes "core" exercises that strengthen muscles in the abdomen and lower back. That's because you need a strong core for balance, posture and everyday movements.

But there's another core muscle group that you probably haven't thought about. New research suggests that a strong foot core might be the key to avoiding painful plantar fasciitis, shin splints, Achilles tendinitis, bursitis and other common foot and leg problems.

OH, MY ACHING FEET!

The Institute of Preventive Foot Health reports that more than three-quarters of all US adults have suffered from foot pain at some point in their lives.

Surprising: Much of the foot/leg pain that is attributed to overuse is actually caused by weakness of the small muscles, known as intrinsic muscles, deep inside the feet.

Latest development: Research now suggests that strengthening the intrinsic muscles by walking barefoot and doing certain simple foot exercises (see next page) can help prevent and treat the common foot and leg problems mentioned earlier.

How's Your Foot Strength?

If you've had plantar fasciitis, shin splints, Achilles tendinitis or other foot/leg injuries in the past, your feet probably need strengthening. *Two tests to assess foot strength...*

• **While standing, rise up onto your toes.** If your feet roll outward, the small foot muscles are not as strong as they should be.

• **While standing, rest a few fingers on a table or the top of a chair for support.** Then lift one foot off the floor and notice how much—and how quickly—the other foot wobbles. If your foot is stable for 30 seconds or more, the small foot muscles are probably in good shape.

Patrick O. McKeon, PhD.

THE CASE AGAINST SHOES

Shoes protect your feet from rough surfaces and harmful organisms and keep your toes warm. But they do not contribute to foot strength.

Millions of people worldwide go shoeless most of the time—and have stronger feet because of it. A study published in the podiatry journal *The Foot* found that modern-day Zulus, who often go barefoot, have the healthiest feet, while shoe-wearing Europeans have the unhealthiest feet.

Explanation: The intrinsic muscles in the feet have sensory receptors that convey important information—about gait, balance, alignment, etc.—to the larger (extrinsic) muscles in legs and feet. Shoes blunt these signals by preventing the muscles from flexing normally.

Result: Without this vital information from the small muscles, the large muscles become overworked and break down more rapidly, leading to possible injuries.

KICK OFF YOUR SHOES!

The easiest way to strengthen the small foot muscles is to shed your shoes and pad around the house in your bare feet. I advise people to walk barefoot as much as they can. (Wearing thin, non-slippery socks is OK if your feet get cold.)

Wearing shoes without thick soles or a lot of arch support (so-called minimalist shoes) also permits the intrinsic muscles in the feet to flex and contract but not as much as walking barefoot.

Examples of brands to try: Vivobarefoot and New Balance Minimus.

Caution: Flexing the intrinsic muscles too much when you aren't used to it can increase foot/leg pain at first. To prevent this, before going barefoot or wearing minimalist shoes, incorporate the foot exercises below into your routine. Then try going barefoot or wearing minimalist shoes for a few days. If you start to develop pain, stop going barefoot or wearing minimalist shoes but continue to strengthen your feet for a few weeks and then try again.

Also: You want more support, not less, when you're dealing with a current injury to allow the tissues to heal. Don't wear minimalist shoes or go barefoot until you've fully recovered—and check first with your doctor if you have neuropathy (a type of nerve damage that can occur with certain conditions such as diabetes) in your feet.

EXERCISING YOUR FOOT CORE

In addition to walking barefoot whenever you can, exercise that is performed barefoot, such as yoga and Pilates, will also strengthen your feet. But for a simple and effective foot core workout, try the following exercises.

Important: Before you begin the exercises, sit down with one foot flat on the ground. Roll your ankle out to lift the ball of your foot off the ground. Then roll your foot the other way to lift your little toe off the ground. Keep doing this until you can sense where the midpoint is between these two extremes. This point is the subtalar neutral, the optimal position for the foot to be in to adapt to the demands placed on it. Repeat with the other foot.

• **"Short foot" exercise.**

What to do: Sit in a chair with your bare feet flat on the floor. Engage the intrinsic muscles by sliding your big toes back toward the heels, but without curling the toes. (You're temporarily making your feet shorter—hence the name of the exercise.) Hold the stretch for about six seconds. Do this eight to 10 times, rest for about a minute, then repeat the cycle two more times. Do the sequence at least a few times a day on each foot.

Note: It can be difficult to get the hang of this exercise because we're not used to engaging these muscles. You'll know you're doing it right when the foot arches rise.

Once you've mastered this movement, you can work the muscles harder by doing this exercise while standing...or by standing on one foot. Studies have shown that people who do this exercise have improvements in balance as well as arch height within four weeks.

●**Quarter roll exercise.**

What to do: Place a quarter under the ball of each foot, just behind the big toes. While standing, rise up slightly on your toes. Try to roll your feet so that your weight is directly over the quarters (or as close as you can get). Hold the position for five to 10 seconds, rest for about a minute and repeat eight to 10 times. Do the sequence at least a few times a day.

As your muscles get stronger, you can increase the difficulty of the exercise by raising your heels higher or by rising up on one foot at a time.

Sore, Achy Feet? Take the Ball Cure

Jill Miller, fitness-therapy expert based in Los Angeles, author of The Roll Model and creator of the exercise program YogaTuneUp.com.

I f your feet get tender and achy, you might be holding stress in your feet, says fitness-therapy expert Jill Miller. Her easy-to-do move releases foot tension and makes for happy feet. All you need is a small, hard ball such as a racquetball—and a wall.

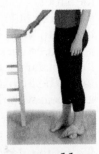

Here's how to tell if that is your problem: You have heel pain, achy arches or soreness in the balls of your feet.

What to do: Stand next to a wall for balance, and place a racquetball under your right foot. Load your weight onto the ball, then move the ball from side to side, and up and down, under the sole of your foot. If you'd like to, you can place your left foot on top of your right foot to sandwich it and massage your right foot from above, helping it to destress, Miller says. Do this

for one minute, then switch feet. Do this at the beginning and end of each day as well as anytime you sense tension building up in your feet.

Important note: If you have persistent foot pain, see a health-care professional.

Photo courtesy of Jill Miller and Victory Belt Publishing from *The Roll Model—a Step-by-Step Guide to Erase Pain, Improve Mobility and Live Better in your Body.* YogaTuneUp.com.

To Fight Chronic Pain, Wear This Under Your Clothes

Gary Kaye, founder and chief content officer, Tech50+, Oxford, Connecticut. Tech50+ covers consumer-electronics–related topics relevant to people over age 50. Mr. Kaye has reported on technology for more than 30 years at NBC News, ABC News, CNN, Fox Business Network and other organizations.

C hronic pain can be insidious. But what if you could relieve chronic pain almost anywhere in your body just by wearing a discreet band on your leg?

There is a new product on the market that makes that claim—and believe it or not, it has received FDA approval.

Anytime there's a way for our readers to get help with chronic pain that doesn't involve dangerous painkilling drugs or other risky or unproven methods, we're all over it. So we took a good look at this product.

It's called Quell, and it's a band that you strap around your lower leg to stop pain you're feeling in your neck, back, shoulder and elsewhere on your body (although it doesn't work for headaches). The device, designed by researchers from MIT and Harvard, has been approved by the Food and Drug Administration as a medical device that can be sold to the public without a prescription for relief of chronic pain. It can be used while you're awake and/or while you're sleeping.

Gary Kaye, the founder and chief content officer of Tech50+, a website that covers consumer electronics–related topics for people over age 50, called our attention to the new device. "It's very good for people who have chronic pain.

Of course, it won't ameliorate the condition that may be causing your pain, but it can reduce the pain you feel." (Kaye has no financial stake in this or any of the devices he reviews.)

AN ESTABLISHED TREATMENT

The basic technology underlying the Quell device has been around for decades—transcutaneous electrical nerve stimulation (TENS). If you've had physical therapy, you may have had TENS—tiny electrodes attached to your body and hooked up to a battery pack deliver a tingling sensation. These neural pulses are believed to release natural brain chemicals that block pain signals.

While TENS doesn't work for every patient, studies show that it can relieve pain in many people with conditions such as chronic low back pain, neuropathy (nerve pain) and fibromyalgia. A recent meta-analysis of randomized clinical studies found strong evidence that TENS is more effective than placebo for chronic musculoskeletal pain and moderate evidence that it is effective for neuropathy. "In addition," the report said, "the general consensus from clinical experience is that TENS helps patients to manage their pain."

HONEY, THEY SHRUNK THE PT MACHINE

With Quell, the technology has been adapted and miniaturized so you can wear it. You strap the band, which contains electrodes, on your calf, adjust it so that it's the right level of tingling for you, and then set it so that it goes on for an hour at a time, followed by an hour off.

You can use it for just an hour or set it for near-continuous use, with a sleep cycle that's a lower intensity so it doesn't wake you up. There's an accompanying Bluetooth app that lets you use a smartphone or tablet to track both your pain—and your sleep, since there is such a close relationship between pain and sleep quality. Quell's battery lasts up to 40 hours, which, since it's used only every other hour, is good for a few days. It takes about three hours to recharge.

SHOULD YOU TRY IT?

Because the FDA approved Quell based on the efficacy of the underlying TENS technology, the company didn't need to submit independent studies showing that the Quell device itself is effective. But an earlier version called Sensus was tested with physicians who used it on their chronic-pain patients, and more than 50% of the patients were still using it six months later, a sign that they were getting relief. According to the company, two-thirds of Quell users take less pain medication and 81% report an improvement in chronic pain. The company also offers a 60-day money-back guarantee in case Quell doesn't work for you. That said, it would be preferable if there were published, peer-reviewed studies of the new device.

If you decide to give it your own personal trial, let your doctor know—especially if you are being treated for a chronic pain condition. That way, you can monitor your progress together and work out any issues as you attempt to reduce your use of pain medications. While this nerve stimulation is generally safe and without significant side effects—one reason the FDA has approved it for use without prescription—it should not be used if you have a cardiac pacemaker, implanted defibrillator or any other implanted metallic or electronic device…if you are prone to seizures…or if you are pregnant. (Nor does it work for every kind of pain, such as migraine pain, although there's another wearable device for that, Cefaly.)

The cost, which at present is not covered by insurance, is about $250 for the device—plus about $30 a month for replacement electrodes. You can learn more at *Quellrelief.com*.

New Painkiller Causes Fewer Addictions

US Food and Drug Administration, Silver Spring, Maryland.

New harder-to-abuse narcotic painkiller has been approved. Targiniq ER is a combination of the narcotic *oxycodone* and *naloxone*, which blocks the euphoric effects of oxycodone. Naloxone is activated if the pill is crushed, snorted, dissolved or injected, but Targiniq still can be abused by swallowing too many pills. Targiniq is approved for use by patients with chronic pain that has not responded to other medications.

CHAPTER 20

Women's Health

How Women Can Feel Sexy (Without Popping a Pill)

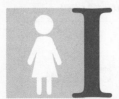f you're a woman, everyone wants to help you with your sex drive.

The medical profession may classify you as having hypoactive sexual desire disorder (HSDD)…aka, low libido. The drug industry wants to sell you its latest pill.

The good news: If low sex drive bothers you, there are better ways than popping a pill to rekindle the flames of desire.

BEYOND THE LITTLE PINK PILL

The pharmaceutical industry is excited about *flibanserin* (Addyi), the first-ever drug approved for low libido in women, but many doctors and mental health professionals aren't so jazzed about it. It doesn't move the desire needle much, and there are worrisome side effects. And did we mention that you're supposed to take it every day…but you can't take it if you drink alcohol?

Even the HSDD diagnosis itself is controversial. "There is no evidence that hypoactive sexual desire disorder is a medical condition," according a report in *Journal of Medical Ethics.* The author documents the extensive marketing campaign that the pharmaceutical industry sponsored to convince physicians that HSDD is, in fact, real—and thus needs to be treated with a drug.

Still, there's no question that many women do struggle with a lack of desire, and that it can have real, sometimes painful, effects on their sense of well-being, as well as on their relationships. If you're dealing with lagging libido—and you can't or don't want to try the new "little pink pill"—what can you do about it?

To find out, we spoke with noted sex therapist Kathryn Hall, PhD, a psychologist in Princeton, New Jersey.

Kathryn Hall, PhD, a licensed psychologist and sex therapist with a private practice in Princeton, New Jersey. She is president-elect of the Society for Sex Therapy and Research, and author of *Reclaiming Your Sexual Self: How You Can Bring Desire Back Into Your Life.* DrKathrynHall.com

LOW LIBIDO IS VERY COMMON AND VERY NORMAL

There are many, many reasons why women lose desire for sex—relationship problems, stress, fatigue, body image issues, hormonal changes in menopause, medications such as anti-depressants, as well as depression itself, Dr. Hall noted. But you don't have to have a reason. Many women don't. *Here's why…*

It's very common for women to lose sexual desire as a relationship progresses over time from lust to love.

"We know from a lot of studies that for many women, desire—their spontaneous lust—seems to wane in midlife," Dr. Hall says. "It's a normal pattern to lose that sort of lustful feeling, and it doesn't mean there's something wrong with you." The truth is, there's no "normal" when it comes to desire and how it plays out. If you don't want to have sex very often, or at all, and that doesn't bother you or your partner (if you have one), that's fine. Your desire, or lack thereof, is only a concern if it's distressing for you or problematic for your relationship.

If it does bother you, on the other hand, Dr. Hall has some suggestions that she's seen work for the many couples she's counseled. *Here they are…*

REKINDLING DESIRE

For women, what often replaces lust is "responsive desire"—getting in the mood after things have already gotten going because her partner has taken the initiative. That's perfectly fine for many couples. But some partners may resent always having to initiate sex. And many women miss the excitement of lust and eventually start to feel like sex is an obligatory chore, something they have to do so their significant others don't get angry. Fortunately, Dr. Hall has seen many patients and couples work with these challenges to improve their sex lives, although she acknowledges that it's not necessarily an easy road. *Here are some of the strategies she believes can help…*

•**Be realistic about sex, but don't give up on it.** Now that you know that a lot of women struggle with a low sex drive, you can work on bringing desire back into your life. "You've made a decision that you need sex in your life

and in your relationship and that you're going to put some energy and effort into it," Dr. Hall says. "It's not going to happen naturally." And that's OK.

•**Have maintenance sex.** "A lot of couples who stay sexual throughout their life span have what I call 'maintenance sex,'" Dr. Hall says. They think, "OK, it has been a while and I don't really feel like it but, you know what? I'm going to put some effort into it because we need sex in our life and in our relationship." Dr. Hall says these couples understand that bad sex happens and boring sex happens, but they still make lovemaking a priority because most of the time sex is satisfying.

•**Set yourself up for success.** The first step is to get out of the rut of feeling that sex is a chore. Start by challenging the belief that you never want to have sex with your partner. Think about the occasions when you enjoy it more, such as when you've just shared a nice time doing something together, and choose those kinds of situations for initiating sex—rather than if it's late and you have to get up early and go to work the next morning, or when you've been fighting.

•**Reengage with your own desire.** You may feel like you want to get sex over as quickly as possible. For many women, that means focusing only on satisfying their partners to get the deed done. Hurry up. You don't need to take care of me. Let's just focus on you. Have your orgasm and then we'll be done. If this sounds like your internal dialogue during sex, try slowing down and paying attention to what you need and want sexually. Put on some clothing that makes you feel sexy. Watch some erotica or, if you've ever used one, get your vibrator out. Have a glass of wine if that helps. Do these things not because you think it's going to turn your partner on, but because it's going to turn you on. And don't forget to clue your partner into what you like. He or she is probably dying to know!

•**Make an effort to initiate sex.** This is probably the furthest thing from your mind, but it may be a big deal to your partner.

Dr. Hall says: "When couples come in to see me, the man will often say, 'Look, I'm always the one that initiates this, and I don't like doing that. I want to be desired.' Of course he does, right?

Men in their midlife want to feel like, 'Hey, I'm still vital and attractive and desirable,' and, if his partner never wants to initiate sex with him, it doesn't feel great." Being more mindful about initiating sex from time to time can go a long way toward making your partner feel physically cherished—and that can only reap benefits for you.

Questionnaire for Libido Pill

Irwin Goldstein, MD, director, San Diego Sexual Medicine.

*F*libanserin (Addyi), the controversial drug recently approved by the FDA to help boost low libido, is designed for premenopausal women with hypoactive sexual desire disorder. This condition is diagnosed based on such questions as, "Are you bothered by your decreased level of sexual desire?" For the full questionnaire, go to *bit.ly/1TWmtMK*. Possible side effects of the drug, which is taken daily before bedtime, include drowsiness and dizziness (and no alcohol is allowed).

Helpful: Since a woman's reduced sexual desire may have caused problems in her relationship, sex therapy may also be beneficial.

No More Hot Flashes!

JoAnn V. Pinkerton, MD, executive director of The North American Menopause Society, Menopause.org. She is professor of obstetrics and gynecology and division director of Midlife Health at the University of Virginia Health System in Charlottesville.

I magine trying to function in the world when, at any moment, you can be randomly dropped into a self-generating sauna. That's what it's like for women who have hot flashes.

While hormone therapy, hands down, works the best for most women, it's not a universal answer. Some women don't want to take hormones because the treatment has been linked to increased risk for breast cancer and heart disease. And hormone therapy is inappropriate for women who have had an estrogen-sensitive cancer or a history of blood clots.

Scientists have begun solving some of the mystery of what causes hot flashes. And research has recently revealed which non-hormonal treatments really help against hot flashes.

SOLVING THE MYSTERY

New research has changed what we know about hot flashes. *Key findings…*

Before: Experts believed that symptoms of menopause lasted only about six months to two years.

Now: Research published in the April 2015 edition of *JAMA Internal Medicine* revealed that hot flashes go on for much longer than anyone thought—7.4 years, on average…and the earlier the symptoms started in perimenopause, the longer they were likely to continue after menopause.

Before: Hot flashes were believed to be an unfortunate but benign "side effect" of menopause.

Now: Recent research from the University of Pittsburgh School of Medicine published in *Obstetrics & Gynecology* suggests that hot flashes may be a marker for more serious disease processes. For example, studies have shown that women who have hot flashes are more likely to have higher levels of triglycerides and LDL "bad" cholesterol, putting them at greater risk for cardiovascular problems. This was true for all women who experienced hot flashes, but the risk was greater for women who had them frequently—on at least three days a week.

Another important study found that women with physiologically measurable hot flashes at night have more white matter hyperintensities—changes in the cerebral white matter (nerve fibers that connect brain cells) that could indicate a loss of blood flow in the brain.

BEST DRUG-FREE THERAPIES

In November 2015, The North American Menopause Society (NAMS) published the results of its review of hundreds of scientific studies focusing on nonhormonal treatments for hot flashes. The goal was to determine which treatments really worked. *In the NAMS review, two therapies stood out as providing significant relief from hot flash symptoms without hormones or other medication...*

• **Cognitive behavioral therapy (CBT).** CBT is designed to help people change their underlying emotions, thinking and behavior patterns. The first step in CBT for hot flashes is relaxation—a clinical psychologist trains women in paced, slow breathing and stress-reduction techniques. Then women talk about their experience with hot flashes and learn how to manage their reactions. For example, instead of thinking, *Hot flashes are ruining my life* or *I hope I don't get a hot flash in the middle of the meeting*, women might learn to change their thoughts to, *Hot flashes are temporary...They only last a few seconds...I know how to handle this.* Over time, negative beliefs recede and the experience is less upsetting.

CBT can take a number of forms—individual or group therapy, or even take-home books or recordings. This is short-term therapy, usually requiring no more than eight hours spread over four to eight weeks.

Studies showed that after CBT, though the number of hot flashes didn't change, about 75% of participating women perceived the hot flashes differently and seemed psychologically better able to handle them. This improvement remained steady even six months later.

CBT is covered by some health insurance, but check with your provider. To find a therapist familiar with CBT, talk with your primary care physician or gynecologist. Or you can search for a therapist in your area by visiting the website for the Association for Behavioral and Cognitive Therapies at *ABCT.org*.

• **Clinical hypnosis.** This is a newer therapy for hot flashes that may provide even greater relief than CBT. You start by getting into a deeply relaxed state. Then the therapist uses individualized mental imagery (such as coolness, relaxation or a safe place) and suggestions to change the body state—in this case, from one that is susceptible to hot flashes to one that is not.

Two studies from Baylor University showed remarkable results from clinical hypnosis. Participants had about a 55% drop in hot flash frequency and a 65% drop in hot flash intensity. Hypnosis has also been shown to improve sleep.

The downside of clinical hypnosis is the effort required. In the study, participants attended weekly training sessions for five weeks and had to practice with an audio recording at home every day. Plus, not everyone can enter the state of deep relaxation necessary for hypnosis. The first step is to find a qualified practitioner through the National Board for Certified Clinical Hypnotherapists (*NatBoard.com*). Before your first visit, ask if the hypnotherapist has experience treating menopause symptoms.

FOR MORE HELP

If you need more help for bothersome hot flashes, see a menopause expert (find one in your area at *Menopause.org* under the "For Women" tab). The physician can do an evaluation of the severity of your symptoms and work with you to find the best solution, whether or not that includes hormone therapy.

Women who have more than seven hot flashes per day or 50 per week, which disrupt their ability to function or sleep, or who experience heavy sweating are often good candidates for therapy. Don't suffer in silence. Ask for help!

Hot Flashes Linked to Heart Disease

Rebecca Thurston, PhD, associate professor of psychiatry, psychology, epidemiology and clinical and translational science at University of Pittsburgh and director of the Women's Biobehavioral Health Laboratory there. She has led several studies on the link between hot flashes and cardiovascular disease.

More than 70% of women experience hot flashes around the time of menopause. Not only are hot flashes bothersome (to say the least)—but research has also connected them with increased cardiovascular disease risk in certain women. In a recent ultrasound study, we found that "super flashers"—women who report at least five or six flashes daily—had significantly thicker carotid artery walls than other women. Other research has shown that the thicker the arterial walls, the greater the risk for heart disease and stroke. Having hot flashes infrequently (an average of four or fewer daily) does not seem to be linked to greater carotid thickness.

"Early-onset flashers"—women who have hot flashes at a relatively early age—also may be at higher risk. In another ultrasound study, we measured how well patients' blood vessels dilated after a cuff was released. Women who first experienced hot flashes at age 42 or younger had significantly worse responses than those whose flashes began later in life. Poor blood vessel responses are associated with the development of cardiovascular disease.

Self-defense: Consult your physician about whether you are up-to-date on cholesterol testing and other cardiovascular screenings. If you smoke, stop. Eat a healthful diet. Exercise regularly. If overweight, commit to a weight-loss plan.

Tomato Juice Relieves Menopause Symptoms

Study of 93 women by researchers at Tokyo Medical and Dental University, Japan, published in *Nutrition Journal.*

Women who drank about seven ounces of unsalted tomato juice twice a day for eight weeks reported a 16% improvement in hot flashes, fatigue and irritability.

Reason for the improvement: Tomatoes contain lycopene and gamma-aminobutyric acid (GABA). Lycopene reduces stress, and GABA helps ease hot flashes.

How to Beat Breast Cancer

Elisa Port, MD, chief of breast surgery at Mount Sinai Medical Center, director of the Dubin Breast Center and an associate professor of surgery at the Icahn School of Medicine at Mount Sinai in New York City. She is author of *The New Generation Breast Cancer Book: How to Navigate Your Diagnosis and Treatment Options—and Remain Optimistic—in an Age of Information Overload.*

One-third of all new cancers diagnosed in women are breast cancers. The American Cancer Society estimated

Sleep Away Urinary Incontinence

Bathroom woes may affect overall health. In a new study of 351 menopausal women, those who were overweight and/or had trouble sleeping experienced more urinary frequency...stress incontinence (leaking urine when coughing, laughing or sneezing)...waking at night to urinate...and urge incontinence (leaking urine when feeling the need to urinate).

Takeaway: Controlling body weight and getting adequate sleep may help relieve urinary problems—and fewer urinary problems may mean better sleep.

Masakazu Terauchi, MD, PhD, chair, department of women's health, Tokyo Medical and Dental University, Japan.

that more than 230,000 cases of invasive breast cancer were diagnosed in the US in 2015.

But no one should let the fear of breast cancer obscure some very encouraging facts. The overall five-year survival rate from breast cancer now is close to 90%. Less than 7% of breast cancers are diagnosed before the age of 40—those diagnosed later in life tend to be easier to treat. Many women with breast cancer will never need highly aggressive (or disfiguring) treatments.

Despite such good news, misunderstandings about breast cancer are common. *Here's what you need to know now...*

•**Lumpectomy often is the best choice.** Many women assume that a mastectomy is the "safest" way to beat breast cancer. It makes intuitive sense that removing an entire breast would improve long-term survival.

Not true. Survival has nothing to do with the amount of additional healthy tissue that's removed during surgery. About 60% to 75% of breast cancer surgeries are lumpectomies, in which only a small amount of tissue is removed. If your doctor gives you a choice, you can assume that the probability of survival for both procedures will be essentially the same.

The advantages of lumpectomy are obvious. The surgery is less extensive and women need less anesthesia, both of which are associated with shorter recovery time—and the breast probably will look much the same as it did before the surgery.

Downside of lumpectomy: About 25% of women will need a second procedure to remove cancer cells that were left behind during the first surgery if clear "margins" aren't achieved. Most patients will require a five-to-seven-week-long course of radiation. And the risk of the cancer coming back is slightly higher (usually less than 5%) in women who choose a lumpectomy rather than mastectomy (1% to 2%). Despite the slightly higher risk for local recurrence in the breast, the survival rates between lumpectomy and mastectomy are the same for women who are eligible for both.

A lumpectomy often is the best choice for tumors that are smaller than 4 centimeters (cm) to 5 cm. Some women feel that they'll have peace of mind only when the entire breast is removed. This can be a valid decision as long as you understand that the medical outcomes are roughly the same.

Of course, there is no "one size fits all," and absolutely, there are cases where a mastectomy is the better choice for an individual patient. For example, most women who are genetically predisposed to breast cancer and test positive for the BRCA genes are at much higher risk for recurrence with lumpectomy alone. In these cases,

mastectomy—and often removal of both breasts, bilateral mastectomy—is recommended.

•**You may respond well to neoadjuvant chemotherapy.** Chemotherapy usually is considered for women whose cancer has spread to the lymph nodes and for those with large tumors. It's typically given after surgery. For certain types of cancer, however, a different approach is highly effective. In this approach, the chemotherapy is given first.

This therapy, called neoadjuvant chemotherapy, is used to shrink a tumor prior to surgery. In some cases, it will allow women who would otherwise need a more extensive surgery, such as a mastectomy, to have a lumpectomy instead. It's also the only recommended approach for women with inflammatory breast cancer, which involves the whole breast along with the overlying skin. It also can be a good choice for women with "triple negative" cancers, which don't respond to hormonal treatments (see below), and those with HER2/neu-positive cancers. In some cases, this treatment shrinks a tumor so much that surgeons can find no residual cancer (but surgery still is necessary to ensure that this is the case).

•**Consider drugs that block hormones.** Between 60% and 70% of all newly diagnosed breast cancers are estrogen/progesterone-receptor positive. This means that exposure to these hormones can increase the risk for a recurrence.

Women with these types of cancers are almost always advised to take medication that reduces their risks. *Tamoxifen* (Nolvadex) is recommended for women prior to menopause. Aromatase inhibitors (such as *letrozole*, or Femara) are used after menopause.

The medications kill tumor cells that might have spread beyond the breast... reduce the risk that cancer will come back in a treated breast...and reduce the risk for cancer in the opposite breast. Women who take them can reduce their risk for a cancer recurrence by 40% to 50%. Patients usually take one pill a day and continue the treatment for five to 10 years.

Important: New research has shown that premenopausal women who take tamoxifen for 10 years usually have a greater reduction in cancer recurrences than those who take it for only five years.

Do You Need Extra Testing? Dense Breast Calculator

Not all women with dense breasts need additional screening for breast cancer. Women with dense breasts have a higher risk for breast cancers, but only 24% benefit from extra screening. A calculator (*Tools.bcsc-scc. org/BC5yearrisk/intro.htm*) from the National Cancer Institute's Breast Cancer Surveillance Consortium can help women ages 35 to 79 decide whether extra screening is warranted. Discuss the results with your doctor.

Karla Kerlikowske, MD, professor in the departments of medicine and epidemiology/biostatistics at University of California, San Francisco, and an internationally recognized expert on breast cancer screening.

The medications can cause unpleasant, meno-pause-like side effects, such as hot flashes and/or vaginal dryness. Tamoxifen also is associated with some rare but serious side effects such as a slightly higher risk for uterine cancer and blood clots, and aromatase inhibitors can affect bone density, which can be a problem for women with osteoporosis. But the side effects usually are minor, and many women feel the side effects are an acceptable trade-off for the superior protection.

WHAT ELSE CAN YOU DO?

Studies have shown that surgeons who treat a lot of patients (more than 50 cases a year) have better results. Ask your doctor to recommend a surgeon who specializes in breast cancer. *Also helpful...*

•**Ask your doctor if being in a clinical trial makes sense for you.** Most clinical trials are conducted by top hospitals and doctors. You'll get very sophisticated (and attentive) care. In many cases, even if you're assigned to a control group, you still will get the same treatment that you would have gotten if you hadn't joined the study. Those in the "active" group will get something that's expected to be at least as good—and possibly better.

Even if your doctor isn't personally involved in a clinical trial, he/she can talk you through the issues, including the pros and cons of participating...where to look for studies that involve your type of cancer...and what the studies are likely to involve.

•**Keep your weight down.** There's no evidence that specific dietary changes affect recovery from breast cancer. However, there is good evidence that maintaining a healthy weight is important, particularly for women with estrogen-sensitive cancers. (Much of a postmenopausal woman's estrogen is produced by fatty tissue.) Women who maintain a healthy weight may have up to a 5% survival advantage compared with those who are obese. Normal-weight women are less likely to get postsurgical infections and blood clots—particularly important for those who take tamoxifen, which slightly increases the risk for clots.

There isn't clear evidence that regular exercise helps prevent breast cancer, but I have found that cancer patients who exercise tend to recover more quickly—and of course, they find it easier to maintain a healthy weight.

Breast Cancer Alert

Jo Freudenheim, PhD, professor of epidemiology and environmental health, University at Buffalo, New York.

Risk of developing breast cancer is 14% higher in postmenopausal women with periodontal disease than in those without the condition, according to recent research. Harmful mouth bacteria may travel into the bloodstream and affect breast tissue.

Many Breast Cancer Patients May Not Need Chemo

Laura van 't Veer, PhD, leader, Breast Oncology Program, University of California, San Francisco Helen Diller Family Comprehensive Cancer Center.
Jose Baselga, MD, PhD, physician-in-chief and chief medical officer, Memorial Hospital at Memorial Sloan-Kettering Cancer Center, New York City.
Stephanie Bernik, MD, chief, surgical oncology, Lenox Hill Hospital, New York City.
Victor Vogel, MD, MHS, director, Breast Medical Oncology/Research for Geisinger Health System, Danville, Pennsylvania.
Presentation, American Association for Cancer Research meeting, New Orleans.

Many breast cancer patients receive chemotherapy they don't need, according to the results of a long-awaited clinical trial.

A genetic test called MammaPrint determined that nearly half the women slated for chemotherapy based on standard clinical assessments didn't really need to undergo the challenging treatment.

After surgery to remove their tumors, breast cancer patients with a MammaPrint score recommending against chemotherapy had a 95% survival rate, said co-researcher Laura van 't Veer, PhD, the test's inventor.

"That's very high, and we showed that it doesn't differ between those who are treated and those who are not treated by chemotherapy," said Dr. van 't Veer, leader of the breast oncology program at the University of California, San Francisco Helen Diller Family Cancer Center.

The clinical trial involved nearly 6,700 women at 111 medical centers in nine countries. It "represents what we in medicine call the highest level of evidence," American Association of Cancer Research President Jose Baselga, MD, PhD, said.

"This study is telling us in a very clear way we can spare many women chemotherapy," said Dr. Baselga, chief medical officer of Memorial Hospital at Memorial Sloan Kettering Cancer Center, in New York City.

ABOUT MAMMAPRINT TEST

Previously, doctors guessed whether a woman needed chemo by measuring the tumor, examining its cells under a microscope, and using genetic testing to determine whether the tumor would respond to hormone therapy, Dr. Baselga said.

The MammaPrint test looks at a panel of 70 genes within the tumor itself to assess its aggressiveness and the odds it will come back without chemotherapy, Dr. van 't Veer said.

"Our test looks under the hood, at the engine of the tumor," she said. "The biology tells more about the tumor than simply examining its size, because you're really looking into the tumor."

MammaPrint has been on the US market since FDA approval in 2007. But, many cancer doctors have waited for the results of this clinical trial to see how well it works, Dr. Baselga said.

Although the results should be considered preliminary until published in a peer-reviewed medical journal, Dr. Baselga said "this is the result we were hoping for."

STUDY RESULTS

In the clinical trial, researchers sorted breast cancer patients into four groups, based on whether MammaPrint testing or traditional clinical assessment recommended chemotherapy.

MammaPrint reduced chemotherapy prescriptions by 46% among the more than 3,300 patients in the trial categorized as having a high risk of breast cancer recurrence based on common clinical and pathological criteria, the researchers said.

Further, just over 2,700 patients who had a low MammaPrint risk score but a high clinical risk score wound up with a 94.7% five-year survival rate, whether they got chemo or not, the researchers said.

Stephanie Bernik, MD, chief of surgical oncology at Lenox Hill Hospital in New York City, said the results of this study were eagerly anticipated.

"If we can select those patients that don't need chemotherapy, unneeded treatment can be avoided and we will be one step closer to making sure treatment for breast cancer is tailored to the individual," she said.

IMPLICATIONS

MammaPrint testing will be particularly valuable for young women with breast cancer, said Victor Vogel, MD, director of Breast Medical Oncology/Research for the Geisinger Health System in Pennsylvania.

Young women have been more likely to receive chemotherapy in standard breast cancer care, even though it can destroy their fertility and leave them open to long-term health problems, Dr. Vogel said.

"In my training, if you had a young woman with breast cancer, she got chemotherapy," Dr. Vogel said. "But now we can be selective, and we know there's a very large number of young women with small hormone-responsive tumors who do not need chemotherapy."

Dr. Vogel said he frequently uses the Mamma Print test in his practice, and found that it helps all patients regardless of how they fare on it.

"It works both ways," he said. "It reassures the people who don't need chemotherapy, and when you get a big score that says there would be benefit, it encourages the patient they're doing the right thing by taking chemotherapy."

MammaPrint is covered by Medicare and is reimbursed by most large health insurers in the United States, Dr. van 't Veer said.

The test is expected to save health care dollars, Dr. Baselga said.

"You are saving all the money for chemotherapy that would be used for no reason, and you are protecting women from chemotherapy that is toxic and they don't need," he said.

info For more on breast cancer treatments, visit the American Cancer Society website *cancer.org* and search "how breast cancer is treated."

Better Breast Cancer Treatment

Timothy Whelan, BM, BCh, professor of oncology, McMaster University, Hamilton, Ontario, Canada.

Radiation of lymph nodes is usually not given to women whose early-stage breast cancer has spread to just a few nodes.

New research: Among women with early-stage breast cancer who had surgery, 82% of those who also had radiation to the breast and nearby lymph nodes were cancer free over the following 10 years, compared with 77% who received surgery alone. Side effects included skin rash, chronic swelling of the arm and inflammation of the lungs.

Family History of Prostate Cancer Raises Breast Cancer Risk

Jennifer L. Beebe-Dimmer, MPH, PhD is associate professor at Barbara Ann Karmanos Cancer Institute and Wayne State University School of Medicine, Detroit. She led a study published in *Cancer.*

A woman whose father, brother or son has or had prostate cancer may have a 14% higher risk for breast cancer. And women with a family history of both prostate and breast cancer have a 78% elevated risk for breast cancer.

Self-defense: Discuss screening options with your doctor.

Overactive Thyroid Increases Fracture Risk

Nicolas Rodondi, MD, head, ambulatory care department, Bern University Hospital, Bern, Switzerland.

Overactive thyroid (hyperthyroidism) has been shown to increase bone fracture risk.

Now: A new study indicates that even mild cases of the disease raise risk as well.

Details: In an analysis of 13 studies involving 70,000 patients, researchers found that there was an elevated risk for fractures in the hips and spinal areas of participants with subclinical hyperthyroidism, especially when the TSH level was under 0.10 mlU/L.

Breakthrough Therapies for Women's Hair Loss

Shari R. Lipner, MD, PhD, an assistant professor of dermatology and assistant attending physician at the New York-Presbyterian Hospital/Weill Cornell Medical Center in New York City. Dr. Lipner is board-certified in dermatology, lectures nationally and has authored numerous research articles and book chapters.

If you were a woman suffering from hair loss 25 years ago, your only option was to cover your head with a wig.

Now: Female hair loss is highly treatable—most cases improve within a matter of months—using a variety of breakthrough therapies.

WHEN HAIR LOSS STRIKES

More than half of all women will experience significant hair loss (more than 100 hairs per day) in their lifetimes. Any woman who has this amount of hair loss should see a dermatologist right away to determine the cause.

Some forms of hair loss can be temporary (see next page), while others are typically permanent unless treated within a year of the start of symptoms. If the follicles remain dormant for too long or if there is scarring, stimulating hair regrowth may be impossible. Treatment works best when started at the first sign of hair loss.

Men who have hair loss tend to get a "receding hairline," while women get an expanding center part. This condition, known as female pattern hair loss (FPHL), is the most common type of hair loss in women.

Self-test: Part your hair in the center. With FPHL, the center part is no longer a thin, crisp line. It is wider—and in later stages, it takes on a Christmas tree appearance with balding "branches" extending out from the center.

FPHL is a chronic, progressive hereditary condition often caused by changes in levels of male hormones as women age. It gets worse over time, and the hair won't regrow on its own. That's why you need treatment.

THE BEST MEDICATION

The only FDA-approved medication for women's hair loss is minoxidil. It has been available as 2% liquid for many years.

Newer treatment option: In 2014, the FDA approved extra-strength 5% minoxidil foam for women.

The 5% foam version has a higher concentration of medication and also causes fewer side effects than the liquid version, which contains propylene glycol—a trigger for allergic reactions in some women. Both versions, however, can cause hypertrichosis, a form of excess hair growth, particularly along the sides of the face.

Caveats: When using either form of minoxidil, it takes at least six months to see hair growth. Also, you must use the product indefinitely—discontinuing it will cause your new hair growth to fall out again. It costs about $40 a bottle and is not typically covered by insurance.

Even though minoxidil is available over the counter, it's wise to consult a dermatologist before using it. The cause of your particular hair loss may require a different treatment. For example, topical steroids or steroid injections are given for hair loss caused by the autoimmune condition alopecia areata. *Finasteride*, which is FDA approved for hair loss in men, is sometimes prescribed off-label for women who have elevated levels of male hormones.

WHEN YOU NEED MORE HELP

While 80% of women in clinical studies can regrow hair with minoxidil, for the unlucky few who can't, there are some new treatments that may be worth considering...*

•**Platelet-rich plasma (PRP).** This procedure is thought to jump-start dormant hair follicles. With PRP, some of your own blood is spun down in a centrifuge to separate platelet-rich plasma. Nutrients are added to the plasma, and the mixture is injected into the scalp with small needles.

PRP is available in some clinics, but it has not been approved by the FDA. While early findings are moderately positive, most practitioners believe the best results are for PRP combined with minoxidil treatment or hair follicle transplants. PRP is not covered by insurance and costs more than $1,000 for a single treatment, which may need to be repeated every three to six months.

•**Laser phototherapy.** With laser treatments, the idea is that light can stimulate hair growth at the level of the follicle. A few small studies have shown good results with no reported side effects, but there are no long-term studies. *Two laser therapies that have been cleared by the FDA...*

•Theradome, which looks like a bike helmet with 80 tiny lasers inside. It is available online for $895 and should be used for 20 minutes at least twice a week for 12 to 24 weeks.

•HairMax LaserComb, which looks like a cordless phone with light-emitting bristles. You turn it on and hold it over one spot on your head until a beep signals you to move it to another location. It is used three times a week. The base model costs $295 and is available online.

•**Hair loss camouflage.** Scalp micropigmentation is a permanent tattoo applied by a trained physician in a stippling pattern on the scalp to fill in areas of hair loss. It effectively disguises areas of hair loss and scars. Cost generally runs from $1,000 to $5,000.

TEMPORARY HAIR LOSS

For about 20% of women who suffer from hair loss, the condition is temporary.

Here's why: Hair can function as the proverbial canary in the coal mine—follicles react to unhealthy body changes before we know any-

*To find a hair-loss specialists, go to the website of the International Society of Hair Restoration Surgery, *ISHRS.org.*

thing might be wrong. Fix the problem, and hair grows back.

Consult a dermatologist to see if one of these conditions could be causing your hair loss…

•**Extreme stress.** A death in the family, hospitalization, moving to a new house or other life-altering change can cause hair follicles to go dormant, and hair falls out several months later. Typically, hair will regrow within a few months, once stress levels are reduced.

•**Weight loss/poor nutrition.** For healthy hair, you need to eat a well-balanced diet. Rapid weight loss, eating disorders and crash diets low in protein can cause hair to fall out. Your doctor may recommend a multivitamin or other supplement if you have any deficiencies and will likely check your iron levels. Healthful eating is all you need to regrow hair, usually within several months.

•**Medical conditions.** Thyroid conditions, scalp infections and anemia can also cause hair loss. Treating these diseases can stop the hair from falling out.

•**Hairstyling** practices. Bleaching, straightening, relaxing or perming can temporarily (or sometimes permanently) damage the scalp and hair follicles.

Women Need to Be Extra Vigilant Against Vision Loss

Prevent Blindness, news release.

Women are a majority of the 4.4 million Americans over age 40 who are visually impaired or blind, according to the national organization Prevent Blindness.

The group said women are at greater risk than men for vision loss from such eye diseases as cataracts, glaucoma and macular degeneration, as well as a condition called dry eye, which is more common after menopause.

Pregnancy can cause dry eyes, puffy eyelids and refractive changes that may show up as blurred or double vision. Pregnant women's vision may also be affected by migraine headaches, diabetes and high blood pressure, according to Prevent Blindness.

The organization also warns that some glaucoma medications may harm a fetus, and advises pregnant women to discuss all medications and any vision changes with their doctor.

Eyes benefit from a healthy lifestyle, including regular exercise, good nutrition and not smoking, the experts said.

Periodic dilated eye exams are the best way to track eye health, and can also detect conditions that affect overall health, such as diabetes and high blood pressure, according to Prevent Blindness.

info The U.S. National Eye Institute has more about healthy eyes at *nei.nih.gov/healthy eyes/*

Got Glaucoma? Skip These Yoga Exercises

Study titled "Intraocular Pressure Rise in Subjects With and Without Glaucoma During Four Common Yoga Positions" by researchers at New York Ear and Eye Infirmary of Mount Sinai, New York City, Medical Faculty Mannheim of the Ruprecht-Karls-University of Heidelberg, Germany, Columbia University Medical Center, New York City, published in *PLoS ONE*.

Practicing yoga can keep you fit and flexible. But if you're one of more than three million Americans with glaucoma, certain poses could put your vision at risk. In a new study of older yoga practitioners (average age 62), including some with glaucoma, four yoga moves significantly increased pressure inside the eye, known as intraocular pressure. *The moves are…*

•**Downward-Facing Dog**
•**Standard Forward Bend**
•**Plow Pose**
•**Legs-Up-the-Wall Pose**

It's normal for eye pressure to increase in these positions even if you don't have glaucoma, and pressure did quickly return to baseline for both groups after they completed the moves. So further research is needed to determine whether this temporary spike increases risk for progression of glaucoma. While the jury's out, however, if you have glaucoma, which is more common over age 65, you may want to avoid head-down yoga positions.

Fortunately, you can find many other energizing and healing poses in the practice of yoga. If you have a teacher, ask him or her to guide you in developing a routine that doesn't put extra pressure on your eyes.

Hiccups Can Indicate A Stroke

Anil Minocha, MD, professor of medicine and chief of gastroenterology, Overton Brooks VA Medical Center, Shreveport, Louisiana, and the author of *Dr. M's Seven-X Plan for Digestive Health.*

Hiccups, those annoying chest spasms, are usually caused by gulping air… drinking carbonated or alcoholic beverages…or stress.

What happens: The diaphragm muscle that separates the chest from the abdomen involuntarily contracts, which causes the vocal cords to close suddenly, triggering the "hic" sound. Most episodes of hiccups are brief and don't require medical follow-up.

Folk wisdom abounds, but certain remedies do cure hiccups.

Examples: Close your ears with your fingers while drinking water through a straw. Biting on a lemon also works!

But if your hiccups are persistent and painful, you need to see your doctor. Hiccups can be a sign of many conditions, including gastroesophageal reflux disease (GERD), kidney disease or a brain or esophageal tumor.

Hiccups, accompanied by chest pain, can also be a little-known early symptom of stroke in women. Other symptoms of stroke that are unique to women may include shortness of breath and whole-body numbness. If your hiccups are painful and unrelenting and you are also experiencing traditional stroke symptoms—such as blurred vision, severe headache, arm weakness, facial drooping, confusion and/or speech difficulty—call 911.

Migraine Frequency Increase Explained

Study of more than 3,600 women led by researchers at University of Cincinnati and Albert Einstein College of Medicine, New York City, published in *Headache: The Journal of Head and Face Pain.*

The frequency of migraine headaches increases as women go through perimenopause, during which hormone levels change and menstrual cycles become irregular. The chance of high-frequency migraines—10 or more per month—increases by 60% during this transition and is highest in the later stage of perimenopause. Hormone therapy may help reduce migraine frequency.

More Older Women Now Living With "Moderate" Disability, Study Shows

Vicki Freedman, PhD, research professor, University of Michigan Institute for Social Research, Ann Arbor.
Amy Kelley, MD, associate professor, geriatrics and palliative medicine, Icahn School of Medicine at Mount Sinai, New York City.
Barbara Resnick, PhD, RN, chair, gerontology, University of Maryland School of Nursing, Baltimore.
American Journal of Public Health, online.

Back in the 1980s, older US women typically lived more years free of disabilities than their male peers did, but a new study shows that pattern appears to be changing.

For older men, the news is largely positive, researchers report: They're not only living longer, but with fewer disabilities.

Good News on Ovarian Cancer Screenings

Currently, most ovarian cancer cases are detected only at an advanced stage.

But: A recent study found a 20% reduction in ovarian cancer deaths when postmenopausal women with no known malignancies or family history of ovarian cancer were screened annually for seven or more years. The screening—an ultrasound and the CA-125 (Cancer Antigen-125) blood test—already is used in high-risk women with certain gene mutations or an extensive family history of ovarian or breast cancer.

Anil Sood, MD, is director of the Blanton-Davis Ovarian Cancer Research Program, University of Texas MD Anderson Cancer Center, Houston.

For women, the picture is different: They've made smaller gains than men have and, in some respects, they've taken a step backward.

Specifically, older US women were more likely to be living with moderate disabilities in 2011, compared with 2004—a reversal in the improvement seen since 1982.

The study defined moderate disabilities as problems with daily activities such as shopping, doing household chores or managing money. For men, the prevalence of those issues dropped between 1982 and 2004, then stayed largely unchanged.

Older women, on the other hand, saw their prevalence of moderate disability decline from almost 13% in 1982, to about 10% in 2004. But by 2011, that figure had risen to 14%, the investigators found.

POSSIBLE EXPLANATIONS

The reasons for the trends are not clear, said study author Vicki Freedman, PhD, a researcher at the University of Michigan Institute for Social Research, in Ann Arbor.

On average, she said, women are at an economic disadvantage compared with men, and that could be one factor. "The next step is to

better understand why this is happening," Dr. Freedman said.

Another expert had a different theory.

Women's higher rate of obesity in more recent decades could also be playing a role, said Barbara Resnick, PhD, RN, chair of gerontology at the University of Maryland School of Medicine in Baltimore. She is also a former president of the American Geriatrics Society.

US men are heavier than they used to be, too. But, Dr. Resnick said, they also typically have more muscle mass and strength than women do, so they may be able to preserve more of their physical function as they grow older.

The findings are based on information from national health surveys of Americans aged 65 and up, conducted in 1982, 2004 and 2011.

Over those years, men started to gain on women in terms of life expectancy, and disability-free life: In 1982, a 65-year-old man could expect to live, on average, another 14 years; by 2011, that had increased to 19 years—with almost all of that extra time disability-free.

For the typical 65-year-old woman, life expectancy rose by only two years, from 18.5 to 20.5 years. And she could expect to live disability-free for one of those extra years, the researchers said.

The increase in older women's level of moderate disability seems to be the main driver, Dr. Freedman's team found. Rates of severe disability—requiring a nursing home or help at home with bathing, dressing and other basic needs—held steady for men and women between 2004 and 2011.

Women are at greater risk of debilitating conditions like arthritis, bone fractures and dementia. But it's not clear whether that accounts for the recent increase in moderate disability among older women, according to Dr. Freedman.

Amy Kelley, MD, is an associate professor of geriatrics and palliative medicine at Mount Sinai's Icahn School of Medicine, in New York City. She cautioned that the increase in women's moderate disability levels was seen over a short time period—from 2004 to 2011.

There could have been similar ups-and-downs between 1982 and 2004, Dr. Kelley pointed out.

That said, she applauded the study's aim. "This is focusing on not just life expectancy, but the quality of people's lives," Dr. Kelley said.

And that, she added, needs more attention in everyday health care, too.

Americans who make it to age 65 typically have a lot of years left ahead, Dr. Kelley pointed out. "So how can we make that time high-quality?" she asked.

Dr. Resnick said it's important for older adults to stay physically active—through a daily walk or light resistance exercise to keep muscles strong, for example.

Dr. Kelley agreed, saying older adults and their doctors need to think beyond controlling "numbers"—such as blood pressure and cholesterol levels. "So you can ask your doctor, what should I be doing to keep up my capacity for daily activities?" she suggested.

But, Dr. Kelley added, it's not up to older adults and their doctors alone.

"Communities need to make sure there are sidewalks that are safe for an older person with a cane," she said. "They need to have community centers that offer opportunities for older [people] to be active."

And "active" does not only mean exercise, Dr. Kelley said. Everyone benefits when older adults have chances to volunteer and otherwise stay involved in their community, she pointed out.

"Older adults have so much to offer," Dr. Kelley said. "As a society, we should make sure the opportunities are available."

What Your Mammogram Reveals About Your Heart

Study titled "Digital Mammography: Screening for Coronary Artery Disease?" by Harvey S. Hecht, MD, professor of cardiology at the Icahn School of Medicine at Mount Sinai, New York City, presented at the 2016 annual conference of the American College of Cardiology.

Digital mammograms detect more than breast cancer—they also may identify early signs of heart disease. The digital machines, which now account for more than 95% of all mammograms, pick up levels of calcium deposits in the arteries inside the breast.

These are generally benign—in the breast. But calcium deposits (calcification) in the arteries that supply the heart are a well-established marker for coronary artery disease—the most common form of heart disease. A chest CT scan accurately measures calcium deposits in the coronary arteries, but it also exposes the patient to additional radiation, so it's not done for everyone.

If you have calcium deposits in your breast arteries, however, you probably have them in your heart arteries, too, finds a new study. Radiologists at the Icahn School of Medicine at Mount Sinai in New York City studied 292 women who were not known to have heart disease who had digital mammograms and chest CT scans in the same year.

Results: Breast calcium accurately predicted coronary calcium. It wasn't a perfect match, but it identified women at high risk as accurately as standard cardiology scores.

So the next time you get a mammogram, ask your doctor if any calcification was visible.

Don't panic if the answer is yes. It doesn't mean you have heart disease. But it could be a wake-up call to work harder to reduce known risk factors such as high blood pressure and high blood sugar. Conversely, if you have little or no calcification, it may help you avoid an unnecessary prescription for a statin.

357

Index